R. B. Duncan, FRCS, FRACS, FAAOA

# CFIDS, Fibromyalgia, and the Virus-Allergy Link
## New Therapy for Chronic Functional Illnesses

D0145527

"**A**s a practical account for both patients and physicians, this book highlights Dr. Duncan's experiences with latency therapy for chronic fatigue syndrome (CFS) and fibromyalgia (FM). In this unconventional text, Dr. Duncan challenges traditional paradigms with the hypothesis that the cause and perpetuation of symptoms of CFS/FM find their roots in an interplay between environmental (toxin exposure, diet, etc.) and internal (allergies, previous infections, etc.) factors, an interaction that leads to reactivation of latent pathogens. Many of Dr. Duncan's patients have improved with the therapeutic approach that he details in this book, and this experience fuels his desire to share the controversial diagnostic and therapeutic methodology that he has practiced over many years. Not unlike other off-stream approaches, such as the treatment of varied medical conditions with recolonization of the large intestine with the right kind of bacterial flora—an intervention that is now getting support from conventional biomedical studies—latency therapy requires a more objective assessment, for which this book offers a structured background and an open invitation. Both physicians and patients will find this methodical and pragmatic account interesting and informative."

**Roberto Patarca-Montero, MD**
Research Director,
E. M. Papper Laboratory
of Clinical Immunology,
University of Miami
School of Medicine;
Author of the *Concise Encyclopedia of Chronic Fatigue Syndrome;*
Editor of the *Journal of Chronic Fatigue Syndrome*

# CFIDS, Fibromyalgia, and the Virus-Allergy Link
## *New Therapy for Chronic Functional Illnesses*

## THE HAWORTH MEDICAL PRESS
### Chronic Fatigue Syndrome, Fibromyalgia Syndrome, and Myalgic Encephalomyelitis

**Roberto Patarca-Montero, MD, PhD**
Senior Editor

*Concise Encyclopedia of Chronic Fatigue Syndrome* by Roberto Patarca-Montero

*CFIDS, Fibromyalgia, and the Virus-Allergy Link: Hidden Viruses, Allergies, and Uncommon Fatigue/Pain Disorders* by R. Bruce Duncan

*Adolescence and Myalgic Encephalomyelitis/Chronic Fatigue Syndrome: Journeys with the Dragon* by Naida Edgar Brotherston

*Phytotherapy of Chronic Fatigue Syndrome: Evidence-Based and Potentially Useful Botanicals in the Treatment of CFS* by Roberto Patarca-Montero

*Myalgic Encephalomyelitis/Chronic Fatigue Syndrome and Enteroviral-Mediated Organ Pathology* by John Richardson

# CFIDS, Fibromyalgia, and the Virus-Allergy Link
## New Therapy for Chronic Functional Illnesses

R. B. Duncan, FRCS, FRACS, FAAOA

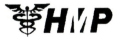

The Haworth Medical Press®
An Imprint of The Haworth Press, Inc.
New York • London • Oxford

Published by

The Haworth Medical Press®, an imprint of The Haworth Press, Inc., 10 Alice Street, Binghamton, NY 13904-1580

Medicine is an ever-changing science. As new research and clinical experience broaden our knowledge, changes in treatment and drug therapy are required. While many suggestions for drug usages or treatment regimens are made herein, the book is intended for educational purposes only, and the author, editor, and publisher do not accept liability in the event of negative consequences incurred as a result of information presented in this book. We do not claim that this information is necessarily accurate by the right, scientific standard applied for medical proof, and therefore make no warranty, expressed or implied, with respect to the material herein contained. Therefore the patient is urged to check the product information sheet included in the package of each drug he or she plans to administer to be certain the protocol followed is not in conflict with the manufacturer's inserts. When a discrepancy arises between these inserts and information in this book, the physician is encouraged to use his or her best professional judgement.

The author has exhaustively researched all available sources to ensure the accuracy and completeness of the information contained in this book. The publisher and author assume no responsibility for errors, inaccuracies, omissions, or any inconsistency herein.

Cover design by Marylouise E. Doyle.

**Library of Congress Cataloging-in-Publication Data**

Duncan, R. Bruce.
    CFIDS, fibromyalgia, and the virus-allergy link : new therapy for chronic functional illnesses / R. Bruce Duncan.
        p. cm.
    Includes bibliographical references and index.
    ISBN 0-7890-1072-0 (hard : alk. paper) — ISBN 0-7890-1073-9 (pbk. : alk. paper)
    1. Chronic fatigue syndrome. 2. Fibromyalgia. 3. Allergy. 4. Virus diseases. I. Title.

RB150.F37 D83 2000
616.97—dc21

                                                                    00-022098

# CONTENTS

# ABOUT THE AUTHOR

**R. Bruce Duncan, FRCS, FRACS, FAAOA,** is Director of the Virutherapy Clinic in Wellington, New Zealand. Dr. Duncan, a Fellow of the Royal College of Surgeons of England and Australasia was also former Head of the Ear, Nose, and Throat Department of Wellington Hospital, New Zealand. He has served as Examiner for the Royal Australasian College of Surgeons and was a Foreign Fellow of the American Academy of Otolaryngic Allergy from 1974 to 1994. Dr. Duncan has published more than a half-dozen professional papers in American journals of otolaryngology.

Dr. Duncan ran a surgical practice in New Zealand. After experiencing CFIDS/ME and a severe grain allergy, he added allergic, and later, viral (microbial) therapies to the clinic.

# Preface

*CFIDS, Fibromyalgia, and the Virus-Allergy Link* introduces a new medical diagnostic and therapeutic area and modality. Read about

1. the benefits of an allergy therapy linked to microbial therapy, in particular, virutherapy;
2. the increasing numbers of young people suffering from unexplained fatigue, muscle pain and symptoms, personality and memory problems (all ages are affected, but it is the eighteen to thirty-five age group who make up 80 percent of the patients); and
3. difficult to diagnose and treat chronic fatigue states and fibromyalgia that often respond to virus-allergy link therapies.

The clinical responses and patients' descriptions during virus-allergy link investigation and treatment suggest the presence of a second immune system involving the body's billions of cells. Latent (hidden) immunity is not detected by laboratory blood tests. Laboratory testing detects the antibodies of the blood and cellular immune system.

Throughout the book, surmises, hypotheses, and calculated guesses developed from fourteen years of clinical experience explain the symptoms and treatment responses of latency immunity. Virus-allergy link treatments stimulate/enhance excretion or detoxing, besides improving body immunities through lifestyle and diet changes. Learn how to treat persistent, fluctuating symptoms and illness following a severe viral infection, a mental shock, or a mysterious slow/rapid deterioration in health and mental activity. Suspect a psychological diagnosis that does not respond to therapy. This book can help parents of schoolchildren with viral allergy-like illnesses, in particular, glandular fever, from which children appear to recover but continue to experience fluctuating symptoms of memory loss and weak, painful muscles. Chapters 2, 3, and 4 describe what I learned from fourteen years observing 2,000 patients and attempting to answer their tens of thousands of questions. My clinical and personal experience of allergy and surgery began forty years ago, followed by personal experience of chronic fatigue immune dysfunction syndrome (CFIDS).

The combination of modern American clinical allergy therapy, serial dilution therapy, and multiple latent virutherapy began in 1985. Over the years, treatment results have continued to improve with modifications of treatments and additions to the range of test extracts. Virus-allergy link advice and latency therapy are safe. No patient suffered permanent provoked symptoms; all provoked symptoms returned to pretest levels. The majority of patients gained further improvement or a return to remembered health.

*CFIDS, Fibromyalgia, and the Virus-Allergy Link* describes a simple, easy-to-operate injection technique and therapy suitable for the treatment of CFIDS/chronic fatigue syndrome (CFS)/myalgic encephalomyelitis (ME) and fibromyalgia. The simple treatment and its low cost will appeal to those unfortunate people who have lost their jobs and become dependent due to subjective, affective, all-in-the-head, chronic fluctuating illnesses. They have no means of financing scientific investigative medicine, and they receive symptom suppression drugs as treatment. Successful latency therapy discards symptom suppression drugs.

Over the years, patients made suggestions that are incorporated in virus-allergy link therapy. Patients should start by matching their symptoms with one or more of the sixteen common symptom groups (p. xxi), then with any of the case notes in the popular Identikit© (p. xxiii). If latent illness is suspected, patients should obtain the advice of their family physician, who can put them in contact with an allergist.

Patients depend on repetition of important advice and facts because of their memory defects and fluctuating levels of concentration. Advice is repeated throughout the book, where appropriate, for readers with CFIDS/ME/latency illnesses who may experience memory, recall, and reading problems. Patients prefer abbreviations rather than long medical words, hence the ABBREKEY© bookmark (p. xix).

Chapter 1 gives an abridged description of latency therapy for medical professionals. Chapter 2 is an account of latency symptoms in different parts of the body. Chapter 3 attempts to answer patients' questions and enhance their understanding of latency treatment. Chapter 4 suggests required home and lifestyle changes. Chapter 5 provides a virus symptom checklist and six important virus-allergy activities. Chapter 6 explains why food restrictions are required and how to accommodate them. It includes over 90 of the most popular and useful recipes used by patients during their recovery.

This book does not include a description of the blood and cellular immunity of the body, the natural immune system (NIS). The lay reader can find excellent accounts of this system in health books on allergies, chronic fatigue syndrome, and autoimmune diseases and conditions. For those interested in an advanced description of the NIS, short texts on immunity are available for students. Popular scientific journals, from time to time, also have excellent articles on the NIS. The concept or hypothesis of the latency immunity system, as presented in this book, attempts to include and explain (1) the many symptoms and illnesses that do not appear to stimulate responses by the NIS; (2) those symptoms considered to have psychological, functional, subjective, all-in-the-head—even neurotic—causes; (3) the many forms of these symptoms and illnesses; and (4) why symptom suppression therapy is prescribed in the absence of any positive findings from laboratory testing or medical technology.

The longer the duration of a patient's illness and the greater its severity, the more marked the provoked symptoms will be and the longer the recovery. There are no quick-fix prescriptions in *CFIDS, Fibromyalgia, and the Virus-Allergy Link.*

*R. B. Duncan*

## The Wall

That damned Wall.
Unseeingly looming ahead.
Always there in the shadows.
Waiting for the unwary.
Each invisible brick a minefield of disaster.
An energy-sapping void.
Of nerve-tingling despondency.
As when a light fuses.
Leaving an empty shell.
Only a blank fogged mind.
And unwilling body.
Crying out for help.
In a silent scream.

I've always had a clear vision of The Wall. It is a physical barrier which I can suddenly hit without warning, and then I'm a shivering, jelly-legged, weak, depressed person, looking for the nearest place to sit down and plan my escape home. It's not such a fear now and nowhere as severe, but the memory remains vividly in my mind.

*Brenda Lofthouse*
*Recovered sufferer*
*from the virus-allergy link*
*illness complex*

# Acknowledgments

Sincere thanks go to my mentors, Bill and Marion Bryan. The work, time, and suggestions of Sue Megann, Jean Rothwell, Sharon Fergusson, Margaret Hale, Alan Rothwell, Ivan Lindoss, and Clare Duncan are much appreciated.

Thanks also go to Christine Lewis and the John Ilott Trust for supporting this publication. I would also like to acknowledge the production staff of The Haworth Press for their hard work and dedication to the publication of this book.

Welcome to Latency Therapy; walk away from Symptom Suppression Therapies.

*Mary, a patient, 1995*

# Introduction

Dear Reader,

Many functional, nervous, and hysterical symptoms, even so-called placebo effects and stress tensions, have real causes. Scientific medicine depends on the results of laboratory tests and technological examinations. Any treatment that does not fit the scientific proof requirements is called *anecdotal*. Successful treatments using anecdotal methods are frequently labeled *placebo effects;* in fact, the two words are bandied about often without justification. You must understand what the term *placebo* means, as it is commonly used by medical professionals when they believe a drug or treatment method has no influence on the body or effect on the related or relevant symptoms. The medical profession believes that patients have such faith in placebo treatment that they unconsciously experience symptom improvement. In time, the improvement reverts to the original symptom level. Patients who suffer a so-called functional illness diagnosis become very resentful; they are convinced the anecdotal virus-allergy treatments helped them greatly or restored them to health.

This book's selection of important anecdotal symptoms with real causes are as follows: (1) food, pollens, inhalants, and mold allergies; (2) molds, bacteria, and their toxins, especially *Candida*-related complex (CRC), *Giardia,* and *Helicobacter;* (3) petrochemical toxicity; (4) the effects of faulty lifestyle and ecology; and (5) the new dimension of multiple latent virutherapy (MLV).

*CFIDS, Fibromyalgia, and the Virus-Allergy Link* brings together all these factors, as well as the functional nervous symptoms and illnesses they cause or aggravate. New concepts and treatment are offered to help your particular nervous or stress tension problems. You can win back your remembered health by contacting a sympathetic physician and complying with the change of lifestyle suggestions for three to four months. During your progress, you will recognize past and present symptoms brought on or provoked by highly diluted solutions of testing substances called *anti-*

---

The author does not support or agree with some of the frequently expressed opinions of clinic patients. A fair and unbiased account of latency illness is presented to the reader.

*gens/latentors.* This book is your treatment and backup guide as you travel through the highs and lows of the preliminary work-up and virutherapy. Modern medicine and surgery have little to offer people with functional symptoms undetected by normal physical and laboratory tests. These patients resent symptom suppression and antidepressant drugs because such treatment often makes them feel manipulated, like puppets.

What started from my suspecting poliomyelitis symptoms in patients with chronic fatigue, food allergies, and CRC problems, in 1984, rapidly escalated to include a wide range of symptoms and diseases associated with molds, bacteria, their toxins, and thirty latent viruses, from adenovirus to common warts.

New *causal medicine* therapy depends on identifying the causes of symptoms, not suppressing them through drugs, suggestion from psychological therapy, or surgery.

## THE INTERACTION OF FOOD EXCLUSIONS AND MLV

Please understand that the variable intensity and type of symptoms are at first due to the food exclusion and mold treatments. MLV brings further aggravations and then a gradual clearing of symptoms. At this stage, the body's immunities and detoxing are improving so you experience days when you feel *great.* It is disappointing when cytomegalovirus (CMV), Epstein-Barr virus (EBV), dengue, or another virus adds a fresh crop of symptoms and increases foul detoxifying odors. Regular saunas and heat therapy boost detoxing, and it is at this stage that petrochemicals are recognized by their chemical odors. Those who previously used recreational drugs are surprised when detoxing reproduces the drugs' typical smells. This is not the time to make a food indiscretion, as improvement may halt for a week or more.

When symptoms are severe, try to resist the impression that the therapy is failing. Tell yourself that if nothing was happening, the treatment would be useless. Conventional medical logic suggests that improvement should continue, as it does with symptom suppression drug therapy, unless there are *side effects.* "Logic is not easily applied to biology and the workings of our mind and body."

## IMPORTANT TREATMENT NOTICE

Before beginning any procedures or advice described in this book, consult your family physician or specialist. The recommendations in this book are not my legal or medical responsibility, for obvious reasons. Symptoms and illnesses that correspond to those described in this book must be supervised by a physician.

Please do not begin any treatment that you may believe is linked with, or derived from, the surmises I advance and discuss in this book. First obtain your physician's advice, as your understanding and interpretation may be faulty, even dangerous, if you proceed.

## ABBREKEY© ABBREVIATIONS ✂

| | |
|---|---|
| ADD | attention-deficit disorder |
| ALA | alpha-linolenic acid |
| ATV | adeno(tonsil)virus |
| CFIDS | chronic fatigue immune dysfunction syndrome |
| CFS | chronic fatigue syndrome |
| CMV | cytomegalovirus |
| CRC | *Candida*-related complex |
| Csd(s) | corticosteroid(s) |
| CSR | change-of-site response |
| EBV | Epstein-Barr virus |
| IBS | irritable bowel syndrome |
| Ig | immunoglobulin |
| IK | Identikit |
| LIS | latency immunity system |
| ME | myalgic encephalomyelitis |
| MLV | multiple latent virutherapy |
| NCM | new causal medicine |
| NIS | natural immune system |
| NSAID | nonsteroid anti-inflammatory drug |
| OCIS | organ cell immune system |
| OWGGs | Old World grass grains (wheat, barley, oats, rye, rice, millet) |
| PCRT | polymerase chain reaction test |
| PMT | premenstrual tension |
| PNT | provocation neutralization test |
| PNA | perennial nasal allergy |
| PVFS | postviral fatigue syndrome |
| RAST | radioallergosorbent test |
| RSI | repetitive stress injury |
| RSV | respiratory syncytial virus |
| SD | serial dilution—provocation or therapy |
| SET | skin endpoint titration |
| SLE | systemic lupus erythematosus |
| SLO | sublingual organ |
| SSD | symptom suppression drug |
| SV | serial vaccination |
| VAL | virus-allergy link |
| v. zoster | chicken pox/shingles |

## INSTRUCTIONS ✂
Cut free the Bookmark.
If mislaid, photocopy.                    !

## ABBREKEY© BOOKMARK

| | |
|---|---|
| ADD | attention-deficit disorder |
| ALA | alpha-linolenic acid |
| ATV | adeno(tonsil)virus |
| CFIDS | chronic fatigue immune dysfunction syndrome |
| CFS | chronic fatigue syndrome |
| CMV | cytomegalovirus |
| CRC | *Candida*-related complex |
| Csd(s) | corticosteroid(s) |
| CSR | change-of-site response |
| EBV | Epstein-Barr virus |
| IBS | irritable bowel syndrome |
| Ig | immunoglobulin |
| IK | Identikit |
| LIS | latency immunity system |
| ME | myalgic encephalomyelitis |
| MLV | multiple latent virutherapy |
| NCM | new causal medicine |
| NIS | natural immune system |
| NSAID | nonsteroid anti-inflammatory drug |
| OCIS | organ cell immune system |
| OWGGs | Old World grass grains (wheat, barley, oats, rye, rice, millet) |
| PCRT | polymerase chain reaction test |
| PMT | premenstrual tension |
| PNT | provocation neutralization test |
| PNA | perennial nasal allergy |
| PVFS | postviral fatigue syndrome |
| RAST | radioallergosorbent test |
| RSI | repetitive stress injury |
| RSV | respiratory syncytial virus |
| SD | serial dilution—provocation or therapy |
| SET | skin endpoint titration |
| SLE | systemic lupus erythematosus |
| SLO | sublingual organ |
| SSD | symptom suppression drug |
| SV | serial vaccination |
| VAL | virus-allergy link |
| v. zoster | chicken pox/shingles |

# Indications for Multiple Latent Virutherapy

Order of frequency of symptoms seen at the clinic:

1. Unexplained mental and muscle tenseness, lack of motivation
2. Unexplained fatigue and sleeping disorders
3. Chronic sinusitis—sinus headache and ear symptoms, such as fullness
4. Recurring "flu infections" or "flulike symptoms" not controlled by repeated antibiotic courses or immunization
5. Skin conditions of one year or longer duration requiring frequent hydrocortisone or corticosteroid topical drug therapy
6. Indigestion, bloating, pain, and "colitis" symptoms (e.g., irritable bowel syndrome)
7. Headaches, migraines, and constant head pain (one that never goes away); considerable side effects from headache medications
8. Recurring eye irritation, mild infection, and visual disturbances
9. Kidney and bladder problems (e.g., urinary tract infections, urgency, pain on passage, and water retention)
10. Depression, moods, sleep disorders, and feelings of being manipulated like a puppet by unknown causes
11. Memory and recall defects, fearful dreams, and "spacing out" mind states
12. Variable pain and weakness of muscle groups, localized muscle spasms, e.g., pressure points or "knots"; chronic low back, shoulder, and neck pain that does not respond to conventional therapies
13. Asthma controlled by symptom suppression inhaled corticosteroids and cromolyn drugs, with sticky, often colored chest mucus
14. In children, variable deafness and sticky mucus in the middle ear, with or without ventilation tubes; failure to learn and reduced physical activities
15. Difficult to manage "overactivity" in children and teenagers, with or without long-term drug therapy
16. CFIDS/ME affecting adults, teenagers, and children, with constant or fluctuating symptoms of nine months or longer duration

Medical Heretics advance medicine
by their choice to THINK DIFFERENTLY.

*A recovered patient*

# IDENTIKIT©

## TRY MATCHING YOUR SYMPTOMS
## WITH THE VIRUS-ALLERGY IDENTIKIT:
## AN INVITATION TO IDENTIFY
## YOUR SYMPTOMS AND ILLNESSES

Use the Identikit to refer back and check out the additional twenty-six alphabetical case histories (pp. xxv-xxxv).

The Identikit (IK) lists body regions and the main symptoms associated with each. The short case notes scattered throughout *CFIDS, Fibromyalgia, and the Virus-Allergy Link* have page references. The more descriptive case notes use alphabetical references. Most short and long descriptions are composites. Personal experiences (P) have disclosure consent.

How will this book help you to understand your symptoms and seek out treatment?

1. Select from the Identikit range the body areas associated with your symptoms.
2. First read the selections from the twenty-six alphabetical references and then read the text references. Study the case notes you identify with for an understanding of latency therapy.
3. Decide if you are prepared to change some aspects of your lifestyle.
4. If in doubt, read the article "Latency Immunity and Therapy: A Clinical Study of Latent Epstein-Barr Virus Incidence in 297 Idiopathic Chronic Fatigue Patients with Plausible Hypotheses" (see Appendix I, pp. 297-299).

Many popular health books offer a diagnostic points/scoring table of signs and symptoms. Check out the Virus-Allergy Scorecard (pp. 114-116) because latency therapy treats a wide range of symptoms, many of which could be due to other causes. Matching your symptoms is a better and more accurate approach than a numbers game.

## INDEX OF SYMPTOMS

Fatigue
B, E, G, M, P, V

Lack of Motivation
I, N, O, R

### Respiratory

Sinusitis
B, F, W

Head Colds
F, T, 37

Nasal Allergy, Pollinosis,
and Therapy
104, 149

Chest Infection
X, 40

Bronchitis
H

Asthma
A, B, J, 41, 43

### The Gut, Gastrointestinal Tract

Mouth, Bad Breath
(Halitosis)
46, 47, 186

Throat
C, 45, 46

Stomach and Indigestion
F, H, U

Colon, Rectum, Anus
U

Irritable Bowel Syndrome
(IBS)
N, T, Y, 229

Microbes of the Gut
W, 98, 104, 138

*Candida*-Related Complex
(CRC)
C, Q, 87, 120, 138

*Giardia*
G, V, 88

*Helicobacter*
T, 48, 51, 138

### The Skull and Brain

Headache
O, 56

Migraine
J, X, 123, 189

Constant Head Pain (Viral)
J, 55, 102

Cannabis
56

Food Addiction
239

Head Injuries
123

Moods
H, L, Y, 121, 127, 208

Depression/Aggravation
E, J, Q, S, X,
58, 120, 180, 204

Memory Problems
C, E, L, Q,
55, 56, 62, 63, 111

Speech and Learning
111, 112

Attention-Deficit Disorder
D, 67, 107, 112, 205

Petrochemicals
88, 139, 157, 161, 186

Sleeping Disorders,
Dreaming
G, Q, 60, 103, 174, 208

Multiple Sclerosis, Sys-
temic Lupus Erythemato-
sus (SLE)
P, 67

### Eyes

Eyelids
72

Conjunctiva and Cornea
72, 149

Retina and Vision
F, T, X, 74

### Ears

Variable Deafness
and Tinnitus
Q

Vertigo and Dizziness
K, U, 75

Glue Ear of Children
D, 76

### Skin

| | | |
|---|---|---|
| Dermatitis/Eczema<br>G, S, 79, 186 | Acne<br>80 | Hives<br>M, 78, 201 |
| Itching<br>72, 104 | Numbness<br>U | Psoriasis<br>S |

### Muscles, Joints

| | | |
|---|---|---|
| Neck Pain<br>I, 82 | Back Pain<br>R, 21, 91 | Muscles, Myalgia<br>E, I, J, K, 46, 85, 91, 123 |
| Joints<br>A, N, Q, 31, 87, 193 | | |

### Genital, Urinary

| | | |
|---|---|---|
| Kidney<br>I, 139, 186 | Bladder<br>Q, S, 99, 100, 111, 150 | Urethra and Prostate<br>S, 96 |
| Water Retention<br>99 | Premenstrual Tension<br>(PMT)<br>H, Z | |
| Fertility<br>P | Lovemaking Problems<br>M, N, T, 99, 101, 102, 190 | Genital Herpes<br>T, 102 |

### Vascular, Hormonal

| | | |
|---|---|---|
| Body Temperature<br>Disorders<br>I, S, T, 169, 189 | Blood Pressure, Hyper-<br>tension<br>Z, 71 | Heart Symptoms<br>F, Z, 71 |
| Obesity<br>169, 184 | Thyroid Sex Hormones<br>I, 99 | Microbes, Viruses<br>117, 120, 177, 193 |

## CASE HISTORIES

## A. Male, Age 68 (P)

Severe asthma 25 years, arthritis 18 years. Childhood pneumonia became asthma at age 8. Asthma went away at age 23 and returned in a serious form at age 45. Two years later joints were stiff and painful. Age 51, food testing and exclusion of allergic foods cleared the asthma and arthritis. Seven years later he stopped food exclusions, and shortly after the asthma and arthritis returned. He preferred symptom suppression drugs (SSDs) for the asthma and arthritis. Peak flow meter readings were 350 to 400 units. Six years later the SSDs were not controlling the asthma and arthritis. Attended the clinic and within four months was off all drugs, with peak flow at 700 to 730 units. CRC, *Giardia, Mucor, Aspergillus,* RSV, rubella, and EBV were significant treatments.

### B. Male, Age 25

Asthma, slowed speech and thought, tenseness, sinusitis, and unexplained fatigue as long as he can remember. Exposure to petrochemicals as a baby brought on the asthma, which has required medication ever since. Attended the clinic three years ago, with peak flow at 300 to 350 on full asthma medication. Molds and house dust therapy improved the peak flow to 550. Exclusion of OWGG foods along with CRC and *Giardia* therapies brought the peak flow to 650. Six viruses provoked improvement; RSV improved the lung function, and brought about return of normal speech and thought. EBV reduced fatigue and muscle tenseness. Nasal polyps retracted, the nose opened up, and five months later no polyps were present in the nose. Has experienced continued good health and mental ability.

### C. Male, Age 12 (P)

Chronic tonsillitis, change of personality, and progressive loss of memory developed over the last three years. Attended the clinic before having a tonsillectomy. Exclusion of poultry, CRC, and sublingual (under the tongue) drops of influenza, RSV, and ATV cleared the infections and restored his pleasant personality. School performance improved and he is a top art student.

### D. Male, Age 5 (P)

A chronic throat and chest infection at age 4 continued for four to five months despite antibiotics. Hyperactivity and marked aggressive behavior prevented him from attending preschool classes. Continuing infections and antibiotics further aggravated the behavior, disrupting his first term at school. Exclusion of OWGGs and CRC therapy markedly reduced some aspects of hyperactivity but had little effect on learning and aggression. Influenza, polio, RSV, and ATV cleared the infection. Hepatitis provocation evoked a severe aggressive response, which was neutralized. Within a month he was well-behaved and began to learn and cooperate. The teacher was amazed at the transformation, which was interrupted when he ate OWGG foods. Automaton hyperactivity (or ADD) people do not remember the disturbed behavior and cannot understand why they are being chastised for it.

### E. Females, Ages 13 to 18

Following glandular fever ("the kissing disease") they developed unexplained fatigue and/or loss of memory. The minimum period was six months. At first diagnosed as functional or psychological, later changed to CFIDS. Schooling and correspondence school were abandoned, as the memory defects prevented reading and discrimination of topography of their streets and neighborhood. Depression and excessive crying brought on suicidal thoughts. One or more food allergies were excluded and therapy involved CRC and greater than eight latent viruses, of which EBV and CMV improved depression and muscle strength; RSV, rubella, and rotavirus restored the memory; and morbilli cleared the muscle pains. All returned to school within four months of starting MLV.

## F. Female, Age Group 21 to 26

Repeated influenza during the winter brought on chronic sinus infection, hyperactivity, and memory problems that became constant. She experienced uncontrollable shaking and tremors, but her thyroid activity was normal. A year later she developed IBS with anal and genital itch, requiring treatment for thrush. She was greatly disturbed at night by racing of the heart (tachycardia). Unusual visual shifting images occurred during dawn and sunset. She expected to lose her job. Exclusion of poultry cleared the hyperactivity. CRC and *Giardia* therapy cleared the bowel symptoms and the anal and vaginal itch. SV with flu shots cleared the chronic sinusitis and recurring flu attacks; polio improved the heart symptoms; and RSV restored her memory and cleared the chest wheezing. Recovery took five months of therapy, helped by the summer weather, and she held her job.

## G. Female, Age 30 (P)

PVFS two and a half years ago confined her to bed. At the same time, two or three small eczema areas appeared and began to extend over most of the body surface. She had constant insomnia, despite spending most of her time in bed. Three foods including dairy and beef were excluded, with reduction of skin itch and eczema. Three molds, house dust, and CRC cleared her chronic sinusitis and further improved the eczema. *Giardia* improved her IBS and joint aches. Mumps relieved the pain in the thigh muscles, as well as the itchy tongue, eyes, nose, and ears. EBV gradually reduced her depression and she lost her "leaden limbs." Amphotericin B by mouth and enema reduced the *Candida* bowel symptoms; Nystatin was ineffective.

## H. Female, Age 35

IBS for ten years, together with depression, unexplained mood changes, incoordination of speech and movements (temporary dyslexia), and unexplained three- to four-day coughing bouts of twenty years' duration. For the last eight years suffered marked PMT lasting five days. Exclusion of sugar and OWGGs cleared most IBS symptoms. House dust, molds, and CRC improved the coughing, but it was finally cleared with whooping cough (pertussis). Five viruses cleared the remaining symptoms: hepatitis stopped the fearful dreams and thoughts; CMV and EBV reduced the mood changes, depression, and incoordination. The PMT improved with SV estrogen treatment shots. She regained normal health within five months of treatment and continues her new lifestyle.

## I. Female, Age 38 (P)

Never recovered from glandular fever nine years ago. Developed CFS. Suffered muscle bruising and aches, sometimes the whole body, at other times in various areas. Was bedridden for weeks at a time with severe neck and back pain, excessive fatigue, and depression, was constantly cold, and unable to do housework or look after the children. Enlarged lymph glands in neck, armpits, and groin varied in size and tenderness. A constant full feeling in the breasts was aggravated by any support garment. Recovery took two years, with many relapses occurring for shorter periods and with less intensity. Short periods of marked muscle weakness, unexplained fatigue, and depression returned her to bed. Within six months she was coping with housework and her three children. Although recovered, she still has EBV relapses of muscle weakness and muscle pains (morbilli) with tender lymph glands. Two foods, three molds, CRC, *Giardia,* and *Helicobacter* were significant. Seven viruses besides CMV for the bladder and kidney trouble and EBV for the depression, fatigue, and muscle weakness were required.

## J. Unisex, Age Group 25 to 35

If you suffered a severe case of measles while an infant or child, you may have latent morbilli encephalitis. A 30 year old with CFIDS had constant head pain and frequent migraines and headaches. The right side of the body was weaker than the left. Other symptoms were mood changes, fluctuating memory and memory lapses, chronic asthma, and genitourinary complaints. Muscle weakness of the lower legs was cleared with CMV and *Cladosporium.* The provocation with morbilli was dramatic, causing a sudden severe head pain, a migraine aura, uncontrolled right arm movements (athetosis), aggravated asthma, deep depression, and crying. The symptoms were relieved, but they returned for ten days as a prolonged delayed provocation. All symptoms cleared. The strength in the right side of the body almost equaled that in the left, and the asthma cleared. A month later, CMV and RSV provocation restored past memory— so active it gave her insomnia for ten days! Six months later almost recovered. Exclusion of OWGGs, CRC, *Helicobacter,* and nine viruses, morbilli, polio, CMV, and EBV were significant.

### K. Male, Age Group 22 to 26

A competitive athlete suddenly developed joint and muscle pains and cramps; he was giddy and could not coordinate his limbs; he suffered from unexplained fluctuating fatigue; and his limbs felt like lead. His peak flow meter readings were 400 to 450. After four years of poor health, he attended the clinic, and a year later his athletic performance and muscle strength were restored, with peak flow at 650 to 700. Dairy and beef products caused revolting halitosis, and CRC, *Giardia,* and five viruses (the principal viruses—glandular fever, polio, and RSV) restored his health and athletic performance.

### L. Male, Age 28 (P)

During the late teens he was careless with horticultural spraying. Seven years ago family deaths brought on a personality change; he avoided people, was constantly tired, and had long depressed periods. He failed to complete his final year at university. A year later he became bedridden for eight months and suffered repeated herpes and shingles infections. There followed a period of slow recovery interrupted by fatigue, self-doubt, and inability to concentrate because of poor memory and recall. Six years later he attended the clinic, experiencing improvement from OWGG exclusion, CRC, and *Giardia* therapy. Dramatic improvements occurred with eight viruses. (The principal ones were EBV, hepatitis, herpes, and v. zoster). Has continued with serial vaccinations of these viruses at eight-week intervals and holds a full-time overseas job.

### M. Male, Age Group 35 to 40

Presented at clinic with four-year history of marked obesity, chronic fatigue, extensive eczema and hives covering most of the body surface, bizarre behavioral changes, memory lapses, and lack of libido and erectile ability. Within five months, the obesity was lost and the skin cleared from OWGG exclusion, CRC, and house dust and mold therapies. The sexual functions returned as the obesity cleared. The irritable bladder and kidney function responded to *Ureaplasma* and *Papillomavirus* (warts), the testicles to mumps, and erection to CMV and *Helicobacter.* He has a fixed allergy to OWGGs, and the slightest amount provokes his eczema and hives.

## N. Male, Age 35 (P)

A rapid onset of CFS following influenza. Other symptoms were arthritis, weak and aching legs and arms, heart irregularity and chest pains, and IBS. Within three years he lost his job because of memory, spelling, and writing problems. Began treatment four years after onset of CFIDS. A good response to exclusion of OWGGs and potato, but improvement plateaued despite CRC, *Giardia,* and *Helicobacter* therapy. Although significant provocations resulted from testing with eight viruses, there was no further improvement until the carpets and underfelt were removed from his house. *Parvovirus,* which is associated with animals, and *Mycoplasma hominis* cleared the arthritis. The previous owners of the house had kept animals locked up inside while they were working. Removal of the soiled carpets and underfelt cleared most symptoms. CMV and *Helicobacter* restored his libido.

## O. Female, Age 36

During childhood nearly died of a herpes-related encephalitis. During her teens obsessive-compulsive behavior developed, and over the next five years CFIDS, headaches, and memory problems affected her ability to hold a job. Over the following ten years the compulsive behavior worsened, with little improvement in the CFIDS. She improved on exclusion of dairy, beef, and poultry products. CRC, *Giardia,* and *Helicobacter,* together with six viruses, in particular, herpes and glandular fever, markedly reduced the compulsive behavior. Her health and personality improved over the following six months, and she has held a job.

## P. Male, Age 40

Trained in organic chemistry and became a teacher. By age 32 had CFIDS, with muscle weakness, lack of libido, and low body temperature. For eight years he was treated for myasthenia gravis (muscle weakness). Began treatment two years ago with exclusion of OWGGs and potato, CRC, and *Giardia,* with significant improvement in energy and IBS. Eight viruses, of which three were significant. Polio, RSV, and CMV improved muscle and memory problems, while glandular fever cleared the remaining CFIDS symptoms. The recovery occurred in "fits and starts." He returned to teaching and has suffered no relapses. A happy event was the return of his libido and the addition of two more children to their family of four.

## Q. Male, Age 48 (P)

A heavy smoker and regular beer drinker suffered severe influenza eighteen years ago and was left with tinnitus and unsteadiness. He continued smoking and drinking despite recurring influenza. Within three to four years he developed fatigue; he often fell asleep at work and after meals but suffered insomnia. His physician diagnosed stress, but he could not tolerate the tranquilizers. He continued to hold a job, but his memory deteriorated, requiring copious reminder notes. Blurred vision and difficulty focusing and a sensation of being "spaced out" convinced him to stop smoking and drinking. Three years ago depression and crying occurred without any reason. Influenza required bed rest for two to three days, during which he experienced aches, pains, and muscle spasms in the legs. Genitourinary symptoms were treated with little benefit by numerous antibiotic courses. Two years ago he took an interest in his illness and, as a result of reading, approached the clinic for treatment. OWGGs and all foods containing yeast and mold were excluded. He began to lose his obesity. CRC, *Torulopsis* (a yeast), and *Giardia,* together with six viruses, brought about a recovery within six months. The muscle spasms were relieved by polio, the muscle pains by morbilli; RSV cleared away the brain fog and improved his memory; herpes cleared the tinnitus and, together with *Giardia* and *Ureaplasma,* restored normal bladder functions. Glandular fever reduced swelling of the neck glands and improved depression and fatigue. Now he has recovered and does not stray from the new lifestyle of regular exercise and tolerated foods. He continued glandular fever shots at two-month intervals for two years.

## R. Male, Age 58

Laboratory worker and researcher. People engaged in laboratory work involving animals are prone to CFIDS (a clinic-related observation). The researcher took early retirement because of memory and recall problems, and the onset of CFIDS with fatigue, muscle weakness, and pain. After four years of poor health in retirement he started treatment with exclusion of OWGGs and two minor foods, CRC, *Giardia,* and *Helicobacter.* The memory and recall recovered with RSV and rotavirus, the muscle and joint symptoms with *Parvovirus,* CMV, polio, and flu. EBV cleared the CFIDS and other symptoms. Two years later a relapse required resumption of virutherapy, including herpes. The relapse cleared within six weeks, and over the last two years his health has been better than at any time in the previous ten years. *Parvovirus, Helicobactor, Giardia,* and *Candida* are transmitted by animals, in particular, through their saliva.

## S. Female, Age Group 45 to 50

The body eczema present since infancy extended across most of the skin surface after a pregnancy. At the same time, she became cold and her hands and feet lost their color for long periods. Over the next fifteen years she experienced periods of depression and her memory recall became progressively worse. Urinary frequency and bladder infections persisted in spite of antibiotics. Improvement came after exclusion of dairy and beef products and OWGGs. The skin improved with CRC and house dust/molds. The skin itch cleared with hepatitis; the genitourinary problems disappeared with CMV, *Helicobacter, Ureaplasma,* and *Trichomonas.* The muscle aches and excessive coldness were relieved by polio, rubella, and *Giardia.* A few small patches of eczema and psoriasis that did not itch persisted. Eight viruses were significant.

## T. Male, Age 48

Twenty-five to twenty-eight years ago resided in Europe/North America/Asia. Contracted severe influenza and then flulike illnesses, leaving him with muscle pains and spasms, fatigue, and sensitivity to cold. Since then his health has deteriorated, with blurring of vision, IBS, and oral and genital herpes outbreaks. Before starting treatment two years ago, the relapses required bed rest for weeks or months. Poultry and OWGGs were excluded; CRC, *Giardia,* and *Helicobacter* began an improvement in health. The response to dengue fever was dramatic. The genitourinary symptoms and herpes were relieved by *Giardia, Helicobacter, Ureaplasma,* and common wart virus *(Papillomavirus).* Polio, rubella, and RSV restored his vision and markedly improved memory and personality. The oral herpes cleared with v. zoster and herpes virutherapy. **Comment:** Although genital herpes may appear to respond to influenza shots, in time, relapses do not respond. Herpes 1 and 2 are more effective, but the best results are obtained when given with v. zoster.

## U. Female, Age 52

Thirty years ago developed strange illness of changing numbness and tingling of skin areas, unexplained fatigue, aching muscles and joints, IBS, chronic sinusitis, and her memory became hopeless. Some years later she developed unsteadiness (Ménière's disease), and nasal surgery was advised to relieve the chronic sinusitis and unsteadiness. This exacerbated the conditions. Two years ago she attended the clinic. OWGGs and pork were excluded. CRC, *Giardia, Helicobacter,* and morbilli improved fatigue and muscle aches. Rotavirus cleared the IBS and constipation, besides stimulating mental activity. Polio and v. zoster relieved numbness, tingling, and the constant head pain. The Ménière's unsteadiness responded to mumps. The chronic sinusitis improved with food exclusions but finally resolved with flu, adenovirus, and RSV, with the RSV improving her memory as well. No relapses occurred during the three years following completion of MLV.

## V. Male, Age 25

Slow onset of fatigue, headaches, joint aches, and muscle pains followed vomiting and diarrhea during a vacation in Indonesia. Sugar restriction improved the joint and muscle pains. Laboratory testing was negative to *Giardia* and intestinal amoebas. During the following year he took three antibiotic courses, quinacrine, metronidazole, with temporary improvement of the IBS symptoms and foul-smelling flatus. The drugs had no effect on the intermittent variable swelling of the neck glands. Treatments over the next three years did not clear the IBS. He attended the clinic and, because of a marked reaction, began a total exclusion of OWGGs. Provocation testing with CRC and amoeba dilutions was negative. Provocation testing with *Giardia* crippled him for two days. Five other viruses gave significant provocations, and as treatment continued, provocation with CRC was positive. Food exclusions and virutherapy cleared symptoms over the next year. The principal viruses were EBV, hepatitis, and rotavirus. He has a fixed food allergy to OWGGs and has been unable to reintroduce them into his diet.

## W. Female, Age 48 (P)

Suffered clinical hepatitis without antibody blood test confirmation. For the next twenty years suffered CFIDS and attended five prestigious medical clinics in North America, which diagnosed her symptoms as "all in the mind." An allergy clinic in Chicago detected allergies to wheat and barley (celiac syndrome). Exclusion of these foods increased her energy and reduced symptoms for many years. The clinic detected evidence of a liver disorder. After two pregnancies her health took a dive, and the chronic fatigue returned, along with aching muscles. Treatment included full OWGG exclusion, CRC, and *Giardia,* and nine significant viruses. Symptoms of hepatitis B were provoked by hepatitis virus, CMV, glandular fever, mumps, and dengue fever. IBS responded to CRC and *Giardia,* in addition to the full OWGGs exclusion. She recovered her remembered health and has remained well for several years.

## X. Female, Age 58

At age 28 developed migraines and other head pains; at ages 38 to 40, repeated lung infections became chronic infective bronchitis; at 50, unexplained fatigue and a constant feeling of coldness, together with deteriorating vision, caused loss of job. Attended clinic three years ago and excluded OWGGs and stopped smoking. Polio improved her appreciation of colors, which now appear brighter and more vivid than she remembers. CRC and *Giardia* improved her fatigue and head pains. The migraines cleared with morbilli, house dust, and three other molds. All these therapies improved her respiratory problems, but Coxsackievirus was the principal virus improving the chest symptoms and relieving the weepy depression and muscle weakness. The chronic infective bronchitis remains under control but is not suitable for operation. Her health is considerably better, but she requires ongoing *Candida* therapy and MLV.

## Y. Female, Age 50 (P)

Acquired DDT pesticide poisoning as a child and teenager in North America. Health began to deteriorate at age 25, with a decrease in physical activity and memory and unaccountable mood changes. The chronic fatigue disappeared during the early years of her marriage and pregnancies and on return was regarded by physicians at several clinics as being psychosomatic. A change of residence brought on severe CFIDS and stopped her social activities. She could not manage the house for weeks on end and developed severe petrochemical sensitivity. Antidepressants and other SSDs were not tolerated. At age 48, removal of natural gas from her home jump-started the recovery. CRC, *Giardia,* and *Helicobacter* markedly improved the IBS and sleepy lethargy. Her response to EBV provocation was dramatic, with four to five weeks of depression and crying, after which she had increasing numbers of days when she felt better than she had for years. Seven other viruses were significant. After removal of the natural gas from her home she gained considerable benefit from saunas. For months she had a chemical taste in her mouth and her body had a chemical smell after the saunas. She resents the twenty years or so of her life that were disrupted by pesticide poisoning.

## Z. Female, Age 56 (P)

During her first year of marriage, at age 25, she developed fatigue, headaches, racing of the heart, IBS, and aching legs. The headaches gradually became more severe and frequent over the following ten years, possibly aggravated by three pregnancies. She developed pelvic inflammation, but the numerous courses of antibiotics were of little use; they aggravated bladder symptoms, and she began to suffer from vaginal thrush. At age 45 she had a hysterectomy, which gave a period of relief, but a CSR brought on giddiness (vertigo), fluctuating blood pressure, and frequent spacing out, with memory problems. She deteriorated until she was unable to cope with daily activities, became depressed, and developed phobias. Within nine months of attending the clinic she was free of most symptoms. Morbilli relieved the migraine, and CMV, the heart symptoms; her remaining pelvic and bladder symptoms responded to *Chlamydia*, CMV, *Helicobacter,* and *Ureaplasma*. She was extremely sensitive to OWGGs, with the smallest amount disabling her for twenty-four hours. Most of the symptoms were further improved by CRC and *Giardia.*

# Chapter 1

# An Outline of Latency Immunity, Indications, Methods, and Treatment

## *INTRODUCTION*

"What is causing my symptoms/illness?" How can you answer a disappointed compliant patient when clinical laboratory tests and medical technology return normal/negative results? A physician's duty is to continue investigations and then refer to psychological medicine. The disappointed patient often chooses alternative health. Before patients investigate these therapies, or if they received no benefit from them, they are suitable for latency therapy.

The extraordinary results described in *CFIDS, Fibromyalgia, and the Virus-Allergy Link* can be duplicated on your problem, subjective, functional, affective, and temperamental patients. Patients are relieved of their anxieties because causes are found for their strange *all-in-the-head* symptoms and illnesses. They are delighted with the reduction, even cessation, of long-term symptom suppression drugs (SSDs), physiotherapy, and return visits to clinics. You have the satisfaction of adding another treatment option, and you retain your patients, who are not likely to move into the alternative health arena.

Fourteen years ago, I suspected that similarly disillusioned patients with posture and body language suggestive of convalescing polio victims harbored polio virus. Provocation with 1:5 serial dilutions of polio gave remarkable responses and recovery for some, although not all. Within five years I acquired eight viruses, protozoa, bacteria, and their toxins. Patients with long-standing (duration of one year or more) subjective illness were accepted by the clinic if they provided a recent work-up by their family physician. The results continued to improve. I presented a paper to the American Academy of Otolaryngic Allergy (AAOA) (1990) in San Diego. The HIV scare (1986-1992) caused considerable patient resistance to virutherapy.

Latency therapy cannot stand alone. It is complementary to established therapies. Latency therapy facilitates specific excretion (detoxing) of excess intracellular latentee (antigen), allowing individual cells to regain normal activities. Latency therapy improves depressed body cell immunity. It does not appear to affect the natural immune system's (NIS) leucocyte activity or antibodies. Latency therapy is a variant of vaccination medicine. *Surmise:* Mass vaccination for the extermination of *poliomyelitis,* while suppressing the active infection, may be replacing it with a latent state of infection.

Active infection/disease and allergens (antigens) involve the NIS's antibody and cellular immunity. Latent infection/disease and allergens (latentors) involve the organ cell immune system (OCIS) as intracellular latentees and excreted latentee antilaten (antibody). The excretion of latentees is accompanied by provoked recognized symptoms and smells. Provoked excretion of latentee antilatens may provoke symptoms but no smell.

Latency therapy is a simple injection technique to uncover hidden intracellular foreign materials from previous infections or exposures. By manipulating each identified antigen (latentee) with serial 1:5 dilution doses, an excretion-provoking (neutralizing) dose is found. A series of treatment shots at weekly or longer intervals from one or more treatment vials gradually reduces the overload of antigen (latentee), and organ cellular activity returns to normal. The descriptions of latency immunity raise numerous problems in describing and explaining the cell immune activity, the reasons for encouraging often spectacular clinical responses, and the various patterns of excretion (detoxing) from different body areas and organs. At first, latency therapy appears to be anecdotal, and the provoked symptoms, a placebo response. The clinic responses, the return of health, and the persistence of recovery impressed patients, leaving them with no doubts about the validity of latency therapy. It remains for interested physicians and virologists to unravel its mechanism.

Latency immunity is the immune response of a group or groups of body cells with varying loads of a similar foreign latentee (antigen). The involved organ cells have a tropism toward the latentor/latentee. Latent, meaning hidden, is the preferred word for an immune activity in many ways distinct from the NIS. Laboratory antibody tests are inappropriate for latency immunity. The expensive polymerase chain reaction test (PCRT) may have an application, but in contrast to the inexpensive serial 1:5 dilution antigen-provoking shots, the PCRT is less accurate and does not provide a neutralizing/treatment-starting dose. The state of viruses responding to latency therapy has similarities to the *inapparent* group of *permissive* viruses. Besides the inapparent group, permissive viruses have *nonpermissive* and latent groupings. The term "latent" is taken from the third group, which could be described as *dormant*. Latency immunity involves every cell in the body, whereas the latent group of permissive viruses is small and receives little comment or mention in microbiology texts. The latent group appears dormant or inactive, whereas latency immunity, although hidden from laboratory testing, is apparent, with functional, subjective, affective symptoms of tropism cell group overload. Provocation brings on immediate and delayed symptoms, often dramatic or severe, until improvement or recovery occurs. Looked at another way, the three groups of permissive viral cell states may be amenable to latency therapy (p. 29).

Latency terms attempt an analogy with the NIS. *Surmise:* The infection or foreign material latentor/antigen enters the body and bypasses the natural immune system during the early stage of confrontation. Latentors are taken up by susceptible (tropism) organ cell groups. The latentor is held as an inactive latentee. If cell immunities are lowered, microbial replication occurs. On recovery, the cell can excrete excess or, if dormant, be stimulated to excrete the overload of latentees. The cell retains enough latentee to act as an immunity template. Susceptible cell groups holding numerous minimal immune templates that do not depress cellular activities do not appear to provoke symptoms or detoxing with provocation testing. Cell groups are provoked and excrete latentees years later by a dilution dose of the virus that entered as an active infection fifty to sixty years earlier, for example, migraine (morbilli) and fibromyalgia (Epstein-Barr virus [EBV]). *Surmise:* The viral templates are transferred from apoptosis cells to replacement cells. Subclinical reinfections occurred during the sufferer's life. Excreted latentee provokes recognized symptoms and detoxes at various body sites and organs when its smell or stench is detected. A latentee antilaten (antibody) is excreted with or without clinical signs and symptoms, but there is no smell. In the past, much importance was given to the characteristic smells of viral and bacterial infections and abnormal metabolic products.

During fourteen years of clinical latency therapy, out of over 2,000 patients, only a handful recovered with a single viral or microbial provocation and serial vaccination therapy. The majority of patients have a principal and several secondary microbial/viral identified causes of their functional latency illness. The complexity of subjective functional illness means that only some of the causes can be identified and detoxed. Every effort should be made to detect causes of functional latency illness. If a patient returns negative viral antibody test results that do not agree with your clinical assessment, turn to latency therapy when the provoked symptoms support your diagnosis and also provide you with a beginning treatment dose.

In latency therapy, stage I, the preliminary work-up scans three to five common foods, five to six inhalants and fungi, including *Candida*-related complex (CRC). Previous allergy test results are reviewed or repeated using provocation. In stage II, the multiple latent virutherapy (MLV) scans selected latentors (antigens) of twenty-five viruses, twelve bacteria and their toxins, and two protozoa. A minority of patients require a more complete food work-up, if suspicious food symptoms persist after the second month of the work-up. As the patient proceeds through the preliminary and virutherapy stages of a latency work-up, other symptoms suggestive of different causes are revealed. At the end of the work-up, if the recovery is not adequate, previous laboratory and technical investigations should be repeated. The average recovery period is six to seven months to two years. Patients who will tolerate prolonged treatment are those who have been disillusioned by previous conventional and alternative therapies they received during the previous year or for longer periods of time. The description of symptoms or illnesses acts as a guide to significant microbial dilutions for therapy. The neutralizing and treatment doses of each microbial varies with individual patients. An example is recovery of memory: CRC, *Listeria, Chlamydia,* respiratory syncytial virus (RSV), polio, influenza, hepatitis, rubella, v. zoster, and EBV. One or more of these microbials have restored or improved memory using latency therapy.

Latency immunity requires clinical rather than research papers to establish its position as a medical therapy. The practical problems of controlled studies for latency illnesses are daunting. Latency does not fit the scientific medicine requirements. Should all medical endeavors be subjected to the "one way" scientific rigor? If so, several useful clinical therapies will remain outside of these artificial limits. Is this why certain allergy techniques, CRC therapy and latency therapy—all successful treatments—are anecdotal with placebo responses? Recommended information sources are as follows:

1. H. S. Krause (Ed.) (1989). *Otolaryngic Allergy and Immunology.* Philadelphia, PA: Saunders Company.
2. R. L. Trevino and H. S. Dixon (1997). *Food Allergy.* New York: Thieme Medical Publishers.
3. W. J. Joklik (Ed.) (1992). *Zinsser Microbiology,* Twentieth Edition. Norwalk, CT: Appleton and Lange.
4. B. M. Hyde (Ed.) (1992). *The Clinical and Scientific Basis of ME/CFS.* Ottawa, Ontario, Canada: Nightingale Research Foundation.
5. J. B. Miller (1972). *Food Allergy.* Springfield, IL: Charles C Thomas.

6. J. B. Miller, C. E. Lee, E. L. Blinkley, and S. M. Hardt (1972). Relief of influenza symptoms by the provocative neutralizing method. *Journal of Medical Association of State of Alabama,* 41: 493.
7. R. B. Duncan (1999). Latency immunity and therapy: A clinical study of latent Epstein-Barr virus incidence in 297 idiopathic chronic fatigue patients with plausible hypotheses. *Journal of Chronic Fatigue Syndrome,* 5(2): 77-95.

A scientific study design of latency raises insurmountable organization and finance problems. Symptoms and signs are intermixed, interdependent, and there are irregular subjective patterns. In addition, (1) short- and long-term fluctuations occur at variable intervals, and (2) the article "Latency Immunity and Therapy" reported that the majority of patients provoked a principal and, on average, five secondary viruses. For the remaining patients, the role of the principal virus changed with some of the secondary viruses at different stages of their recovery. For example, at first, symptoms and smells lasting three to eight weeks suggested influenza; then for a similar period symptoms and detoxing suggested hepatitis; then a further change suggested cytomegalovirus (CMV)/EBV. Following a period of recovery or marked improvement in health, a relapse suggested one of the three was the principal virus, and occasionally a fourth was responsible for the predominant symptoms and smells. Most latency illness is complex, with multiple fluctuating causes and symptoms.

## MATERIALS

The extracts for the preliminary work-up, inhalants, foods, molds, including CRC, are readily available through commercial firms. The selection of foods should include wheat and rice, egg or chicken, milk or beef, potato or tomato, and corn. Other foods can be added later, depending on local food preferences. Select the 1:20 concentration. House dust, *Alternaria, Cladosporium,* mixed grass pollens, ragweed/weed mix, *Mucor,* and *Aspergillus* are 1:20 concentration. The *Candida* concentrate is a mix of *C. albicans, C. Tropicalis,* and other yeast species, such as *Torulopsis glabrata,* may be in the mix. *Giardia* and *Helicobacter* complete the basic preliminary work-up set.

MLV work-up requires influenza, polio, morbilli, hepatitis, and possibly CMV. Processed viral solutions may be available from commercial laboratories that culture viruses. The viral vaccination preparations may be safely used if they have expired and are treated with heat to denature the viral protein. Using Phenol 0.4 percent adds to the denaturing process.

Influenza vaccine and serial dilution provocation and treatment were initiated by Dr. J. Miller over twenty-five years ago. The 1 milliliter (ml) of influenza vaccine used as a concentrate provides a considerable quantity of 1:5 dilutions, probably sufficient for testing of forty to fifty patients and the treatment of twenty to thirty patients. The denatured viral protein does not appear to deteriorate over the following two years.

### Treatment Station Supplies

1. Sterile rubber cap vials; 2 ml for treatment and 5 ml for testing solutions.
2. Sterile disposable syringes with or without fitted needles. Inexpensive ½ to 1 ml syringes suitable for clinic skin provocation tests. One or more boxes of 100 quality gauge 28 to 29½ ml syringes supplied to patients for home therapy. Twenty-five to fifty 3 ml syringes and twenty to thirty 15 ml syringes.
3. A normal saline dilutant with preservative in liter packs. Sterile treatment vials prefilled with dilutant, 2 and 5 ml, are available.
4. Trays for holding the 5 ml testing vials.

These supplies are available from commercial allergy supply houses.

Stationery supplies include clipboards, test sheets for patients and the technician's notes, electric timers, a small mirror, and books or magazines, one of which should have simple large print, as well as suitable children's toys and coloring books for different ages, but no felt pens.

Testing solutions of individual antigens (latentors) are diluted 1:5 from concentrate, i.e., ten treatment vials from $5^1$ to $5^{10}$ dilutions. CRC and most viruses are diluted to $5^{15}/5^{20}$ (refer to Serial Dilutions Chart on p. 36). First label ten or fifteen vials with the antigen and dilution number. Fill testing vials with 4 ml of dilutant, draw up 1 ml concentrated antigen, and mix three to four times in vial number one. Draw 1 ml of vial number one's mixture and place in vial number two, mixing three to four times. Continue in like manner to vial dilutions $5^{10}/5^{15}$. CRC is diluted to $5^{22}$. The starting dose is $5^7$ for men and $5^8$ for women and children. The injection or shot is 0.05 ml. For skin whealing it is 0.05 ml inhalants or 0.10 to 0.15 ml for foods (skin endpoint titration [SET]). The injection for whealing and provocation is intradermal. Provocation injection is 0.10 ml subdermal or subcutaneous. Sublingual drops are used for children, 0.10 to 0.15 ml, adding six to eight drops of glycerine sweetener. The dose is drawn up in a syringe and slowly dropped onto the tip of a teaspoon. The antigen and glycerine mixture is placed under the tongue of the child who sits on the parent's knee. The technician kneels before the child because it is difficult to place the drops from a standing position.

An emergency resuscitation kit of medications, face mask, and oxygen cylinder is mandatory for all allergy testing. Cushions are supplied for those with back problems and the occasional apprehensive person who suffers a vasovagal attack. Have a large plastic bowl on hand for vomiting. Do not test/provoke a food or inhalant that caused a marked or alarming reaction in the past. A no-responsibility form is required from all patients undergoing latency testing and therapy.

Family health clinics should add a latency therapy unit as an alternative option to symptom suppression drug therapy. The latency unit employs a registered trained nurse for every six to eight patients referred daily. The unit is situated in a pleasant, naturally well-lit room, as appointments last up to four hours. During the testing, patients are encouraged to read from a selection of allergy and ecology health books. Questions are encouraged, and those the technician is unable to handle are referred to the physician. Successful/satisfied patients are quick to spread, by word of mouth, the advantages of a latency unit within the community.

Reorder concentrates from the original supply company unless responses are disappointing. Expensive standardized antigens are not necessary. Food, inhalant, and mold replacements are compatible with exhausted concentrates. Bacterial, protozoan, and viral concentrates can vary from replacement supplies. The replacement concentrate dilutions do not need standardization with the expended dilutions because provocation, not skin whealing, is significant. The dilutions of antigens (latentors) remain sterile for long periods, unless no preservative is used, in which case they should be replaced at six- to eight-week intervals. Those solutions with an antiseptic could be changed at three months, but if few patients are treated at the clinic, replace them at twelve- to eighteen-month intervals. The 2 ml treatment vials are posted in a letter envelope at standard rates. Exhausted treatment vials are not refilled.

For detailed instructions refer to references 1 and 2 on p. 4, *Otolaryngic Allergy and Immunology* and *Food Allergy.*

## *TECHNIQUE*

The needle technique (SET) was developed by Miller for food immunization. Latency therapy requires the needle technique, and sublingual drops for children. When a large skin whealing occurs, measure and record the neutralizing dilution. The patient takes the testing sheet home and inspects the wheals in 8, 12, and 15 to 24 hours (h) during the following day. The test sheet shows the order of injections from one to twenty. Skin markings can blur or be accidentally washed off. The needle prick marks are present and are counted on the arm from above to the delayed whealing injection. For example, the patient notes there are no skin wheals, only a little redness around each prick mark on going to bed. The following morning a wheal or inflammatory response may have appeared. If the ink markings are blurred, the patient counts the prick marks from the top of the arm and notes whether the eighth prick mark has a wheal. Number eight on the testing sheet is house dust $5^2$. The patient notes house dust $5^5$ and $5^7$ have enlarged since the previous evening. The finding is reported to the clinic. Delayed skin responses are accurate indicators of sensitivity. Delayed skin whealing and erythema does not occur with viral testing unless it is a response to materials in the culture medium, e.g., viruses grown on eggs.

The starting testing dose is $5^2$ or $5^3$, if there are no active or present symptoms suggestive of the virus to be tested. If symptoms and case history are suggestive, testing starts at $5^4$ or $5^6$. After an interval of 10 to 15 minutes (min), the dose is decreased by two dilutions. A provoked symptom or sensation occurs and is recognized by the patient. It is cleared or neutralized by continuing two decreasing dilution steps (see also reference 1, p. 4). The patient usually experiences a feeling of well-being with neutralization of the symptoms. If no provoked responses occur on reaching $5^7$ or $5^9$, the next antigen is commenced. Patients with severe symptoms, especially muscle weakness from CFIDS/ME and those with severe asthma are started on high dilutions, e.g., $5^{20}$, $5^{15}$. The strength is increased by two or three dilutions until provoked symptoms occur, e.g., at $5^{12}$. The provoked symptoms are neutralized by returning to weaker dilutions, e.g., $5^{20}$, $5^{18}$, $5^{16}$, $5^{14}$, $5^{12}$, with provocation at, for example, $5^{14}$ giving neutralization. (Refer to harmonic effects in reference 7, listed on p. 5.)

Use one antigen at a time. For safety, resist using two or more at the same time, as provoked responses are confusing, and occasionally very severe. Interference with and modification of provoked immediate and delayed symptoms caused by the effect of one virus on another give confusing or negative responses. The same virus on testing gives an immediate symptom or sensation recognized by the patient, but the delayed provocation may be a different recognized sensation or a combination of the immediate plus different recognized symptoms. At first it is difficult to assign symptoms and sensations to viral provocation, immediate or delayed, unless they are clear-cut and obvious. Table 1.1 on regional

TABLE 1.1. Regional Symptoms and Frequently Provoked Latent Microbes

| Symptom/Region | Significant Latent Viruses | Latent Bacteria | Latent Molds/Protozoa |
|---|---|---|---|
| Nose | Influenza, ATV, RSV, Rhinovirus, Polio, Herpes I, *Papillomavirus 4*, Hepatitis | *Chlamydia, Pseudomonas, Helicobacter, S. albicans, S. aureus, M. pneumoniae* | CRC, *Mucor, Aspergillus, Giardia* |
| Bronchus/Lungs | Influenza, RSV, Polio, Morbilli, Mumps, V. zoster, Herpes I, ATV, Rhinovirus, CMV, *Papillomavirus 4,6,* Coxsackievirus | *Chlamydia, Legionella, M. pneumoniae,* Pertussis, *Pasteurella, Helicobacter, Pseudomonas* | CRC, *Mucor,* Aspergillus, *Cladosporium, Alternaria, Cryptococcus, Giardia, Trichomonas* |
| Mouth/Tongue/Throat | Mumps, Herpes I, V. zoster, CMV, Hepatitis, Dengue, EBV, Rubella, ATV | *Helicobacter* | CRC, *Giardia, Trichomonas* |
| Stomach/Intestines/Colon | Hepatitis, Mumps, Polio, ATV, CMV, Rotavirus, EBV, *Papillomavirus 4,6* | *Helicobacter, Listeria, Legionella, Mycobacterium,* Paratuberculosis, *C. difficile* | CRC, *Giardia, Trichomonas, Cryptosporidium, Blastocystis* |
| Headaches/Migraine | Morbilli, V. zoster, Influenza, Polio, CMV, Herpes I, *Parvovirus,* Rubella, ATV, EBV | *Listeria* | CRC, *Giardia, Trichomonas, Mucor, Aspergillus* |
| Moods/Depression/Memory/Dreams | Influenza, Hepatitis, Polio, Morbilli, RSV, Herpes I, CMV, Dengue, EBV, V. zoster, Rotavirus, Coxsackievirus, Mumps | *Listeria, M. pneumoniae* | CRC, *Giardia, Trichomonas, Mucor, Aspergillus* |
| Heart/CV System/Vascular Spasm | CMV, EBV, Polio, Rubella, Mumps, Influenza, RSV, Coxsackievirus | *Chlamydia, Helicobacter, Ureaplasma* | CRC |

TABLE 1.1 *(continued)*

| | | | |
|---|---|---|---|
| Eyes/Vision/ Eye Itch | Rubella, Mumps, ATV, Herpes I, V. zoster, Influenza, RSV, Morbilli, Polio, Dengue, Hepatitis | *Chlamydia* | CRC, *Alternaria, Cladosporium* |
| Ears/Hearing/ Tinnitus/Vertigo | Influenza, RSV, V. zoster, Morbilli, Hepatitis, Rubella, Mumps, ATV, Herpes I, *Papillomavirus 4,6* | *M. pneumoniae* | *Mucor, Aspergillus* |
| Skin | Influenza, Hepatitis, Polio, Morbilli, Rubella, Herpes I and II, V. zoster, Mumps, RSV, EBV, *Papillomavirus 1,4,6* | *Chlamydia, Staphylococcus aureus* | CRC, *Trichophyton, Epidermophyton, Cryptococcus* |
| Muscle Pain/ Spasm | Influenza, Polio, CMV, EBV, Dengue, Rotavirus, Morbilli, Rubella | *Chlamydia, Listeria, Ureaplasma* | CRC, *Giardia* |
| Joints | Mumps, Coxsackievirus | *Helicobacter, C. difficile, M. hominis* | *Trichomonas* |
| Genitourinary/ Kidney/Bladder | CMV, Herpes II, Hepatitis, Mumps, EBV, *Papillomavirus 14,16* | *Helicobacter, Ureaplasma, Chlamydia* | CRC, *Giardia, Trichomonas* |
| Sleeping Disorders Somnific | EBV, CMV, Hepatitis, Influenza, Morbilli, V. zoster | *Helicobacter* | CRC, *Giardia* |
| Insomniac | RSV, Polio, Rubella, Rotavirus, Mumps, *Papillomavirus* | *Chlamydia* | |

*Notes:* ATV is now more commonly known as adenovirus; *C.* = *Clostridium*; *M.* = *Mycoplasma*; *S.* = *Staphylococcus.*

symptoms, Figure 1.1 on tender and pain-sensitive sites, and descriptions of conditions (see Chapter 2) will aid an understanding. Maintain a clinical record of individual virus provocations and a range of definite or suspected provoked responses. The patterns for the clinic become apparent after 100 to 200 patients are tested.

People over the age of fifty-five, those with chronic latency symptoms, and those debilitated by latency illnesses may not provoke whealing or immediate symptoms during testing. If this becomes apparent during the testing session, they are given an explanation. All patients expect immediate reactions because of immunoglobulin E (Ig E) type techniques. Some become annoyed or frustrated at the end of the testing. They may forget what they were told at the clinic and fail to phone the following day. The clinic must contact patients two to three days later, as unrecognized provoked symptoms may have occurred. Some elderly people will dismiss the consultation as a waste of time or money. Do not continue to treat these patients because compliance is suspect, the result will probably be a failure, and they will voice their dissatisfaction throughout the community.

Older people and those suffering chronic, often disabling, illness lose their ability to excrete. Until nonspecific or specific latency therapy stimulates excretion (detoxing), testing for provoked symptoms may be negative. Once detoxing starts up, antigens (latentors) previously tested with negative responses are retested and provoke delayed symptoms.

*Surmise:* Food immunization technique suppresses symptoms by using strong dilutions of foods (e.g., $5^1$ to $5^5$). It is mediated through the blood and cellular immune system with an increase in antibodies to foods. Latency responses occur with higher dilutions (e.g., $5^5$ to $5^{15}$). There is no antibody response. A PCRT occasionally detects the latentor (antigen). Latency immunity is associated with delayed provoked symptoms and excretion detoxing. I questioned hundreds of patients who had mixed responses with food immunization therapy. At no time did any detect excretory or detoxing smells. Latency therapy may not be associated with provoked symptoms and smells. A latentor-antilaten complex (antigen-antibody) is postulated. Patients may not detect smells because of adaptation of their sense of smell to what is being excreted. Ask the patient for a confirmation of detoxing smells by a relative or friend.

Antihistamines are stopped four to six days before testing. Corticosteroids, antidepressants, and nonsteroid anti-inflammatory drugs (NSAIDs) are stopped, if possible, four days before testing. Patients must disclose the drugs they are using. Patients who do not disclose their medicinal or social drug use will, in time, raise the suspicion of the physician, when an expected pattern of provocation and recovery does not occur. The presence

FIGURE 1.1. Comparison of Fibromyalgia Tender Point Sites and Latency-Provoked Pain-Sensitive Sites

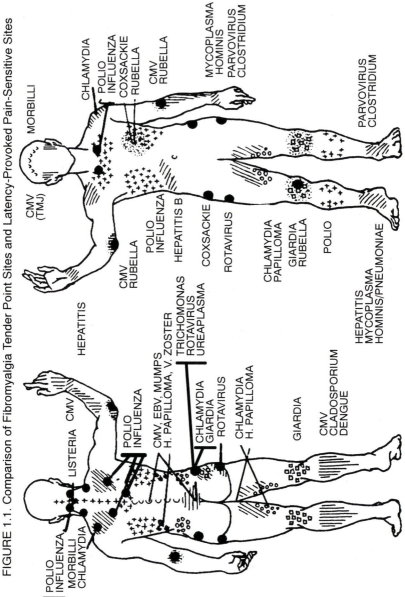

of medical drugs means few or no immediate provoked symptoms, although they may not interfere with delayed provoked symptoms. A case history pattern suggestive of food allergy, i.e., to Old World grass grains (OWGGs), and symptoms of CRC and no test provocations requires an empirical decision to totally exclude grains and treat CRC. If the patient agrees and the empirical decision is correct, after six to eight weeks, provocation testing is resumed and reliable provoked responses appear. As the patient's condition improves, a gradual withdrawal of drugs begins. The withdrawal is complete three to four months later. Detoxing of chemicals and drugs may give a chemical taste and leave a chemical smell in the bedding and underwear.

### Syringe and Sublingual Drop Therapy

Treatment doses are 0.05 ml, with no buildup of doses, e.g., from 0.05 to 0.5 ml. Progressive dosage strength applies to strong dilutions, but with weak or high dilutions, e.g., one part in several hundred thousand, millions, or billions, increasing the dose does not improve provocation and excretion. When there is no response after two or three weekly shots, the vials and an explanatory note are returned by the patient. A personal contact and interview may be necessary before the new treatment vial dilutions are made. Eventually, after two or three vial changes, dilutions $5^4$ to $5^5$ fail to provoke. It is assumed the organ cells of the body will not excrete any more latentees. The patient no longer experiences symptoms due to that latentee. Patients with CFIDS/ME, severe asthma, and other debilitating chronic conditions will detox and experience relief for two, three, or more weeks with $5^{22}$, even $5^{25}$. They are unable to increase the treatment strength and so continue with a treatment shot once every three or six weeks for months or years. I cannot explain this effect. Improvement is usually sufficient for them to rejoin the workforce. Laboratory testing of blood and cellular immunity is normal, so it may represent a failure of latency immunities to recover.

Treatment vials and dropper bottles contain one to four individual viruses at their empirically determined treatment dilution. Viruses are grouped together when they provoke symptoms that are similar or involve a particular organ or body surface. Examples are as follows:

1. Asthma: influenza, polio, morbilli, *Mycoplasma pneumoniae,* and *Legionella.*
2. Respiratory infection and glue ear of children and adolescents to age fourteen: sublingual drops with influenza, RSV, adeno(tonsil)virus

(ATV) (now more commonly known simply as adenovirus), *M. pneumoniae,* and *Pseudomonas aeruginosa.*
3. Nonspecific urinary tract infections: CMV, *Ureaplasma, Papillomavirus* (2, 4, 16), *Chlamydia, Helicobacter, Giardia,* and *Trichomonas.*
4. Irritable bowel syndrome and dysbiosis of the intestinal tract: hepatitis, polio, rotavirus, ATV, mumps and *Papillomavirus, Candida albicans* and *C. tropicalis, Giardia, Helicobacter, Escherichia coli,* and *Listeria;* supplemented by drug therapy for helminths (worms).

Patients with a condition provoked by four or more latentors require one vial for every three latentors; for example, six provocations for a patient with asthma would call for two treatment vials. Dysbiosis of the intestinal tract requires a virus vial and a bacteria/protozoa vial.

When relief is patchy or insufficient from the preliminary work-up or other therapies, (e.g., homeopathy, food immunization, acupuncture, etc.), latency therapy may enhance the combined treatment result. Latency symptoms and therapy reach all areas of the body. Latency treatment of the brain and muscles gives superior responses. A prognosis to predict the amount of relief from allergy and latency illnesses is difficult, but the exception is young people who suffer a rapid loss of memory. As detoxing and symptoms diminish, the interval between treatment doses is gradually increased to three to six weeks. Children and adolescents complete their excretions by four to five months. Long-term seriously ill and elderly patients require six to nine months. Patients with persistent or relapsing unexplained functional illnesses, e.g., CFIDS/ME, of several years' duration, require twelve to eighteen months before recovering a useful level of health. Long-term chronically ill patients acquire many latentees over the years. It is not possible to detect all of them, especially if the patient acquired some in a tropical third world nation. *Surmise:* Serial dilution provocation of the malaria parasite protein could ease or clear residual fluctuating symptoms of a past active infection of malaria. Compliant patients obtain worthwhile relief, but a return to remembered health is not possible until more is known and understood about latency illnesses. Chronic latent symptoms from EBV, CMV, mumps, CRC, *Giardia,* and *Staphylococcus aureus* require treatment shots at four- to six-week intervals for two or more years.

## SYMPTOMS AND SENSATIONS
## OF PROVOCATION TESTING

Provoked responses are classified as follows:

1. Immediate: these occur at the clinic and for two to three hours after the end of the testing session.
2. Delayed: these occur three to four hours after leaving the clinic and continue for the next 18 to 24 h.
3. Extended delayed: symptoms occur one to three days after provocation testing.
4. Prolonged delayed: symptoms occur three to six, even eight, days after provocation testing.
5. Shadowing symptoms: these occur during any of the immediate or delayed responses.

### Immediate Provoked Responses

Such responses occur at the clinic during the 10 or 15 min period after a provoking shot or sublingual drops. Microbial, particularly viral, provoked symptoms commonly occur after the fourth or fifth provoking shot ($5^7/5^9$). This is a feature of the latency response. Nearly all provoked symptoms are neutralized or clear spontaneously before patients leave the physician's office. Patients recognize the provoked symptoms, even though the physician or technician may consider them bizarre, such as a constricting band around the head, or the loss of color vision—the room turns black and gray.

> The patient experiences sudden depression, crying, or a Jekyll-and-Hyde personality change with $5^5/5^7$. Neutralization with $5^{10}$ dilution is given at once. Continue with neutralization until symptoms are relieved, e.g., at $5^{12}$, $5^{14}$. Neutralization is often dramatic and a relief to both patient and technician. The treatment dose is $5^{13}$. If the unlikely situation arose that neutralization is inadequate and an anaphylactic-like response is suspected, the appropriate amounts of adrenalin, antihistamine, heparin, and corticosteroid are administered.

The immediate provocation of recognized symptoms and their neutralization gives patients confidence that their functional symptoms have causes. When the symptoms recur at home during the delayed phases, the patients do not resent them but are instead satisfied with the latency finding. MLV flares or relieves a wide range of symptoms (see Table 1.1 and Virus Families in chapter 5). List symptoms often associated with a virus. The symptoms range over the organs of the body and mind. A particular virus may relieve a symptom, but its complete clearance requires two or more viruses in the treatment vial. Patients comment, "It is not a single virus that helped my recovery; I needed the other viruses' boosting effects." A symptom in one patient caused by a principal virus and one or more secondary viruses may not have the same cause in another patient. This is confusing. The same symptom in another person could be cleared by three viruses, each one having a different degree of effect. The next patient with the symptom could have four effective viruses, including two that were significant for the first person. Very occasionally, a symptom of importance for the patient clears with a single virus shortly after starting virutherapy. The symptom recurs some time later despite therapy and is then cleared by another virus. These patterns invite critical comment.

As the patient's age increases, the intensity and variety of provoked symptoms decreases, although exceptions do exist. Delayed symptoms occur no matter what the age. It is not unusual for patients over the age of sixty-five to have four or five provocation testings without any provoked symptoms. But when patients are contacted two to four days later, they report changes in their body routine, improvements or aggravation of mental activities, and weakening or increasing strength in their limbs. People expect wheals will appear after skin testing. They are disappointed when whealing does not occur with the virus provocation. If there is no whealing, no improvement or aggravation of provoked symptoms during the consultation, they consider such treatment a waste of time and money. If they will not accept an explanation, it is better to stop treating these patients.

### Placebo Effect

When the physician suspects a placebo effect, the investigation is abandoned. Medical professionals should restrain from making a diagnosis of placebo effect until a period of therapy elapses. Latency therapy is often effective where other modalities failed. Another approach to the placebo effect is to continue latency provocations. False placebo effects occur during MLV. A food immunization technique to relieve marked provoked symptoms is to increase strengths of neutralizing shots. Avoid this method with latency therapy, as it is not a symptom suppression technique. Latency placebo effects are infrequent but should not be dismissed. A diagnosis of placebo effect requires the discipline of latency immunity, not scientific medicine concepts.

### Shadowing Symptoms

Before describing the management of delayed provoked symptoms, the obscuring effect of shadowing needs to be explained. X virus provocation brings on (1) symptoms that are associated with the X virus; (2) other symptoms appear suggesting other viral causes. The X virus treatment shots are given; the X virus symptoms are provoked for longer periods and in time clear. The non-X symptoms may continue to be provoked or are of short duration. As the testing proceeds, these symptoms are found to be caused by one or more latent viruses and to respond to specific detoxing. Develop a questioning approach to certain atypical symptoms appearing with a virus provocation. Record the symptoms in the patient's case notes. Shadowing symptoms are not usual with food provocations. They are more likely to be present with CRC and other molds if provoked symptoms occur. *Giardia* may provoke symptoms that are better relieved by other protozoa, e.g., *Trichomonas*. Shadowing symptoms occasionally occur with bacterial provocations. Three to six months of clinical experience is enough to recognize suspicious shadowing symptoms.

## Understanding Shadowing Symptoms

The first shadowing symptoms may appear with influenza provocations, although not all provoked symptoms will later be attributed to influenza. Record the symptoms in the case notes. When testing proceeds to neutralization, some symptoms disappear, but not all; for example, mild mood and bowel symptoms persist. Later, you recognize these symptoms during provocation by other viruses (delayed shadowing symptoms). The remaining prolonged provoked symptoms are probably due to influenza. No one pattern can explain a particular viral provocation; for example, one patient may develop a shadow headache, and another does not provoke a similar headache but experiences shadow IBS symptoms. Shadowing symptoms are common, and I estimate that one-tenth of those tested do not have shadowing symptoms. Symptoms relieved by influenza virutherapy shots or drops are due to influenza. Influenza shots will not provoke or clear shadow symptoms caused by other viruses.

Symptoms occurring after treatment doses may include minor shadowing symptoms that do not last for more than 1 or 2 h, whereas provoked symptoms due to influenza may persist for 8 to 48 h. Shadowing explains why treatment results occur when one virus, e.g., influenza, is used as a serial vaccination to treat symptoms caused by other viruses. This therapy could be called "reversed shadowing," requiring strong dilutions, e.g., $5^1$ to $5^5$. Time spent detecting a particular virus that provokes shadowing symptoms gives superior treatment results. Shadowing symptoms occur frequently with influenza, EBV, herpes, hepatitis, and RSV. When provocations with influenza provoke marked symptoms, suspect serious MLV illness despite the unremarkable case history.

Provoking two or more viruses at the same time confuses identification of shadowing symptoms. Sometimes shadowing symptoms are enhanced. In contrast, inhalants and foods are tested in batches of three or four similar antigens. This technique is used with skin endpoint titration (SET). MLV is different. I know of no adequate explanation for shadowing. It seems to occur naturally when influenza sweeps through a community. Those infected have a wide range of symptoms, including a few typical shared symptoms. By contrast, individual animals of a virus-infected in-bred laboratory community develop a restricted range of symptoms of similar intensity. *Surmise:* Shadowing may be the result of organ cells holding several viral latentees, and the stimulation of detoxing of one latent virus provokes detoxing of other latent viruses held in the cell. Latent viruses are considered to be held in the cell cytoplasm, not incorporated in the nucleus's chromosomes. Shadowing symptoms are less frequent in children. Anecdotal observations by mothers describe shadowing symptoms following sublingual dosing of their children.

EBV is the last virus to be provoked because of the severity of its symptoms, which are increased or aggravated by shadowing symptoms of other latent viruses. The severity of the provoked symptoms may be reduced by prior identification and detoxing of all significant latent viruses affecting the individual. By the time EBV is provoked, the shadowing symptoms of treated viruses are greatly reduced, exposing EBV latent symptoms and detoxing smells. A musician patient, who suffered severely from detoxing of EBV and other latent viruses, called EBV the conductor of the viral (latent) orchestra (p. 180). Before EBV is provoked, some shadow EBV symptoms will be recognized among provoked symptoms of an unrelated viral or protozoa excretion/detoxing (for a description of EBV latent symptoms see p. 172 and Table 1.1). Provoking EBV immediately following the completion of the preliminary work-up causes severe, distressing detoxing symptoms, which prevents the recognition of other significant latent viruses. Do not provoke EBV at any stage of latency therapy until all other provoking is completed.

### Delayed Provoked Symptoms

MLV-provoked symptoms are not confined to the allergy testing room. Symptoms may be neutralized, but when patients leave the clinic, these return as delayed provoked symptoms. If not neutralized, they continue for hours or days. Allergists avoid provoked symptoms by using the whealing response from skin scratch and prick tests, SET skin whealing neutralization, and laboratory blood tests (e.g., RAST, ELISA, ALCAT). I have in the past used these techniques, but experience suggests that serial provocation technique gives better results. Persisting or annoying provoked symptoms are cleared or reduced by Trisalts when neutralization is not effective. The three stages of delayed provoked symptoms may be associated with shadowing, although this is minimal compared to the marked shadowing occurring with an immediate provocation. Impress upon patients how important it is to record delayed responses or any unusual symptoms or effects, even though they may not consider them to be delayed responses.

Delayed symptoms may escape from neutralization while the patient is on the way home. Depression, excessive fatigue, visual disturbances, and loss of muscle strength are hazardous. Increasing fatigue, memory disturbance, and inability to think could cause the patient to "crash" upon arriving home and retire to bed. If you suspect that the patient has incomplete neutralization of provoked symptoms or that the neutralization is likely to be short-lived, suggest that a friend or family member/taxi take them home. A mother who provoked to morbilli and hepatitis had terrible problems driving home after collecting her three young children from her mother's house.

Neutralization of symptoms following clinic testing may disappear after the evening meal. If symptoms worsen it is best to go to bed. Some will have a restless night with vivid dreams provoked by the viruses given during the testing session. Some may experience frequent urination, even passing of motions (bowel movements) during the night. Others may enjoy deep, relaxed, satisfying sleep—"the best sleep for months." On waking some experience residual delayed provoked symptoms that clear after breakfast or during the morning. Occasionally patients will call the next day because delayed provoked symptoms reappeared in the late morning or early afternoon. If patients experience symptoms or sensations that did not occur during the clinic testing, they should record them in the Neurotic Notebook (patient diary). Patients may experience no further symptoms until a treatment injection or drops again provoke the symptoms. If they are not provoked by the first, second, or third shot at weekly intervals, the treatment vial should be returned for strengthening of the dose. Patients with long-standing debilitating illnesses and those older than sixty to sixty-five years may not suffer immediate provoked symptoms at the clinic but experience delayed symptoms from which treatment doses can be deduced.

### Extended Delayed Provoked Symptoms

These symptoms are less frequent, continuing on from delayed symptoms into the third to fifth day after the clinic testing. The symptoms have varying intensities and can cause absence from work. Mild jaundice, diarrhea, or constipation may occur. Other distressful symptoms are a persistent headache, recurrence of migraines or aura, spacing out, depression, mood changes, aggravation of dermatitis, and urethra and bladder symptoms. Many of the important pretreatment symptoms return. If headaches or other symptoms are causing distress or marked depression, call the patient to the office and attempt to neutralize the symptoms. Neutralization may persist and give restful sleep. Within two to three days, the extended delayed symptoms should clear.

> A woman suffered a thirty-year history of unexplained fatigue, constant headache, migraine, and tension headaches. She was provoked and relieved by three different viruses. Two viruses continued into the extended delayed symptom period, and the constant headache continued into the prolonged delayed symptom period, eventually clearing after ten days. The viruses were influenza and v. zoster. Morbilli caused the constant headache and migraine.

It is not unusual for patients to experience some symptoms in one or more of the three delayed symptom groupings.

**Note:** If v. zoster provokes symptoms and they are neutralized by a treatment dilution, a later provocation with CMV may reproduce the symptoms in greater intensity, eventually giving a longer period of symptom relief. This is not a shadowing response, as both the v. zoster and CMV are provoking and relieving symptoms.

### Prolonged Delayed Provoked Symptoms

These symptoms appear briefly during or after viral provocation at the clinic and return with a vengeance five to eight days later. The symptoms vary in severity for the next two to seven days. They result from detoxing, which is often strong smelling. At first, I made no connection between the testing and the severe delayed symptoms. In time, a connection between *Giardia* and EBV became obvious. Some physicians will not accept the concept of a prolonged delayed response because of the absence of NIS-specific antibodies. Prolonged delayed symptoms are a reliable guide to treatment dosage, e.g., starting dose for *Giardia* and *Trichomonas* is between $5^{10}$ to $5^{18}$; for EBV and *Papillomavirus*, $5^{15}$ to $5^{22}$. It is safer to begin with high dilutions because stronger dilutions, especially of EBV, can temporarily disable the patient and bring on uncontrollable crying and fluctuating depressions. When severe symptoms are present, I contact a relative or friend who visits the patient two or three times a day and contacts the office to report on the patient's condition. Patients who live alone are encouraged to move in with friends or relatives. Prolonged delayed symptoms may mimic a bacterial infection crisis, a frequent occurrence before the antibiotic era. Latency-provoked symptoms and detoxing increase to a climax with profuse sweating, smells, and sometimes a mild fever. Patients experiencing depression and a sense of foreboding or impending dissolution may require a home visit. When clearing of symptoms begins, within a few days, patients return to normal and sometimes report an elated sensation of "feeling better than ever before." Patients who experience the crisis regard it as a turning point in recovery from CFIDS/ME and fibromyalgia. What is occurring? Is this the response of the NIS or the latency immunity system (LIS)?

### The Strike-Back Response

About one in every 120 patients experiences a severe prolonged delayed response, lasting several weeks, even three or four months. It is important that the physician understands how to manage this difficult condition, which was called "EBV Strikes Back" by a patient.

> Shirley, age 24, an invalid ex-hospital employee with CFIDS/ME of two years' duration, seemed on the road to recovery after eight weeks of therapy. The last provocation session included EBV. Within four days the CFIDS/ME returned, and for the next three months she experienced fluctuating depression, crying, and a stinking detoxing. Suddenly she had restoration of remembered health before her illness, followed by a further relapse of a few days. She made a dramatic recovery and had a new office job six weeks later.

**IK**   Two women in their early thirties with chronic lower back pain, unresponsive to orthopedic and physiotherapy treatments over many years, endured the strike-back response from first CMV and then EBV, with lesser symptoms from polio. A follow-up two years later reported little or no back pain, a clearing of the fibromyalgia tender points, and extreme skin sensitivity areas. Best of all, they were able to sleep through the night.

The unsuspecting patient provokes mild to moderate symptoms during EBV provocation. After four to ten days, a prolonged delayed symptom pattern begins and merges into the strike-back response. Some patients provoke symptoms at the clinic and immediately move into a strike-back pattern of severe detoxing and symptoms, which continues for two to three months. The opposite effect has occurred with morbilli and RSV. During the provocation testing at the clinic, patients become alert, elated, and active. The stimulation continues, rather than wearing off, and patients enjoy a standard of health equal to or better than what they remembered before their illness began. No further treatment is required, but any suggestion of a relapse is treated with appropriate virutherapy. Continuing strike-back symptoms and detoxing alarm and depress patients, who need frequent reassurance. Friends or relatives are asked to visit the patients several times a day and report back to the clinic. After four weeks, home visits are made or the patients are brought to the clinic, and an attempt at neutralizing the symptoms may give several hours of relief and confirm in the patients' minds that there is a cause for the strike-back symptoms. Patients who "survived" the strike-back response and recovered contact and watch other patients. Their experience encourages the sufferers to continue to tolerate the symptoms and detoxing.

During strike-back symptoms, all treatment shots are stopped, but the food exclusions, supplements, and nystatin medication are continued. Relapses after recovery from strike back are prevented or controlled by starting up treatment shots of $5^{18}$ to $5^{20}$ to $5^{24}$ dilutions at increasing intervals from three weeks to eight or ten weeks over the next eighteen to twenty-four months. All strike-back patients who were contacted two or more years later reported a return to normal or near normal health. Strike backs for periods of two to three months occurred with *Trichomonas, Giardia, Papillomavirus* 6, CMV, and EBV.

Delayed responses are very important in estimating treatment doses for molds, bacteria, protozoa, and viruses. Keep in mind that symptoms, patterns, and responses of patients may differ in some minor details from these descriptions.

## *LATENCY THERAPY: FIVE EXAMPLES*

In this section, fatigue, pain, fibromyalgia, headaches, and asthma are described in more detail. The information supplied here—the patterns or order of provocation, anticipating which latentors are provoked depending on the symptom pattern, and any with aggravations of detoxing or provoking—can be applied with confidence to other symptom complexes/conditions that are not included in this section, e.g., dermatitis, urogenital, special senses, and neurological conditions. A manual on latency therapy is in preparation for physicians interested in exploring the possibilities of latency therapy for functional and subjective symptoms. When considering descriptions of latency therapy, remember that it cannot stand by itself;

it complements other effective conventional/alternative therapies, except those associated with symptom suppression techniques and drugs. During the work-up, introduce latentors with caution. Before provoking the patient, refer to the appropriate sections and note the allergy and microbial latentors associated with the symptoms (see Table 1.1). At first, the limited selection of latentors/antigens (see 3. on p. 14) restricts the range of symptoms and conditions that will respond. As more latentors are added to the testing trays, former patients can be contacted to return for additional provocations. From time to time, provoke with phenolated N/Saline or N/Saline at any stage of the provocation, e.g., headache and muscle aches: morbilli provocation; $5^2$—nil; $5^3$—nil; $5^5$—nil; $5^7$—marked symptoms; $5^1$—N/Saline—no change in symptoms; $5^7$—symptoms; $5^9$—reduced symptoms; $5^{11}$—neutralized. Very infrequently is there an aggravation of symptoms, but no comment is made to the patient, and during another provocation, the N/Saline is again introduced. Only a handful of patients, out of the hundreds treated over the past fourteen years, have been suspected of feigning their symptoms or placebo effects. A criticism is inability to reproduce provoked symptoms at a later date. If the repeat testing occurs within a few days, it may have a neutralizing effect, but confidence is restored if the treatment vials provoke similar symptoms. Some patients were denied treatment for two to three months and were again provoked at six- to eight-week intervals, with provocation of similar symptoms, although the intensity varied. Always provoke with phenolated N/Saline during the first testing session, as a phenol allergy may be present. It is difficult and expensive attempting to treat people with phenol allergies. Other sterilizing chemicals are available in diluting solutions. For further advice, refer to commercial allergy supply houses. Those sensitive to sterilizing agents should be referred to allergists who use normal saline dilutions.

### *Fatigue Patterns*

Fatigue (Latin): weary. Weary (Old English): having strength or patience exhausted.

Fatigue is said to be the predominant symptom of CFIDS/ME; or is it? When the CFIDS/ME patients' limbs or back muscles refuse to respond to their voluntary control, is this fatigue? Patients describe overwhelming lack of motivation (or mañana), an "inability to get up and get going." Lack of motivation is equated with fatigue. Latency illnesses have fluctuating symptoms, and at times one or another symptom will predominate, e.g., chronic pain.

Question patients about their fatigue and whether they experience different fatigues. The fatigue of active infection may be different from that of latent infection. Other fatigues described by patients are associated with behavior, such as fatigue with depression or after overactivity, or fatigue with certain detoxing symptoms and smells. Various types of fatigue with subtle differences are associated with the following:

1. Foods and grass pollens.
2. Dust and molds.
3. *Candida, Giardia,* and *Trichomonas.*
4. Latent bacteria, such as *Listeria* and bacterial toxins.
5. Latent viruses.
6. Nutritional deficiencies.
7. Suspected hidden or diagnosed organic illness.
8. Petrochemical toxicity and the toxic effects of xenodrugs (man-made chemical compounds).

Patients are encouraged to record their different fatigues or fatigue patterns.

The onset of a relapse months or years after recovery may be heralded by recognized smells, unexplained feelings of coldness, and remembered fatigue. If appropriate measures and treatment are started immediately, there will be a reduction in intensity and duration of the relapse. Patients recognizing the onset of fatigue may correlate it with influenza or a food indiscretion, etc. If a short period of an unidentified fatigue occurs during an immediate or delayed provocation of symptoms, it is probably a shadow effect. A prolonged fatigue effect, often neutralized with other symptoms, is due to the latentor being provoked. Shadow fatigue occurs with the herpes virus group, polio and Coxsackievirus, OWGGs and grass pollens, *Candida, Aspergillus,* and *Mucor.* Patients are able to relate a previous mysterious fatigue to what is occurring during the present provocation. When an unidentified persistent or fluctuating fatigue is not neutralized by latency therapy, consider referral to a physician for exclusion of the early onset of an organic illness.

Idiopathic fatigue patterns spontaneously disappear as the patient returns to remembered health. An idiopathic fatigue is not influenced by latency provocations until two or more latent viruses are identified. A persistent fatigue pattern cleared when viruses A, B, and C were provoked and treated. It did not matter in which order the three viruses were provoked (e.g., B, A, C or C, B, A), for there was no relief until virutherapy with the three. Be guarded with fatigue prognoses. If a persistent fatigue clears unexpectedly, make an effort to identify one or several latentors. Avoid "pep pills" and antidepressants, if possible, while investigating and treating fatigue. Reduce caffeine, food, and drink to a minimum. Exclude alcohol and cannabis.

### Idiopathic Pain, Tenderness, and Extreme Skin Sensitivity

A severe influenza infection leaves painful memories of symptoms. The illness may have been one for which no cause was found. The influenza was an active infection; the illness with no cause was probably latent. Patients with these symptoms are thoroughly investigated before attending the clinic. Latency therapy is an option that should only be tried when other therapies have provided little or no relief. Before beginning the work-up, explain to patients how their symptoms may change and why pain may increase during provocation and detoxing before improvement occurs. After the preliminary work-up, begin provocations with influenza if symptoms persist. If the patient suffered severe influenza and questioning suggests many of the symptoms could be caused by latent influenza, start with high dilutions, such as $5^{12}$ to $5^{15}$. Strong dilutions, such as $5^2$, will provoke severe or unbearable muscle and head pains. It is difficult to convince a fibromyalgic patient that the severe symptoms provoked by the influenza shot signify that influenza is an important cause of his or her illness. Fortunately, you may be able to neutralize or greatly reduce the patient's pain and resistance to your explanation.

When body pains are provoked by several latentors, patients will identify the subtle differences between pains. Once severe pain is provoked, complete the provocation and neutralization, if possible. Do not continue testing with other latentors known to provoke pain, such as morbilli, polio, v. zoster, *Giardia, Chlamydia, Legionella,* and *Listeria,* for the next three to four weeks. The herpes group of viruses is associated with severe pains, so provoke the individual viruses at extended intervals; for example, do not provoke with CMV immediately after v. zoster is tested. They have similar pain responses to provocation. A painless provocation with CMV may disappoint patients, but the two herpes viruses provoked consequently could give *some* prolonged/extended delayed symptoms. Once patients accept one or more causes of the pains and symptoms are identified, most agree to further provocation and painful detoxing. It is a trying time for the physician and clinic personnel persuading patients to continue compliance. Introduce doubtful patients to former patients who experienced the work-up and recovered.

### Fibromyalgia

Patients with low back pain and tender points suffer prolonged detoxing as improvement becomes obvious by two to four months, with considerable pain relief by six to eight months. Young people experience sudden improvements with a few viral provocations and treatment shots after completing the preliminary work-up. NSAIDs are necessary when pain and symptoms are marked but are gradually withdrawn as improvement continues. If physiotherapy is tolerated, temporary relief continues for 5 to 10 h after treatment. An aggravation of symptoms follows, and then relief for a varying period. Detoxing of smells may occur during the treatment and intermittently for the next 12 to 24 h. Detoxing is encouraged through the use of heat pads and hot baths following the treatment. Those with severe pain and symptoms will not tolerate saunas at this stage.

The American College of Rheumatology compiled a chart of tender points. A correlation of tender points with certain viruses, bacteria, and their toxins became apparent twelve years ago. The patient and his or her physiotherapist identify the site and duration of the tender points. Consult Figure 1.1, and start with the patient's less painful tender points. Begin provoking with a latentor that provokes or relieves the particular tender point. Once the less painful tender points are reduced or relieved by treatment shots, provoke the important tender point, which by then will be less painful. Food allergy pain areas are not listed, as most are general or diffuse and are identified during the preliminary work-up. If there is any doubt about food allergy and fibromyalgia, ask the patient to do a five-day water fast, with the reintroduction of two foods a day. Keep the patient under supervision until the fast is completed. One woman, after completing a water fast, discovered that a constant severe pain in her tailbone area (coccyx) was caused by potato.

### *Headaches, Migraine, and Tension Head Pains*

Do not be prevailed upon by a "quick fix"-minded patient to exclude the preliminary work-up. Foods and inhalants are common causes. Carefully assess previous "complete food investigations" performed by other clinics. If an important provoking food remains hidden, the outcome of the work-up will be disappointing or a failure. The work-up and therapy may be successful, but if later relapses occur during the fall, inspect the patient's living conditions. Obtain the list of latentors from the description of headaches given in Chapter 2 (see pp. 53-57). Respect the rule that if one viral latentor provokes a severe headache, do not use another with a reputation for provoking headaches later in the session. It is surprising how many people with unexplained head sensations have suffered or, after testing, appear to have suffered a head injury in childhood. A typical patient complains that one side of the body is weaker or that he or she is left-handed because the right side is weaker. Test to confirm whether the patient is left- or right-eye dominant. It is not uncommon for patients who thought they had stronger left limbs to discover after the work-up that their right limbs are stronger. With the improvement in strength comes better coordination and balance. Some provoked responses have been alarming to patients. They experience a premonition of a vasovagal attack or athetosis-like movements of the limbs on the weaker side of the body. Patients may suffer sudden headaches, visual distortions, temporary blindness, tinnitus, and depression/crying. Past moderate to severe head injuries are provoked with weak (high) dilutions of morbilli, influenza, v. zoster, CMV, and EBV. Continue provocation with increasingly stronger dilutions until provoked symptoms appear (see p. 66). Latent viruses such as RSV, rotavirus, polio, rubella, and coxsackievirus are provoked in head injury patients. Another cause of chronic headache is childhood vaccination reactions. If reactions are confirmed by the mother, or the infant nursing notebook, obtain pertussis and provoke with a weak/high dilution, such as $5^{12}$. Patients who provoke extreme responses and recover with loss or diminution of headaches are advised to have a further neurological work-up.

Latency therapy identified and treated previously untreatable constant background head pain that is not influenced by the preliminary work-up and appears to be due to latent viruses, especially morbilli. This constant headache is always present and is not influenced by pain suppression drugs. Other head pains and migraines may also be present. Constant head pain is not yet an accepted diagnosis. A history of a strange childhood illness suggests undiagnosed encephalitis. Marked provoked responses are common. Record accompanying body language and behavioral changes. If provoked responses become emotional and exhausting, the treatment session is stopped. If neutralization is effective, the patient takes a vial of neutralizing doses to repeat neutralization if delayed symptoms recur at home. Keep in close contact with the patient for four to six days in case prolonged delayed symptoms should occur. You have a grateful patient for life when you relieve constant headache.

### Asthma

The object of latency therapy of asthma is to reduce or cease using symptom suppression asthma drugs, in particular, the corticosteroids (Csds). Patients are encouraged to reduce, if possible, the level of drug dosage before attending the clinic for testing. Do not provoke any foods known or suspected to have aggravated patients in the past. Patients are always curious as to why they have these marked reactions and often insist that you should test them for, of all things, peanuts and soy products. To do so is inviting a calamity. If they keep insisting, suggest they do a five-day water fast after the work-up is completed. By that time, they are usually much improved, or the prospect of no food for five days is enough to dampen their enthusiasm.

It is surprising that most asthma patients attending the clinic test positive for OWGGs and grass pollens. Be cautious when testing for OWGGs, or if patients have been tested previously and found to be positive to wheat, do not retest; insist instead on total OWGGs exclusion, including rice. The high incidence of OWGGs food allergies means CRC is present and responsible for many of the patients' symptoms. Ask patients to record two or three daily peak flow readings, and a final reading if they wake in the early morning hours. Peak flows are recorded for months in the neurotic notebook. If a provocation causes breathing distress that is difficult to neutralize, stop provocations and hold the patient in the clinic for 2 to 3 h. During provocation, asthmatics may bring up large quantities of colored and clear mucus with excessive coughing. Have plenty of paper towels on hand. When the patients stop coughing, ask them to do a peak flow; the marked increase will make them feel that the distress was worthwhile.

**IK**    Just before the evening meal, an asthma patient who was provoked during the morning phoned and accused me of giving her gastroenteritis. Three or four hours after getting home she began retching and coughing. Up came large quantities of multicolored thick mucus and fluid. She passed two motions. Toward the end her voice was husky and she was exhausted from the repeated retching. She finished the phone call by telling me what she thought of my professional standing. I then asked her to do a peak flow. After an interval, a far more friendly voice told me that it was the best peak flow she had ever done. I suggested that the retching was the body's way of emptying the chest. In preantibiotic days, physicians used an emetic, syrup of ipecac. She made a remarkable recovery with total OWGG exclusion, treatment of CRC, *Aspergillus,* and influenza. I could not determine whether any other significant viruses were present because she refused to have any more provocations.

Latency therapy of asthma requires a large selection of latentors, which is not possible when starting a clinic. Many of your asthma patients will obtain a moderate to considerable response and will probably be happy to return for further provocations when you add to the selection in your testing trays.

**IK**    A woman office worker was pleased with the help she received from the latency therapy eight years previously. She returned for further testing and received more improvement. She was freed from drug therapy by *Legionella* provocation and therapy. It confirmed what she and I had long suspected: that she acquired a sick building syndrome illness from a previous job. If latency evidence of *Legionella* is eventually recognized by legal hearings in courts, much of the present discontent with sick building illness/syndrome decisions will resolve. *Legionella* could be spread through a building's air conditioning system from the lungs of a worker with latent *Legionella*, who is an avid gardener who uses garden peat and animal manures.

## PERSISTENT INFECTIONS AND LATENCY THERAPY

Microbiology texts describe persistent infectious activity as:

1. Nonpermissable: organ cells tolerate infecting virus and release small amounts of virus; antibodies and interferon mop up the escaping virus, protecting nearby cells from infection.
2. Latency: cells appear to be infected by a virus, but none is found.
3. Inapparent infection: virus production is so minimal it is difficult to detect the presence of viruses.

The term latency therapy is intended to include these three groups and a postulated fourth clinical group with symptoms and smells that are excreted or detoxed by nonspecific methods (e.g., saunas) and specific latency therapy shots.

The following observations/concepts and surmises arose from fourteen years of latency provocation and therapy:

1. Inapparent/latent infection is not considered in the clinical management of immunity depression.
2. There are no laboratory tests, with the posssible exception of the PCRT, and no effective therapy other than SSDs.
3. There exists an extensive reservoir of inapparent foci in organ cells, consisting of microbial parasites, their toxins, allergic or toxic food particles, "difficult to excrete" metabolic products, and xenotoxins, including SSDs. The term *latency immunity* is selected to include the whole range of latentors, latentees, and organ cell immunity. It differentiates between body cells holding excess latentees and the blood cellular system, the NIS.

4. There is a considerable need for latency therapy for certain functional/subjective illnesses. Latency provocative testing and therapy are available to patients with low budgets for medical services.

5. The latency group of functional illness could include many undiagnosed, difficult to treat, and psychological conditions, possibly accounting for 10 to 15 percent of patients attending family health groups or clinics.

6. Inapparent foci are more numerous and widespread in the organ cells of sick people, and they are not distributed evenly; for example, with fibromyalgia, high concentrations could be present at or in tender points. Latency provocation and therapy suggest this occurs with *Chlamydia* and CMV, and EBV infection of muscle cells. Other muscles of the affected person appear normal, suggesting viral tropism. In a similar manner, areas of the brain may have neurons with high levels of foci. Such areas could be those bruised by head injury or damaged by past infections.

7. Many foci were established years ago in long-living cells; other foci develop with the present illness. Cells undergoing apoptosis are consumed by neighboring and newly formed cells. It is suggested that the latentees of the apoptotic cells are taken up into the cytoplasm of adjoining cells, thereby continuing an inapparent infection. An example is *Candida*-provoked detoxing in a patient with a history of ten or more years of *Candida* symptoms. The musty-smelling detoxing continues for three to five months. Does latency therapy detox the more recently formed foci first, or do all foci participate in the gradual latentee detoxing?

8. New inapparent foci are formed by active infections in patients with past apparent or subclinical mental shocks, trauma, unrelated infections, and petrochemical toxins, lowering the overall body immunity and facilitating foci formation.

9. *Surmise:* The foci are located in the cytoplasm and nuclei of the cells. The foci are multiple organ cell immunity templates. Each cell may hold a variety of different foci, suggested by clinical responses. Some organ cells may hold a single focus.

10. When the excess load of latentee in cell foci is reduced to normal immune template levels, the cells resume normal activity and recover their functions, e.g.,,, the retina and pancreas islet cells.

11. The terms presently used for permissive infection of cells should be revised if latency illness and immunity turn out to be important bodily activities.

12. Latency therapy may be able to release the chronically ill or under-performing patients from SSDs and other suppression therapies. Clinicians who are not afraid of treated, inactivated viral materials, and who are interested in the "slow fix" therapy of chronic and subjective illness, will be intrigued and surprised with the results of latency therapy.
13. A chronic illness may be given a diagnosis and treatment, but the response is often disappointing. The patient may be harboring inapparent or latency infections that elude the NIS investigation. The PCRT requires body fluid or biopsy material often not readily available. After a trial of conventional therapy the patient should be offered a latency investigation.
14. Latency/organ cell immunity is a basic cell immunity activity. At some time in evolution, a blood system was grafted onto the latency tissue fluid system, so both are separate in a way, yet interdependent.

Inapparent viral infections are difficult to locate because the infected cells release so little viral material. *Surmise:* Lifetime resistance following childhood viral infections stems from inapparent foci of infection persisting throughout life. There is a constant or intermittent shedding (detoxing) of viral material. "Not surprisingly, latent and apparent or inapparent persistent infections may cause chronic and sometimes also progressive disease" (Joklik, 1992, p. 840) (see reference 3 on p. 4).
*Surmise:*

1. Provocation of important latent or inapparent foci of infection stimulates excretion (detoxing) from millions of affected body cells holding an excess of that identical latentee.
2. During the excretion process symptoms are provoked or neutralized, usually accompanied by typical latentee smells.
3. When the real extent and numerous types of inapparent foci are recognized, latency will be regarded as an important organ cell immunity.

**IK** Vera, age 42, suffered rheumatoid arthritis with moderate disability and deformity of hands and feet. After seven years of fruitless treatment she attended the clinic. Excluding OWGGs helped her headaches and IBS. The joint pains and stiffness were at first aggravated and later relieved. Other useful latentors were *Candida, Aspergillus,* influenza, rubella, CMV, and *Parvovirus.* From the ages of 7 to 15, she kept cats in her bedroom. Over the years she and her partner worked with horses and other animals, so it was no surprise when *Clostridium difficile* (tetanus is caused by a *Clostridium* species) provoked severe joint swelling, pain, as well as restricted movement of the affected joints and her spine, with frequent stinking diarrhea. After four days of detoxing she experienced "a wonderful improvement" of her joints and IBS. There was no change in the bony deformity of the joints. The treatment shot was *C. difficile* $5^{18}$, which provoked joint symptoms for one to two days and then improvement.

The morning after the fourth provocation shot of *C. difficile* $5^{18}$, she and her partner discussed business for 30 to 45 min. She was detoxing from her lungs, which gave an offensive halitosis. Four hours later, her partner, who had not missed a day's work for years, came down with joint aches, pain, stiffness, IBS, extreme tiredness that required bed rest, and frequent watery diarrhea. During his twenties he had worked with horses and probably acquired high levels of *Clostridium* in his motions. Horse dung contains *C. tetani.* The partners slept in separate rooms the night before the breakfast meeting. *Surmise:* Detoxing of the *Clostridium* latentee acted as a provocation when inhaled by her partner, resulting in a day and a half off work and *Clostridium*-like symptoms. Parents have reported that while they were using their treatment dose at home, another member of the family, usually a child, would be temporarily indisposed.

## ADDING LATENCY THERAPY
## TO THE PRACTICE OR MEDICAL CENTER

1. Expensive apparatus, laboratory findings, and medical technology contributed little to a diagnosis of latency symptoms/illness.
2. Select the first patients from those who complain of viruslike symptoms. They will have received a full work-up and undergone symptom suppression therapy. The manner in which you interpret "stress" symptoms will determine whether you use latency therapy.
3. A suitable selection of microbial antigens is CRC, *Giardia,* influenza, polio, hepatitis, RSV, and herpes or v. zoster. For the preliminary work-up: wheat, milk or beef, egg or chicken meat. Inhalants: grass pollen mixture, house dust mite mixture, *Alternaria* or *Cladosporium, Mucor* mix, and *Aspergillus* mix. After three months experience, add *Helicobacter, Chlamydia,* morbilli, rubella, CMV, ATV, and EBV. Later additions should include *Papillomavirus,* type 4 and 6, *Papilloma,* type 14 and 16), rotavirus, Listeria, Legionella, dengue, and any

unique infection present in the local environment, such as Rocky Mountain spotted fever *(Rickettsia)* and eastern equine encephalomyelitis (arbovirus).

4. Otolaryngologists and physicians with an interest in allergy may already have an adequate selection of antigens to complete the preliminary work-up, to which microbial/viral solutions are added. I suggest that the physician should work with the allergy nurse or technician to provoke and neutralize between forty and sixty people before the nurse/technician takes over testing.

5. An allergy questionnaire provides a useful assessment of lifestyle and home ecology, if the patient is honest. When the preliminary work-up and the first MLV provocations are disappointing or negative, request a home inspection.

6. Attempt to curb the enthusiasm of the patient or his or her disappointment regarding immediate provoked responses. Expect from time to time that provoked prolonged delayed symptoms will appear up to two weeks after testing. A difficulty is the patient losing interest if delayed provoked symptoms do not occur after three or four days.

7. Adding multiple latent viruses to your practice enables you to convert many of the partial failures to satisfied patients. Over the years patients estimated their additional improvement obtained from latency therapy. An average figure is 30 percent. The 30 percent includes any benefit they experienced from reduction or withdrawal of symptom suppression drugs. Two to six months after the work-up is completed, contact patients and ask them for their assessment of overall improvement.

8. The medical center may decide not to support an inhalant, food, and mold allergy clinic. If the physician is allowed to establish an MLV unit, make enquiries of local physicians, allergists, or otolaryngologists who conduct diagnostic provocation neutralization allergy testing. Refer your patient for food provocation of immediate or delayed symptoms; inhalant provocation and injection therapy; and mold provocation and injection therapy. On completion of the preliminary work-up, the patient returns to your office for provocation testing of selected viruses and bacteria. Limiting the selection of antigens for the preliminary work-up controls costs. After six months or a year, the encouraging results of latency therapy are presented. The medical clinic manager may agree to fund the preliminary work-up testing.

9. The American Academy of Otolaryngic Allergy conducts courses for basic allergy training using provocation and skin wheal endpoint titration (SET). The AAOA promotes food immunization therapy, but for reasons already stated, symptom suppression allergy technique interferes with latency therapy.

### Procuring Microbial Antigens/Latentors

1. Vials or ampoules of individual commercially prepared vaccine doses.
2. Viral culture laboratories, commercial or university departments of virology.
3. The American-type culture collection—a catalog of animal and human viruses.

The contents of a single-dose ampoule/vial or equivalent from a multi-dose vial are diluted 1:5 as described on pp. 5-7. A vial of influenza, 1 ml dose, when diluted 1:5 gives 5 ml and the number two dilution, 25 ml. A starting provoking dose of number two is 0.05 to 0.10 ml, making the $5^2$ starting dose a 1:500 dilution. Dilution of 1 ml of the polio oral vaccine is undertaken in a similar manner. The polio vial can be held until expired or for two years longer. Place the unopened ampoule or vial in 55°C to 60°C for 30 min (pasteurization). The dilution fluid, normal saline with 0.4 percent phenol, has a denaturing effect on the viral protein. Influenza and polio were the first virus dilutions to be used fourteen years ago at the clinic. To date, there have been no deleterious effects or persistent provoked symptoms from their use. The benefit of the few viruses used during that period was immense: regained normal muscle strength and coordination; improved chest expansion and diaphragm movement, much appreciated by asthmatics; clearance or marked improvement of neck and upper back muscle spasms; relief of neck and back pain and the associated frontal headaches; the cessation of nightmares, crashing, accidents, sensations of floating or falling in space; and improvements of mental impairment, including mood and behavior, memory, and alertness.

The benefits described in this book resulted from simple, relatively inexpensive use of the latency immunity response. Cautious physicians may wish to send a selection of commercial vaccine vials or viral concentrates for gamma irradiation sterilization. It is not necessary to use the particular strain of the current influenza or hepatitis epidemic. If a positive antibody test is obtained and the virus type determined, any other type or strain of that virus, or several types, if combined as a vaccine, will be suitable for therapy. The individual typing of viruses is not important because antibody responses are absent when latency illness is present. It is suggested that the effectiveness of expired influenza vaccine dilutions may result from their strains provoking excretion of similar influenza strains that were epidemic at the time the vaccine was manufactured. Patients recognize the provoked symptoms from a past illness, often as far back as early school days. On contacting their mothers, they are told similar symptoms followed a childhood illness or vaccination.

The commercial catalogs of available vaccines indicate which companies to approach, but remember, you only need a small supply. Vaccines that failed after being approved by the Food and Drug Administration (FDA), may still be available, e.g., the RSV vaccine. Certain restraints and conditions of use will apply to these vaccines. Patients suffering long-duration CFIDS/ME and fibromyalgia experienced provoked symptoms and marked detoxing, muscle weakness, jaundice, severe mental depression, loss of memory, etc., from viral provocation doses of $5^{22}$, even $5^{26}$ dilutions. It is incomprehensible that such extremely high dilutions, by themselves, could provoke the marked delayed symptoms and the amount of detoxing smells. The provocation appears to stimulate detoxing of organ cells holding excessive levels of the same or similar viral latentees. The severity of prolonged delayed provoked symptoms suggests it is a biological activity that starts from minuscule amounts of latentees, provoking more and more organ cells to excrete some of their excess latentees until the susceptible organ cells have completed detoxing. Patients described it as "like a wave coming in to a steep beach; it starts as a small wave and then suddenly peaks and breaks with all the symptoms you know so well" (see The EBV Strike-Back Response, in Chapter 5, p. 179). For the first three to four years of latency therapy, patients agreed to hundreds of laboratory antibody tests. However, the study was abandoned because very few tests gave positive antibody results. The positive results that were obtained, in most cases, had no correlation with the symptoms the patients were experiencing. A patient provoked with virus and experiencing symptoms and smells associated with a virus did not produce antibodies to that virus weeks or months later. These observations, if correct, suggest a distinct latency immunity activity.

Physicians introducing latency therapy to their practice will be fascinated with treatment results. In time, they may wish to report their clinical results but may have difficulty getting them accepted by the scientific medicine-orientated journals. The author would be pleased to hear from other physicians interested in virutherapy who obtain similar results to those described in this book.

The physician/allergist/virutherapist is in company with the psychiatrist at the end of the therapeutic line. All are dependent on a prior physical and diagnostic work-up by physicians and surgeons, based on laboratory and medical technologies, to exclude organic illness and disease.

Serial Dilutions Chart

| Vial | To the Power of 5 | Dilution |
|---|---|---|
| 1 | $5^1$ | 1 in 5 |
| 2 | $5^2$ | 1 in 25 |
| 3 | $5^3$ | 1 in 125 |
| 4 | $5^4$ | 1 in 625 |
| 5 | $5^5$ | 1 in 3,125 |
| 6 | $5^6$ | 1 in 15,625 |
| 7 | $5^7$ | 1 in 78,125 |
| 8 | $5^8$ | 1 in 390,625 |
| 9 | $5^9$ | 1 in 1,953,125 |
| 10 | $5^{10}$ | 1 in 9,765,625 |
| 11 | $5^{11}$ | 1 in 48,828,125 |
| 12 | $5^{12}$ | 1 in 244,140,625 |
| 13 | $5^{13}$ | 1 in 1,220,703,125 |
| 14 | $5^{14}$ | 1 in 6,103,515,625 |
| 15 | $5^{15}$ | 1 in 30,515,578,125 |
| 16 | $5^{16}$ | 1 in 152,587,890,625 |
| 17 | $5^{17}$ | 1 in 764,939,453,125 |
| 18 | $5^{18}$ | 1 in 3,824,697,265,625 |
| 19 | $5^{19}$ | 1 in 19,123,486,328,125 |
| 20 | $5^{20}$ | 1 in 95,617,431,640,625 |
| 21 | $5^{21}$ | 1 in 478,087,158,203,125 |
| 22 | $5^{22}$ | 1 in 2,390,435,791,015,625 |
| 23 | $5^{23}$ | 1 in 11,952,178,955,078,125 |
| 24 | $5^{24}$ | 1 in 59,760,894,775,390,625 |
| 25 | $5^{25}$ | 1 in 298,804,473,876,953,125 |

# Chapter 2

# Common Symptoms and Illnesses with a Link to Latent Viruses and Allergies

Multiple latent virutherapy helps or complements accepted treatments. It is given when all other treatments or investigations fail to return the person to remembered health. It is not a "magic bullet" treatment, nor can it work alone. This book enables you, the patient, to check your symptoms against typical case histories.

## NOSE AND CHEST CONDITIONS

### Head Colds and Chest Infections

**IK** "Why do head colds and chest symptoms linger after two or three courses of antibiotics?" "Why can't I get rid of the yellow, brown, greenish crusts and mucus from my nose or chest?" "Is there no way I can give up the drugs for my asthma, as I hate using them?" I have heard these questions hundreds of times at first clinic attendances. The common names for chest and nose illnesses are really "grab bags" of symptoms, and any one symptom may have several causes. It is best to retain the well-known names, but you should have an open mind about causes and treatments, as some symptoms will not go away; you may have them for life, but at a manageable level. After the ecology, allergy, infectious, and chemical components are attended to or controlled, little, if any, medication is needed. Furthermore, the medication works much better on the remaining annoying symptoms and at a lower dosage.

A scientist who recovered from postviral fatigue syndrome (PVFS) and memory problems could not get rid of a persistent cold in his nose and chest. He tried several latent viral treatment vials, some of which helped his memory and moods (RSV, hepatitis). Eventually his nasal "colds" cleared using adenovirus and influenza.

Do not put up with perpetual nose or chest flu or head cold symptoms. Your family physician or *allergist* will be interested in helping. You could ask, "Do I have an allergy to the house dust mite?" You will not be given another series of antibiotics. Symptom improvement may not occur until you have finished the preliminary work-up period. You cannot rush the recovery of your immune responses. The grass pollen season aggravates the symptoms of those with the flu or year-round (perennial) allergies. The weed and mold seasons have a similar effect, but your allergist will know all about local conditions.

Children respond faster to the preliminary work-up. Here are some useful tips: Regular nose blowing is needed to clear away sticky mucus and to open the nose for breathing. Keep the bedroom temperature fairly constant, between 15 and 20°C during cooler weather. Have your child sleep on a modified hammock bed or a raised bed, with the head and chest elevated between 5 and 10 degrees. Breathing is improved because of less nasal congestion and increased chest capacity. Less effort is needed to expand the chest, and the diaphragm muscle does not have to work against the organs and intestines of the abdomen. Children with teething problems will have increased nasal mucus, coughing, and ear symptoms. These teething symptoms are often relieved by successful allergy therapy and virutherapy.

### Nasal Allergies

Foods, house dust, and dust mites are common causes of nasal allergies. Perennial stuffy nose is caused by food or mold toxins coming from within the body via the blood. The stuffy nose does not respond to Csd nasal sprays because long-term use of Csd and cromolyn lower the immunity of the nasal lining, making it easier for microbes and viruses to infect the nose. Seasonal stuffy nose is more likely to be caused by inhalants that alight on body surfaces, e.g., pollens, mold spores, and dust particles. An old treatment was to cauterize the nose with a hot wire, an electric spark, or by freezing, but symptom relief decreased with increasing treatments. The repeated damage to the nasal lining caused crusting and blocking, with CRC, *Aspergillus*, *Mucor* mold, *Giardia,* and *Chlamydia* infecting the nose. Allergy and MLV may restore function to these damaged stuffy noses. (For viruses found in the nose, see Table 1.1.)

## *Pollinosis*

**IK** "My nasal spray inhaler does not work since I got this flu (or head cold). I am full of yellow and green thick mucus and cannot breathe." It is hard to know where the pollen hay fever stops and the flu or head cold begins. Pollen hay fever is aggravated and much more difficult to treat when virus infections or CRC, *Giardia,* and other microbes are living in the nose. The yellow and green mucus needs an antibiotic course followed by nasal pollen drops and MLV with influenza, adenovirus, RSV, CRC, the green bacteria *Pseudomonas,* or other viruses to prevent recurrence. Symptom suppression Csd nasal aerosols or depot injections of prednisone are best avoided because, although they give great relief, they may cause the appearance of symptoms elsewhere in the body (change-of-site response [CSR]), leading to, for example, wheezing, asthma, or IBS. Ask your physician for non-Csd drugs, and if these do not control symptoms, seek an allergist. Normal saline sprays wash away the pollen grains that lodge in your nose and break down the thick mucus. Next season, ask your physician if pollen shots should be tried. Remember to stop eating Old World grass grains (OWGGs) if your grass pollen hay fever is severe and difficult to control.

## *Sinusitis*

"Can you help my sinuses?" I am often asked. "Probably, if I know what your problems are," I reply. "Sinus" means different things to different people. If you suffer from sinus problems you may have read about the many causes and the great range of symptoms. Sinusitis is the most common complaint of all people coming to the clinic since it was founded. Many of the headaches thought to be caused by sinus problems cleared with MLV (see Table 1.1). Many successfully treated patients had previous treatments that gave relief for one to six months before a relapse occurred. They suffered electrical hot-point or freezing cauterizing of the lining of the nose and/or one or more unsuccessful operations. They all wished they had not agreed to any nasal surgery for chronic sinusitis until they had been seen by an allergist and had investigated MLV. Any remaining symptoms have a very good chance of clearance from surgery. The responses of people with "untreatable" sinusitis and failed nasal surgery are success stories for allergy, CRC, *Giardia, Helicobacter,* mold, and multiple latent virutherapy. Patients with chronic sinusitis provoked to a wide range of latent viruses, in particular, influenza, polio, RSV, ATV, and herpes.

Asthmatics and "chronic sinusitis" sufferers using inhaled Csd and cromolyn aerosols notice, within weeks of beginning treatment, that the clear nasal and chest mucus becomes colored, yellowish, brown, and sometimes green. The peak flow readings increase or become normal. The medication opens up the nasal airways and air tubes (bronchi, bronchioles) of the lungs by reducing inflammation of the lining membrane. The downside to inhaled Csd and cromolyn therapy is the suppression of the epithelial immunoglobulin (Ig) A secreted by the lining membranes. (Ig A eliminates microbes entering airways.) The Csd-treated air tube linings now harbor viruses and microbes and are unable to mount a natural immunity response to them. The preliminary work-up and MLV enables many asthmatics to stop their inhaled Csd aerosols. They retain the improved peak flow readings, and the mucus of the nose and chest usually returns to a clear or white color.

### *Bronchitis and Asthma*

Muscle spasm-relaxing drugs, Csds, and cromolyn preparations are inhaled to reduce inflammation and to protect the allergy mast white cells of the blood. So effective is drug control that bronchitis and asthma sufferers are allowed to eat what they like, have animals in the house, and not worry about home ecology or the condition of the workplace. The bronchitis and asthma sufferers whom I see are no longer satisfied with symptom suppression treatment. They read reports of asthmatics dying from strange viral illnesses and thick mucus plugging the air tubes after using inhaled Csds for fifteen or twenty years. Many are worried about long-term use of these drugs. They want to know more about their asthma and its real causes.

The aim of treatment is to (1) identify allergic foods, in particular, OWGGs; (2) reduce or stop the use of inhaled Csds, thereby raising the chest lining immunity levels; and (3) remove the infecting molds and bacteria, *Mucor, Aspergillus,* CRC, *Helicobacter, Giardia,* and *Legionella* from the membrane surfaces of the air tubes. Patients experience a feeling of well-being and easy breathing, with a fluid/watery mucus, when infecting molds and latent viruses are treated.

**IK** One asthmatic said, "The most satisfying improvement from my treatment is gently bringing up normal clear mucus from my chest in the morning." Sticky mucus caused her great distress and terrible coughing bouts for thirty years. Although antibiotics helped at first, for the past ten years they caused irritable bowel syndrome and brought on vaginal thrush. Excluding OWGGs cleared IBS symptoms.

Latency treatment has little effect on multiple latent viruses in the lung lining and air sacs (alveoli) when inhaled Csds continue to be used. *Alternaria* and *Cladosporium, Mucor,* and *Aspergillus* molds are important aggravating causes of asthma. They are widely distributed on trees, on lawns, in soil, and in our buildings and homes, for example, in potted plants. *Alternaria* and *Cladosporium* produce immense quantities of windborne spores. *Mucor* and *Aspergillus* molds invade the moist linings of our body when immunities are depressed. Provocation with individual molds allows patients to experience symptoms they recognize. Your allergist will know the important local molds.

Bring your peak flow meter and your treatment diary (the Neurotic Notebook) to the testing room. Record changes in your peak flow readings. If low readings, the bronchial tubes are blocked; if high readings, they are open. Do a series of peak flow readings when you get home from the clinic, during the evening, and the following day when delayed responses occur. Continue peak flow readings two or three times a day throughout the work-up. Suspect molds are in your nose and chest when you blow crusts from the nose and mucus lumps or balls are coughed up. The yellow and green colors are from the bacteria, and the brownish, black speckling is caused by the molds. Many people experience dramatic improvement during testing. Remarks such as, "My chest has never felt better or freer," add to the surprise because the improvement happens so quickly.

**IK**  So excited was one woman with her newfound energy that she spent a night on the town. The following day ended in the emergency room, but this time she recovered rapidly. The asthma disappeared at the end of the clinic work-up.

Before inhaled Csds therapy it was unusual to get provoked chest symptoms from *Mucor* and *Aspergillus*. Nowadays, all asthmatics who use the inhalers for six to twelve months experience provoked chest symptoms. Attempts to culture chest mucus are negative for molds. The mold provocations are negative six to ten weeks after cessation of Csd inhalers. The fine mold spores contain mycotoxins. Recent work shows that the microscopic spores enter the smallest air tubes, the terminal bronchioles.

Bronchitis and asthma frequently flare up with influenza outbreaks in the community. Instead of receiving a yearly influenza vaccination, which so often aggravates bronchitis and asthma sufferers, use the influenza treatment vial from the clinic. Take a yearly course of six to eight shots, at three-week intervals from fall to late spring. The most common cause of chronic coughing, despite a full work-up, is the presence of whooping cough (pertussis) in the lungs and larynx. It is the occasional whoop at the end of a coughing bout that raises suspicion. Tell your allergist, who will then provoke you with dilutions of pertussis bacteria. Small pockets of whooping cough bacteria remain after the antibiotic course, and in time the cough and whoop start up again.

### Asthma and Latent Viruses

Can we be sure latent viruses are in the lungs of people with bronchitis and asthma? The medical literature (e.g., in microbiology texts) reports virus genomes are found in the lining cells of infected and inflamed air tubes of the lungs. Bronchitis and asthma patients are provoked with twenty viruses because latent viral presence in the lungs cannot be predicted by routine laboratory cultures and tests. Unlike provocation latency therapy, the expensive PCRT may provide a useful answer, but it gives no indication of the treatment or dosage. It may be difficult identifying one virus from another during provocation because of "shadowing effects" (see Shadowing Symptoms in Chapter 1, pp. 16-18):

1. Respiratory syncytial virus has had curious provoked effects on over half the asthma and bronchitis patients seen in the clinic. They feel an itch or irritation deep in their chests. The next provoking shot causes them to cough up mucus or to feel as if they are swallowing lots of mucus. The peak flow reading increases by 50 units or more. So dramatic have the improvements been that many say, "My chest has never felt better or freer!" I comment, "There is more improvement to come when you start virutherapy."
2. Polio affects the intercostal muscles between the ribs and the diaphragm muscle complex. Increases of 50 to 150 units in the peak flow occur from improved chest and diaphragm action.
3. Morbilli, v. zoster (chicken pox), and herpes are important latent viruses in many people with "intrinsic" asthma. There is no way of predicting which viruses will provoke symptoms in an asthmatic (see Table 1.1).

Do not let your allergist forget to test for CRC, *Giardia, Helicobacter, Chlamydia,* and *Pasteurella. Mycoplasma pneumoniae* and *M. hominis* are microbes between a bacterium and a virus. They prefer to live in the cell lining of the nose, chest, and sometimes ankle and wrist joints. Serial vaccination (SV) reduces the amount of mucus and pus associated with bronchitis, emphysema, and chronic sinusitis.

**IK**    A woman with severe asthma made a dramatic drugless recovery after virutherapy with respiratory syncytial virus. Added bonuses were a happier personality, improved memory, and increased output at work. She is convinced that RSV alone was the cause of her years of suffering.

Another woman obtained sudden relief of chronic asthma after provocation with morbilli. As an infant she nearly perished from morbilli encephalitis (viral brain infection).

### How Do Molds and Latent Viruses Affect Our Lungs?

Provocation testing identifies symptoms of bacteria, molds, and latent viruses in the lungs of asthmatics who cough up clear and colored mucopus. The latent viruses appear to depress the activity of our air sacs (alveoli). The preliminary work-up with molds, house dust mites, foods, and bacterial toxins at first decreases and then improves peak flow readings. The thick, sticky colored mucus gradually becomes clear and fluid. The improvements level off three to five weeks after the preliminary work-up is completed. Although the peak flow readings are improved, often markedly, most people cannot climb stairs, walk up hills, or play sports. Virutherapy maintains or improves the peak flow. Within another two to six weeks asthmatics are delighted to carry out these strenuous activities without using the Csd inhaled drug, yet their peak flow readings do not change.

What has happened? *Surmise:* The molds disappear from the air tubes, which function better and give improved peak flow readings. The excess latent viruses are detoxed from the cells of the air sacs (alveoli), which regain their lost activity. There are improvements in the air sacs' interchange of oxygen and carbon dioxide between the air and the blood. The raised levels of oxygen in the blood improve many bodily functions, including increased detoxing from other organs. Aggravations and relapses can occur, so do not throw away your asthma drugs. Always carry an inhaler of salbutamol (beta-2-agonist) with you for the first one to two years. The detoxing of molds and viruses causes halitosis. The partners of asthmatics confide to me that the mold and virus smells are strong and sickening during this period.

*The clinical results suggest that an important cause of fatigue and lowering of immunities is latent viral infection of the alveoli, depressing the transference of oxygen and carbon dioxide.*

CFIDS/ME and "mañana" motivation patients provoke to several of the lung viruses. I surmise from clinical observations that the air sacs are harboring latent viruses *without any chest symptoms*. Virutherapy increases their activity, and patients feel warmer, with red, not bluish, lips and pinker skin. Mental activity and mood changes improve.

An attack of influenza temporarily reverses these improvements, but use of the neutralizing influenza shots from the treatment vial at 12 h intervals over the next two days *staves off the flu* (see Chapter 4, pp. 169-170). You feel as if you are developing active influenza. You dread an aggravation of your symptoms just as they seem to be improving. You can start the first treatment shot or wait until you are sure you are coming down with the flu. Note the time when you take the shot. The symptoms may lessen, even go away, but start to return in 12 h time, when another shot is taken. Repeat two more shots at 12 h intervals, when you should be free of the flu. If it is still around, chances are the infection will be mild. My experience suggests that 85 percent will stave off the flu. Active influenza brings fellow travelers to attack you: adenovirus, RSV, *Chlamydia, Mycoplasma pneumoniae.* You may recognize their symptoms, as you will experience them while being provoked at the clinic. Your treatment vial will contain these microbes, and the shots will provide better relief than influenza alone. Read the exciting story of Dr. Joe Miller's discovery of influenza neutralization (Miller, 1989).

The narrowing of an asthma patient's air tubes by inflammation, muscle spasm, and increased sticky mucus causes distress and a lowering of the peak flow measurement. White blood cells called eosinophils and Ig E antibodies have long been considered the main cause of air tube changes. Dr. H. Oettgren and others (Boston) recently upset the accepted explanation by showing that white cells are present, but not Ig E blood antibodies, when they induced asthma to a mold in Ig E-deficient mice. Asthma drugs are promoted on the assumption that they stabilize the eosinophil white blood cells and neutralize any Ig E. Oettgren's team's findings warrant a reinvestigation of the activities of asthma drugs. What happens in mice may not happen in people (Mehlhop et al., 1997).

Clinical responses in asthmatics suggest that the eosinophil, Ig E, and Ig M responses (NIS) are not always present (e.g., allergic foods that aggravate asthmatics may not stimulate Ig A and Ig M antibodies in the blood). Many clinicians believe non-Ig E and non-Ig M allergic foods are far more important than allergic foods stimulating blood antibodies. Latent viruses do not stimulate blood antibodies, yet they can markedly improve peak flow readings, alter chest sensations, and change sticky chest mucus to near-normal or normal watery mucus. They do not form reacting skin wheals at the site of injection. Researchers should consider repeating the Ig E-deficient mice experiment using viruses known to infect the lungs of mice. Alternatively, the bronchial or air tube secretions from people treated successfully, using these methods, need reviewing.

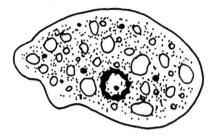

## THE MOUTH AND BOWEL (INTESTINES)

### Mouth, Tongue, and Throat

The lips, mouth, and jaw are busy parts of our body. They are fertile fields for allergies, petrochemical reactions, microbes, and viruses. Microbes multiply on abrasions from chewing, allergies, and viral lesions, increasing pain and inflammation. Allergic itching and burning are aggravated by latent viruses.

**IK**   A chronic allergic condition of a patient's lips was diagnosed as an allergic reaction to citrus, but, despite improvement, it persisted when citrus was excluded. It finally cleared with herpes and v. zoster virutherapy.

The hot burning tongue that defies treatments, nutritional supplements, and investigations will often respond to the preliminary work-up and virutherapy. Herpes simplex is a common virus lesion occurring when the person's immunities are temporarily lowered. Many persisting or recurring abscess and mouth ulcers respond to virutherapy. Most lip and mouth viral lesions come and go so quickly that by the time you are in the physician's office, there is nothing to be seen. It is best for you to record what you see when the pain is present. Use a mirror, light source, and the handle of a tablespoon to observe your mouth, tongue, and throat. The dry uncomfortable mouth has thick sticky mucus and a reduction of saliva. Mumps, herpes, v. zoster, EBV, CMV, virutherapy, and treatment with CRC and *Helicobacter* can restore a moist mouth. Latent mumps and EBV persist in salivary glands in the cheeks and under the lower jaw, causing fluctuation of the sore mouth and glands with decreased saliva and dry mouth.

**IK**    Persistent or variable throat pain at the midline on the back wall of the throat suggests food and inhalant allergies, CRC, and, in particular, latent viruses. The back wall of the throat is sore, at times painful, itchy, with a burning sensation, and is irritated when eating. Many women (very rare in men) feel a constriction in the throat about the level of their breastbone. Victims are tired and irritable and become resigned to their condition because all the treatments and investigations are normal. The one consolation is that they "do not have cancer."

There is always somebody attending the clinic who has had one or two tonsil operations and a series of throat cauterizations, even a "sinus" operation. EBV, together with other minor viruses, is the main cause of the throat disability. The sore throat, at different times, moves between the back of the nose to the lower throat, behind the voice box, and lower in the esophagus. It can last two to three days, two to three weeks, or two to three months, but it always clears for a period and then returns. Adenovirus causes tonsil and adenoid enlargement, with small gland enlargement in the neck. When a bacterial infection of the throat is present, the neck glands enlarge and become painful. In the past, chicken pox (v. zoster) caused severe sore throats in children. I have relieved adults of chronic sore throats using v. zoster virutherapy, twenty to forty years after the childhood infection. When hepatitis is present the throat itch mimics allergy.

**IK**    Glandular fever (EBV) affects the throat as an active or latent viral infection. Neck, armpit, and groin glands are enlarged and tender. It hurts to move the legs, and the arms can barely be lifted above the head because of the pain in the armpits. It is no wonder a typical symptom of EBV is "My arms (or my legs, or both of my limbs) are heavy as lead. I cannot climb the stairs (or hang out the wash)."

EBV virutherapy is cautious, as it takes three to eight months for the throat to recover. Two or more of the other viruses are included with the virutherapy dilution. If you have been to the tropics, arbovirus (mosquito-borne) or dengue fever is suspect. I question older children about the type of sore throat they are suffering. If it is similar to the viral sore throat of adults, then I advise against an operation, in spite of the obvious tonsil enlargement. Most adults treated successfully at the clinic had one or more blood antibody tests for glandular fever (EBV). They were *all negative,* giving the impression that active viruses were not the cause of this throat condition. Recognizing the concept of latent virus sore throat should lead to a marked reduction in surgical procedures performed on adult throats.

Bad breath (halitosis) is said to come from the teeth, tongue, nose, mouth, and stomach. But what if all of these have been checked out and the bad breath continues? Some food allergies cause bad breath that clears when the food is recognized and excluded. Another type of bad breath, with a different smell, is caused by detoxing of latent viruses. You need only enter the bedroom of somebody suffering from a severe case of influenza to smell the virus in the air. Such bad breath resists all fashionable and "scientific" oral hygiene potions. The relief of untreatable bad breath through virutherapy is a social "miracle," patients tell me.

**IK**   Another "stinker" is the fecal (dog or pig motion) smell of latent *Legionella.* Asthma and chronic bronchitis sufferers with constant or intermittent fecal breath clear their halitosis and improve their peak flow readings with *Legionella* serial vaccination. Other causes are *Clostridium, Trichomonas, Listeria,* and hepatitis.

**IK**   A male patient, age 40, had a permanent tracheostomy after severing his windpipe during a car accident twelve years previously. The halitosis from the tracheostomy was musty during CRC provocation/latency therapy; changed to a fecal stench during *Giardia* latency therapy. There were no stomach complaints.

## Teeth

The nooks and crannies of the mouth and teeth are wonderful places for microbes to feed on the leftovers of our meals. A greater variety of organisms can be found in these areas than anywhere else in the body. Fortunately, our immunities and saliva protect our living tissues from being attacked—not so our dead or damaged tissues, such as tooth root stumps or a dead or filled tooth. The potential peril from dead teeth is chillingly described by Dr. H. Huggins, the dentist who championed the danger of amalgam fillings in people who suffered from untreatable/unexplained chronic illness conditions (Huggins, 1993).

How do you know a dead tooth, a filled tooth, or a tooth with an apicoectomy (removal of a dental root apex), is a danger? You cannot rely on X rays because side views are obstructed by the adjoining teeth. Tapping, hot and cold exposure, or electrical stimulation does not always detect latent infection in the tooth or its ligament.

**IK** My phone rang at 4:30 am. A woman's voice described the awful dental pain in the teeth supporting her upper and lower bridges. She was attending the clinic because of CFIDS/ME and was slowly responding to food exclusion and MLV. Her last appointment was two days ago, when she gave an immediate provoked symptom to *Helicobacter* and rotavirus. She reported a cat pee odor to her urine. I dropped in on a friend as he was preparing for the morning clinic. He handed me an oral microbiology text. I was relieved to read a description of Campylobacter (a related bacterium to *Helicobacter*), which occurs in many mouths around dead teeth. Three hours later I neutralized most of her dental pain with *Helicobacter* $5^{12}$. The four teeth bearing the upper and lower bridges were painful and obviously dead. It took three months and three antibiotic courses from her dentist before she agreed to their removal. Within the next two months, her halitosis disappeared, all pain and tenderness cleared from her jaws, and she responded to the MLV.

A professional woman in her forties gradually developed CFIDS/ME and was disabled for four years. She had two expensive dental bridges and five suspicious teeth. At her yearly checkups her dentist assured her the teeth were healthy. Suddenly one tooth bearing the bridge became extremely sensitive and relapsed each time she finished an antibiotic course. Her CFIDS/ME worsened. Dental X rays showed no change. She struggled with persistent halitosis. A physician advised removal of all the dead teeth, including the bridges. Following removal, her symptoms markedly increased over the next seven to ten days and then recovery began. To her amazement, within six weeks, the CFIDS/ME symptoms cleared.

The *Helicobacter* dead tooth test provocation is simple to administer and, if positive, convinces most patients. Other provoked *Helicobacter* symptoms may accompany the tooth pain, for example, tiredness, indigestion, muscle aches, and increased amounts of urine with a cat pee odor. Antibiotic courses for dead teeth fail because they cannot reach the organisms in the dead tooth ligament or infected dentin tubules of the tooth. The pain in the tooth occurs during horizontal sleep, two to three days after the provocation.

## Dental Plates

An upper dental plate hides and protects the microbes in our mouth. A coated tongue, suggesting the presence of *Candida Albicans* and *C. tropicalis,* often occurs with white patches of *Candida* on the bony roof of the mouth. Twice a day, remove the plate, wash it, dust nystatin powder on the upper contact surface, and replace it. Take the nystatin dose after attending to the upper plate. Within three to four days, the roof of the mouth is clean.

Many people do not return for a yearly check of their dental plates. They are surprised when told the dental stump is infected, although they agree that they have experienced an increase in bad breath, mouth ulcers, and herpes. The *Helicobacter* dead tooth test provocation located a hidden infected tooth stump and bone fragments (sequestrums) that were removed with benefit.

The symptoms of temporomandibular joint pain syndrome may be relieved following CMV virutherapy. Patients have commented on improvement in tolerating dental plates following CMV virutherapy for other symptoms or fatigue.

### Stomach, Intestines, and Colon

Modern medicine and food research have greatly reduced chronic gastroenteritis and bowel infections in developed countries. One problem, irritable bowel syndrome (IBS), persists. IBS is a massive Western world problem, a major cause of sick leave, and accounts for up 50 percent of gastroenterologists' practice. Medical technology, including X rays, fiberoptic endoscopy, cultures, and clinical examinations appear to be normal or near normal. Yet the pain, contractions, bloating, and difficulty with motions continue or are controlled by SSDs.

Think about these facts. A gram weight of motion or feces has ten billion organisms or microbes. We have more organisms in our bowels than cells in our body. We provide them with a protected environment and a plentiful food supply when we eat allergic foods. The digested allergic food protein is intermixed with its carbohydrate and fat. Most of the allergic pap is rejected by the absorbing surface of our intestines. The bulk of the allergic food passes down into the lower bowel, where it becomes a feast for the organisms living there. The calories of allergic foods are used up by molds and microbes, not by our bodies.

But we have overlooked another large community of guests, the latent viruses of the gut. In many ways they are just as dangerous, as their activities are unrecognized and hidden. Viruses, besides living in the cells of our gut lining, infect the organisms in our bowels (see pp. 180-183 in Chapter 5).

The cells lining our intestine, enterocytes, can convert double sugars (sucrose) to single sugars, glucose and fructose, that are absorbed. Microbial toxins from the "1,001 gut friends" can disrupt the enterocytes. Allergic foods depress enterocyte activity or cause stunting of the cells, rapid turnover, or minute ulceration and bleeding of the gut wall. These changes starve the body of simple sugars and allow toxic materials to pass through the leaky gut, placing strains on the NIS. The irritated and damaged gut lining responds by increasing mucus production.

Did you have an endoscopic examination and biopsy? Were you told the findings were normal, or that you did not have celiac disease? It is confusing because your symptoms disappeared after excluding OWGGs. The early research on celiac disease, such as that by Dr. Haas of New York (see Gottschall, 1994), found that a severe wheat allergy may not damage the cells lining the gut, but found other food allergies caused similar celiac gut damage changes. Before agreeing to an expensive technological medical work-up, if your symptoms suggest an OWGG allergy, do a complete exclusion for one to three months. Should symptoms persist, see your physician. If the examination reveals nothing, consider a virus-allergy investigation.

When you consider that the total surface area of the intestinal lining is equal to half a tennis court, it is not surprising that virutherapy for irritable bowel syndrome is complicated. Patients with IBS often require four changes of their treatment vial dilutions. The reduction of latent virus activity in the bowel lining appears to decrease abnormal permeability, or leaking, of the gut lining. Long-standing irritable bowel syndrome can clear with treatment using two viruses, but in most cases, it is a combination of the organisms listed previously (see Table 1.1, pp. 9-10). As improvement occurs, the drug dosage is reduced. Patients are warned not to suddenly stop their drugs.

Would any physician or surgeon have predicted there was a bacterium living in the lining of the stomach? Stomach acid is supposed to sterilize our food and any descending mucus from our nose and chest. No wonder the medical profession refused to take seriously the clinical discovery by Dr. Barry Marshall of Perth, Australia. It took years before his discovery was accepted, but, thanks to the media, few people have not heard about *Helicobacter* as a cause of chronic indigestion and stomach duodenal ulcers. The scientific medicine "mind-set," not healthy skepticism, caused the delay. Antibiotics do not eradicate *Helicobacter*, which is adept at developing resistance. The active *Helicobacter* symptoms have been driven underground as latent symptoms or turn up some weeks or months later as a reinfection (see pp. 95, 100). *Helicobacter* infection stimulates excessive formation of stomach acid but, in time, leads to exhaustion of the acid-forming cells. The marked reduction in stomach acid or its absence is called achlorhydria. With no stomach acid, the digestion is disrupted, resulting in aggravation or onset of IBS. If you have a burning sensation in the bladder, chest, or nose, suspect *Helicobacter,* even if laboratory reports are normal. *Helicobacter* toxins make you cold and tired. OWGG allergies encourage *Helicobacter* and make treatment difficult.

**IK**   Previous operations to remove segments of the colon resulted in a colostomy. During the provocation neutralization test (PNT) with *Helicobacter,* the chronic burning sensation in the intestines was relieved. Within twenty minutes the clinic was filled with the sickly smell of cat urine. The patient dozed off, making further testing impossible. He had a dramatic recovery on completion of the full viral work-up two months later.

Crohn's disease of the lower bowel was an oddity, even a rarity, forty to fifty years ago. It presented as a surgical emergency when it caused obstruction of the bowel. It is now a frequent and important cause of colitis. Recent reports are of children, eight to ten years of age, developing Crohn's disease. Changes to our diet and the increased use of sulfur and other chemical preservatives have much to do with this frightening development. *Mycobacterium paratuberculosis* is found in the scarring lesions of the colon caused by Crohn's disease. Provocation of the bacteria provokes and may improve bowel symptoms. A majority of clinic patients with Crohn's Disease have OWGG allergies. Clinical symptoms and responses to provocation suggest there are two types of Crohn's disease: (1) an early diffuse infection of the lower gut lining that (2) later develops one or more of the diffuse areas into a scarring lump. When the lump reaches 1 to 2 centimeters (cm) in size, it can be found with an endoscopic examination and biopsy. Most undiagnosed lower bowel symptoms are treated with SSDs. *Surmise:* Early diffused Crohn's Disease in IBS patients is aggravated by SSDs, such as sulfasalazine.

Virutherapy clears irritable bowel symptoms that began after a severe viral infection. The important viruses are polio, hepatitis, mumps, CMV, rotavirus, and EBV. Important molds and bacteria are *Candida, Giardia, Trichomonas, Helicobacter, Listeria, Legionella,* and, if the person has visited tropical countries, *Entamoeba.* Always treat for worms (Webster, 1996; Wright, 1990).

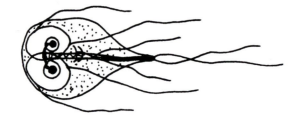

### Carbohydrate Control and Diabetes I and II

For the past twenty to thirty years, it has been fashionable to blame hypoglycemia for a range of unexplained symptoms and, more recently, to blame cholesterol for threats to heart and blood vessels. Recent clinical findings suggest that limitation of fat in the diet is questionable advice for those with raised cholesterol. Hypoglycemia is better understood. Who would have suspected the two conditions are related through the actions of insulin and glucagon hormones? Insulin reduces blood sugar to normal levels and increases the storage of fat in fat cells. Glucagon has the opposite effect, raising low blood sugar to normal levels and mobilizing fat from fat cells.

Many hypoglycemia symptoms dwindled, even disappeared, as patients moved through the preliminary work-up and MLV. At the end of the work-up they are prepared to accept some of their symptoms are due to hidden latent microbes and toxins, while other symptoms are the effect of hormones on sugars and fats in their diet. Children tolerate moderate to large amounts of sugar in homemade meals and in junk and fast foods. Carbohydrate control is a well-tuned balance between the two hormones. They regulate the body's use of glucose and fat, fat accumulation, and behavioral changes. The high blood levels of insulin required to cope with a "sugarholic" diet eventually upset the sensitivity of the body's cell responses to insulin, causing a person to become insulin resistant. As insulin production is increased, normal blood cholesterol levels, control of fat storage, and other body activities and behavior are disrupted. This is the cost of controlling blood sugar levels to protect brain activity and functions. The nerve cells of the brain and their protecting astrocytes will not tolerate changes above or below normal blood glucose levels.

Disaster strikes if an active virus infection such as mumps kills insulin-producing cells and suppresses insulin production in others because of the overload of latent mumps virus. The remaining unaffected cells are unable to keep up with the demand for insulin. The glucagon hormone is no longer restrained and causes reduction of fat storage and body weight loss (type I diabetes). Rubella, Coxsackievirus, influenza, rotavirus, and CRC toxins can damage insulin-producing cells. When controlled type I diabetes symptoms begin to fluctuate and medication dosage changes, suspect that surviving inactive insulin-producing cells are present.

Type II diabetes occurs when the insulin-producing cells no longer keep up with the excessive demand for insulin of a high sugar and carbohydrate diet, or insulin resistance. The glucagon hormone takes over and, in a worst-case scenario, promotes fat loss and excessive amounts of acid ketones that may result in a life-threatening crisis. Type II diabetes is controlled by a carbohydrate-regulating diet, sometimes supplemented by medication, even insulin shots. Type II diabetes is said to be inherited, a genetic defect, and, no doubt, some geneticist will discover the diabetic genes. Many people with type II diabetes have OWGG food allergies, which also tend to be inherited. Communities that do not eat OWGGs or processed sugars/foods do not suffer from diabetes, obesity, high blood pressure, or heart attacks. There is more to type II diabetes than diet control and medication. Besides the common association with OWGG food allergies, people with this condition frequently provoke symptoms that reveal latent mumps, Coxsackievirus, and other viruses. Virutherapy improves control of type II diabetes, even leading to withdrawal of medication.

You have probably read the experts' advice: "Strict adherence to a low carbohydrate diet is the cornerstone of all diabetic therapy." The concrete walls of this long-held dictum should be reinforced by the cornerstones of total exclusion of OWGGs; adequate CRC therapy; reduction of overloading of insulin- and glucagon-producing cells by latent microbes and toxins; and adequate, appropriate, nutritional supplements. Type II diabetes treatments have not eliminated long-term complications, e.g., blindness. It is logical and practical to test the teenage children of diabetic parents for food allergies, in particular, to OWGGs, and, if facilities are available, for the presence of latent viruses.

## HEADACHES, MOODS, DEPRESSIONS, DREAMS, AND MEMORY

### Headaches and Migraines

It continues to surprise me how many people with "allergic" tension headaches and migraines experience viral provocation with one or more latent viruses. The investigation starts with the preliminary work-up. Special attention is given to detecting bacterial or petrochemical toxicity. Those of you with a long history of headaches are asked to observe and record changes in the patterns before and during treatment. An improvement after virutherapy may temporarily relapse when a drug therapy is stopped—in other words, a drug withdrawal symptom. Nearly all drugs used to treat headaches are "man-made" or xenochemicals. Because they are not natural compounds their activity can mimic petrochemicals. There is no reason why latent viruses should not be in brain cells, for HIV has been found in neurons of AIDS victims' brains.

Patients tell me they suffer from several headaches. I provoke their various headaches using different viruses. But the type of headache brought on by morbilli in one person may be quite different from the headache another suffers. There is a general pattern, but not a specific pattern, and no standard headache response to individual virus provocation. When multiple viruses are involved, one virus is dominant for a period of the virutherapy and then another takes its place. The reliance on drugs and psychological therapy to relieve headache, in particular, "tension" headache, should decrease when MLV is an accepted treatment. The wide range of mental effects provoked and relieved by MLV calls for a reassessment of accepted psychological concepts and therapies. No longer can untreatable headaches or common head sensations, such as a band constricting around the head, be branded neurotic or "all in the head." *Listeria* toxin or latent infection causes severe, even crippling, headaches, a stiff neck, and memory loss (see p. 56).

People who experienced worthwhile relief from headaches due to allergy and petrochemical toxicity agreed that virutherapy gave them additional freedom from the headaches, a clearer head, a better mind, and improved memory. Patients were delighted when their "get up and go" motivation returned, as they had not experienced it for years while taking SSDs. Some lucky people told me they suffered no more severe headaches or mood changes from the day the significant virus was provoked and its virutherapy started. I cannot explain why this occurs. Do not get enthusiastic and suddenly stop headache drugs. They may be suppressing other symptoms besides headaches, and a sudden withdrawal can cause symptoms to recur. Latent viral headaches are often associated with mood and personality changes. Sudden drug removal can make life very difficult and stormy. Be careful if you are prone to depression and suicide. Be sure your physician knows about these serious symptoms when he or she suggests you start reducing your drug intake. Once off the drugs, do not throw them out; keep them in the medicine cabinet so they are available to help control relapses.

Constant latent viral headache is a new class of head pain. It responds poorly, if at all, to symptom suppression drugs. A continuous pain in the head, one that varies a little but is always there—when you wake in the morning and go to bed at night—suggests latent viruses are in the neurons of the brain. The background pain continues even when you have other headaches and mood changes. If previous thorough work-ups are negative, virutherapy may be very effective. Most sufferers' medical histories included an undiagnosed/severe infection or a marked reaction to childhood vaccinations. Some had suffered head injuries.

**IK**   A woman was relieved of a forty-year-long constant head pain. Morbilli was the main virus of the three that cleared her head of all symptoms. She later returned to Europe, and her elderly mother reminded her she had morbilli at age eleven and "had never been the same girl after that."

If on the day you are scheduled for a virus work-up you develop a severe migraine, unless you are fully disabled by it, keep your physician's appointment. Chances are, virus provocation will neutralize the headache. It is a wonderful and dramatic experience. Tension headaches with tender head, neck, and shoulder muscles often accompany migraines. Such muscle spasms respond to provocation and virutherapy with influenza, polio, morbilli, herpes simplex 1, CMV, and EBV. Head and face pains attributed to the temporomandibular joint pain syndrome respond to virutherapy, in particular, CMV.

**IK**   A young woman described postviral fatigue syndrome (PVFS) symptoms to me and, during the second visit, confided that she was terrified that her untreatable headaches, failing memory, and poor motivation would end her employment. Before her illness, she was respected for her abilities. If she lost her job, she worried she would lose the friends she had made. The work-up greatly improved symptoms, including repetitive stress injury of her forearms and hands. RSV brought back her memory within ten days of the provocation, astounding her family. She was able to complete her pretesting and treatment day's work in three to four hours. A year later the company laid off 10 percent of its employees, but she was promoted to head of her section.

## Listeria

Latent viruses join up with bacterial and mold toxins to depress our memories. *Listeria* is feared as a dangerous, often lethal, disease of food poisoning. Latent *Listeria* is a cause of undiagnosed memory loss, severe crippling headaches, as well as spasms and pain of the neck muscles. The *Listeria* bacterium is small enough to penetrate our organ cell walls to become latent. This occurs during a bout of food poisoning, which tends to linger for weeks, without any positive laboratory findings. Those who suffer from repeated headaches, severe stiffness and pain in the neck, and memory loss or suppression should request a provocation with *Listeria*. Clinic patients with these symptoms complete the work-up before being tested for *Listeria* and EBV. The detoxing and serial vaccination treatments are continued for four to six months to prevent recurrences. The detoxing symptoms are almost unbearable at times, probably due to other latent viruses being stimulated to detox. Latent *Listeria*, similar to CRC, turns its hosts (you?) into sugarholics.

**IK**    For six years he had put up with severe headaches that did not respond to drug therapy, as well as a neck stiffness that was almost a spasm, a pain at the base of his skull, and IBS. Preliminary work-up (PW) and MLV improved the IBS and his fatigue, but not the headache, neck spasm, pain at the base of the skull, or memory loss. During provocation with *Listeria*, he lost awareness of where he was and what he was required to do during the testing. The dazed state was neutralized by *Listeria* $5^{10}$. That night and the next day, a severe delayed provocation kept him in bed. He returned to the clinic, and the symptoms were partly neutralized for 4 to 6 h. He decided to put up with the detoxing, which continued for four to five days, then gradually improved over the next three weeks. During this time, his wife recognized the smells of *Candida, Helicobacter,* and hepatitis. With the disappearance of the *Listeria* symptoms, his memory returned to almost the preillness level. Three or four weeks later, EBV was provoked, and in six months time, he was fit and well.

## Cannabis/Marijuana

Cannabis facilitates the entry and accumulation of latent viruses, and it increases the activity of latent viruses already present in the nervous system. Many younger people tell me they used the drug for short periods of two to three months. Weeks or months later they developed recurring headaches. Others with headaches before using cannabis now experience additional headache patterns with mood changes. Taking cannabis while suffering from a viral infection, especially influenza, aggravates headaches and mood and behavioral changes. Many unsuccessfully tried to stop cannabis but could not tolerate the crushing headaches of withdrawal. I advise the preliminary work-up and MLV, at the same time slowly reducing the cannabis intake.

**IK** A man who used marijuana for four years completely stopped it seven years ago. For the past five years he suffered variable CFIDS/ME. Two months after the PNT and virutherapy he noticed strong marijuana smells during several of the sauna treatments. Cannabis toxin was still present in fatty tissues after seven years of abstinence. Cannabis toxin is difficult to detox and is a long-term cause of lowered immunities.

When patients inform me of previous cannabis use, I provoke the cannabis symptoms after the foods and house dust. The sooner excess latent cannabis is detoxed, the quicker the response to the PW and MLV.

Two patients, in the thirty-five to forty age group, reached a plateau of improvement. On questioning, both revealed previous cannabis use. One for four years until seven years ago and the other for twelve years until nine years ago. Provocation with cannabis $5^{12}$ brought on mild cannabis sensations and the clinic room filled with the typical smell, which came from their lungs. They continued to detox cannabis smells for the next six to eight weeks, with three saunas a week and serial vaccination of $5^{12,}$ which was reduced to $5^7$. After four to six weeks of testing, the treatment was resumed. From time to time over the next six to eight months both would notice, or be told by their partners, that they were detoxing cannabis.

### Moods

The preliminary work-up often provokes moods or relieves them. Variable or complex moods suggest several latent viruses are present. Patients and their partners are reticent about describing mood changes, fearing they may offend each other. It is difficult to write down how you feel during a mood, but try to record the strange things that are occurring. Remember, you may be manipulated by latent toxins and viruses in your brain. Once you understand what is happening, you may detect that you suffer from several different moods. Provocation will enable you to identify a latent virus for a particular mood. When you are suffering from moods, your recall and immediate memory may be poor or absent. If you have moods, explain to your children and partner that you believe you are being manipulated by a toxin. They will understand and not worry about your behavior. You are more likely to be convinced of provocation and neutralization when latent viruses reproduce the moods and symptoms you know. Later, if moods come on, they can be turned off (neutralized) within a half hour or less by using the treatment dose of the suspected virus. Most symptoms from provocation of viruses are of the delayed type. The herpes group of viruses may not bring on moods until four to seven days after provocation.

CRC moods are most difficult to treat, especially if there is a severe "burn off" of other symptoms when therapy begins. It is not unusual for the moods to be "all-encompassing," in other words, to completely take you over so you are unable to do anything. Moods from food allergies are less severe but will aggravate the CRC moods. Premenstrual tension (PMT) moods that do not respond to conventional therapies may respond to the PW and MLV. If a PMT headache and mood occur on the day you are due at the clinic, phone to cancel, unless the physician suggests you come in for neutralization. The temporary use of antianxiety, antidepression SSDs give adequate relief of swinging mood changes during detoxing. Provocation and skin tests have equivocal results when SSD dosage is medium to high. Before starting therapy, you will be asked to markedly reduce or forego the use of SSDs, if possible. You will need the support of a sympathetic psychologist during PW, MLV, and antidepression drug withdrawal.

### Depressions

Depression is the eighth most common reason for attending the clinic. Those who are successfully relieved of their depressions report a variety of reasons for their recovery. All are keen to discontinue their drugs, although the drugs were helpful for long periods. They feel insecure about the ability of the drugs to help them in the years ahead and are now painfully aware of many of the toxic side effects.

**IK**   "I knew my depression changed at times, but mostly it was an uncharted mystery. At first the antidepressant drugs smothered the peaks and valleys, but as therapy lengthened, increased drug dosage made me feel I was not my old self. During the preliminary work-up and virutherapy testing, I noticed many depressions came on suddenly following the testing session. It was not the depression pattern I knew, a gradual worsening, or a gradual improvement. I am now little bothered by depression or moods. Antidepression drugs do not seem logical to me."

Depressions are graded as tolerable, serious, and dangerous. Depressed people seeking allergy and virutherapy investigation are carefully checked before starting treatment. They are asked to bring a friend or relative to the clinic during testing. The relative should be close at hand for the next four to five days after testing. People with depression problems are not good fighters and need support from the physician and those close to them, honest information, and openness about therapy. They should not be discouraged if MLV provokes aggravation of symptoms, requiring resumption of anti-depression drugs for short periods.

Body heating by saunas, sun saunas, or hot-water baths may bring on depression until the last of the petrochemicals are detoxed. Petrochemicals, molds, toxins, and latent viruses are excreted singly or together in no particular order during the length of the treatment. It is dangerous to eat a suspected or known allergic food, alcohol, sugar, and honey while the investigation is proceeding. Sudden depression may follow. CRC is nearly always present, especially if there is an important food allergy, such as to OWGGs. Since the 1850s, clinicians have reported that three to four months after viral or influenza epidemics, there is an upsurge in postviral depression states and unexplained increases in suicides rates.

Recent concern about teenage suicide overlooks "the difficult to treat" deep depression and floods of tears from detoxing of glandular fever (EBV) and, to a lesser extent, CMV, hepatitis, and CRC. The EBV smell in the urine, motions, sweat, breath, fingernail/toenail quicks, even in collected tears, is clinical confirmation of detoxing of the virus despite negative blood antibody tests. There will be other causes present. It is not unusual for successfully treated adults to recall past bouts of severe depression and floods of tears accompanied by suicidal thoughts. The appearance of suicidal feelings during detoxing and recovery requires caring relatives, a sympathetic psychologist, and the virutherapy clinic staff to keep in contact with the patient for reassurance and support. Treatment of depression is difficult, or impossible, when the patient cannot comply with the requirements of a lifestyle change or has a history of previous drug use/dependence (see Can-

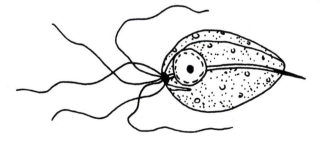

nabis/Marijuana, pp. 56-57). Viruses responsible for mood and depression symptoms are hepatitis, dengue, polio, RSV, morbilli, CMV, herpes, and especially EBV.

### Latency Dreams

The activities of a sleeping brain are diagnostic of latent disease. An excess or the detoxing of latent toxins and microbes stimulates dreams. Typical latency dreams or nightmare patterns are caused by individual agents. Latency dreams are outside of the psychological arena. Dr. Freud had major problems with dream interpretations (Buchwald et al., 1996). Try not to worry about dream subjects that persist in your memory. Dreams caused by excess latent viruses and toxins contain distorted facts and images. After you complete the virutherapy work-up, cruel or terrifying dreams disappear. All available testing viruses are capable of provoking unpleasant and/or pleasant dreams. Hepatitis, polio, and EBV provocation bring on vivid, alarming dreams; RSV, elated and happy dreams; CMV, erotic dreams, dreams with babies and children, and ferocious animal dreams. It is not unusual, after a vivid latency dream, to wake up drenched in perspiration. The "burn-off " symptoms from CRC, poultry, and OWGGs, especially wheat, provoke severe and alarming dreams.

**IK**    "I know when I am in for a bout of latency illness. My headache, head confusion, [and] the pressure worsen; my fibromyalgia springs to life; and my old scary dreaming starts up again. My partner complains of the old body smells, and my fingernail quicks stink."

The nature of dreams changes with better recall, when most of the excess latent virus is detoxed and recovery is under way. Men with excess latent hepatitis experience dreams involving cruelty to others, such as people beating, and shooting, or even stabbing, loved ones. Women with excess latent hepatitis suffer terrifying dreams, such as being beaten up, chased, or even raped. People were so ashamed of having such dreams that only when similar dreams were provoked did they admit to past experience of such dream sequences. You can imagine their relief when they found a cause. Polio-related dreams involve, for example, falling/floating in space, crashing into a cliff, going over the side of the road into a ravine, waking up screaming as the airplane is about to crash, or being overcome by smoke and fire. The polio dream pattern involves active roles for men and passive ones for women.

**IK**    "Ever since I can remember, I get fearful 'falling in space' dreams that wake me up. The polio provocation at the clinic, and each polio detoxing shot brings on the dream. I am sure it is caused by latent polio virus, because my mother remembers I was off-color for a week after my polio sugar lump, thirty-plus years ago."

EBV-provoked dreams feature depression, feelings of hopelessness or despair, close friends or relatives dying, or attempting suicide, with floods of tears and uncontrollable sobbing on waking. Patients experience suicide preparation dreams. There is little difference between men and women with EBV depression dreams. Viral dreaming is aggravated by sadistic videos, television thrillers, and violent novels.

**IK**   His twelve-year illness began with influenza, quickly followed by an illness resembling glandular fever. For years he was in and out of bed. The laboratory tests for liver function were always abnormal, but no cause was found. Sleep was disturbed by aggressive dreams, two or three sessions of dreams a night. One was a terror dream that was always accompanied by pain in his liver area when he woke, but not during the day. MLV confirmed that the dreams and liver pain were probably due to hepatitis B virus.

People are loath to report unpleasant dreams when they phone about the other provoked symptoms, so they are asked whether unpleasant dreams have occurred. For example, if asked, "Are you being chased by someone with an axe?", women will often admit to having such a dream. On the other hand, men experience dreams in which they are doing the chasing. When they wake they are sexually stimulated and often report ejaculation discharges. Fortunately, most people stop dreaming or have the occasional happy, pleasant, or loving dreams when they recover. Months later, a relapse is preceded by one to three nights of the old scary or cruel dreams.

Latent viruses and other toxins are able to provoke terrifying and horrible dreams. *Surmise:* (1) Those who carry out mindless violence and cannot understand why they do it, or cannot even remember their actions, have excess latent viruses in their brains. (2) Women's and teenage girls' vivid sexual dreams, especially those caused by latent hepatitis, CMV, and EBV, are recollected as real events during psychological sessions (recovered memory movement). I reviewed fifty books and texts on dreams written by psychologists and behavioral scientists. Not one of the indexes listed *virus*. Is it not time for psychologists and psychiatrists to reassess their concept of dreams as psychological processes—to let go of Freud's coattails?

### Memory Loss and Recovery

The return of memory and mental ability is the priority for people with CFIDS/ME. All other disarranged body functions can wait. Memory loss caused by viral illnesses may be a sudden, gradual, or an undulating pattern with slow deterioration. Memory recovery is the reverse pattern, but the person who experienced a sudden loss can recover memory in a wavelike manner. Literature and opera have many heroines who lost and then recovered their memory, just at the dramatic moment, to solve the plot! Sudden loss of memory and recovery is usually ascribed to psychological causes. Clinic patients recovered their memory from treatment with CRC, *Listeria*, *Chlamydia*, RSV, polio, influenza, hepatitis, rubella, v. zoster, and EBV. Portions of memory return during immediate or delayed provocation and after two to three virutherapy shots. A general pattern is sudden return of memory of names and details at the workplace; then some hours or days later memory of the position of objects and personal things in the house returns; after varying periods, the details of the town's shopping center and neighborhood roads return; followed by visual memories of faces and figures of relatives and friends together with their names. This process continues until most of the memory returns—for fortunate people, usually of a younger age group, until full memory returns. Once virutherapy shots are underway, memory chunks of varying size will return over a period of a few weeks.

**IK**   A patient, over the age of fifty-five, had a reasonable recovery of memory and continued with his managerial position. He contacted me fifteen months later, disappointed that certain sections of his memory had not returned despite virutherapy. On checking the old notes, I noticed that I had overlooked hepatitis. Happily, hepatitis provoked most of the remaining lost memory over a period of two to three months.

People recall a virus infection suffered in the past, often years ago. Weeks or months later the memory starts to be affected. Generally, the memory was recovered, but years later it suddenly deteriorated for no apparent reason. Loss of memory for recent events and facts is a leading cause of job loss and financial insecurity for people so affected. Patients with memory problems may not be able to complete a physician's questionnaire. One recovered woman, months later, asked to look at her questionnaire and was surprised by some of the responses she had filled in and what she had omitted. If your memory is affected, you will not remember what your physician said when you return home. This is why the Neurotic

Notebook is so important. Jot down symptoms when they occur, not two or three hours later. If you want to get the most help from your physician, conscientiously record your symptoms in your Neurotic Notebook (see Chapter 4, p. 156).

Fluctuations in memory occur less often during the preliminary work-up when foods, molds, pollens, and dusts are provoked. The therapies will be of little use to you if you are deficient in vitamins and trace minerals. Those who believe nutritional supplements help them should continue taking them. A common experience is waking up in the middle of the night and not knowing where you are, bringing on fear and panic (CMV is the principal cause of this disorientation). Getting your memory back is exciting, for you can read books again and remember what was on the pages you have just read. The risk of relapse is greatly decreased by continuing MLV and other treatments, sometimes for a year or two. Nearly all who attend the clinic have at some time in the past been given antianxiety or antidepressant drugs. Most report little or no improvement in memory retention. For some, it seemed to stabilize their memory, but they noticed a decrease in the effect as the months went by. Others benefited for years, but on questioning them, they admitted that they did not feel their memory was as good as before the illness or drug course was started. Some are convinced their three- to five-year antidepressant therapy caused the loss of portions of their memory.

**IK**   A boy, age twelve, developed memory problems and PVFS eight weeks after a vaccination. Visual memory was markedly affected, so he could no longer attend school. After two years of negative investigations and therapies, he attended the clinic and obtained a full recovery. The important viruses were RSV, polio, and influenza. He attended school again after having been unable to understand his lessons for a year and a half. Other patients with memory losses are listed in the Identikit (see pp. xxiii-xxxv).

**IK**   A young woman recovered recent memory. Vivid recollections of activities she could not place in her past life kept returning at odd times. She explained what was happening to relatives and friends who stood by her during the illness. They assured her these events had really occurred in the past. She sought out friends who had been with her and discussed what they did and studied photographs. In this manner, she reconstructed much of her lost past four years. Today she recalls events if asked about them.

An interesting comment from such a patient was, "Memory needs to be taken away from psychology and given a reassignment." A business management consultant, after recovery of memory, remarked, "Allergy, CRC, chemical toxicity, ecology, and virutherapy should be given a nationwide trial." Unfortunately, such a trial would not be "scientific." Laboratory tests are not devised for latency immunity. Little or no response from the preliminary work-up and MLV is an indication of the need for psychological assessment and therapy.

### The Preemptive Syndrome

If you suffer from unexplained tiredness, mañana motivation, or CFIDS, you have many symptoms that seem very real to you but are diagnosed as subjective or functional. The family physician finds little or no clinical evidence on examination, and the laboratory tests and X rays are normal. You are given treatment for stress or psychological conditions, consisting of antianxiety or antidepressant drugs, even a psychological assessment and therapy. The SSD therapy and psychological methods may relieve the symptoms for varying periods, ending in mild or marked relapses. Further visits to the family physician suggest a bias toward a subjective, functional, or stress explanation of your symptoms. Your suspicions are confirmed by the items on the prescription, or a visit to a psychiatrist who supports the family physician's diagnosis. All the while you are insisting the symptoms are real and you want to find the causes. After the treatments fail, further visits result in change of the SSDs or their dosage, depending on toxic side effects or changes in your symptoms.

Patients attending for a PNT and MLV at the clinic speak of a discussion with their family physician that resembled the folowing:

**Family Physician:**  Ms./Mr. B, your blood tests and examinations are normal, and the report from the psychiatrist supports a stress or neurotic personality diagnosis.

**Ms./Mr. B:**  Doctor, you did suggest that the symptoms could be due to viruses. What sort of viruses could be affecting me, and could I have one of the antiviral drug courses?

**Family Physician:**  The blood tests show you have no viral problems, and, anyway, the drugs are very toxic and are reserved for serious viral illnesses.

A diagnosis of neurosis suggests mental illness, a serious and alarming shock for you, the patient. The patient reluctantly accepts the SSDs and psychological treatment, for nothing else seems to be available. The treatments fail and the family physician and specialists are no longer trusted. An alternative medical therapy, usually advice on food allergies and nutritional supplements, gives moderate to marked symptom relief that persists for six months or more, or provides continuing improvement/reduction in the level of symptoms.

Some weeks or months later you seek relief from symptoms or an illness unrelated to the "functional" condition. After an examination, you are dismayed by a pep talk from the physician about pulling yourself together, and you notice that the prescription includes an antianxiety drug. You are annoyed because the family physician is not receptive to your explanation of the successful alternative therapy. The benefit you obtained from this therapy is dismissed as a placebo effect. This further annoys you, as it is obviously a very poor excuse for their useless drug therapy. The family physician or specialist is no longer trusted. You know you do not have a psychological or neurotic illness.

You request a change of family physician, and your case notes are transferred. At the first or following visits, the second family physician preempts the treatment offered by prescribing antianxiety drugs. The second family physician has studied your notes, which included the old lengthy reports on stress, psychology, and psychiatry. Because some of the new symptoms could be subjective, and the previous family physician considered you as having a neurotic personality, a preemptive assessment is made of a functional personality. You are upset by the second physician's preempting your symptoms and by the excuse of a placebo effect for the successful alternative treatment. You believe the new symptoms or condition had little, if anything, to do with your first illness, which responded to alternative therapy. You resent the functional diagnosis and what it implies.

Patients who experience this type of consultation, treatment, and advice believe their old records of stress, neurotic, and psychological diagnoses preempted the physician's diagnosis. The past five years have seen a large increase in the number of patients with stress and subjective symptoms, resulting in a huge increase in the use of antianxiety and antidepressant drugs. The associated costs are of concern to government health departments and medical insurance companies. Yet neither the medical profession nor the health agencies have attempted to explore why allergy and alternative treatments are often successful in relieving patients' symptoms. A welcomed advance has been the acceptance of acupuncture by many medical professionals. Many patients attending the allergy virutherapy clinic report 20 to 50 percent, or more, improvement from alternative health therapies. These patients persisted with treatment even though improvement later decreased to 20, even 10, percent. These patients do well at the clinic, where they discover the real causes of many of their symptoms.

A women's action group is lobbying for the following changes in health information privacy codes:

1. Legislation to enforce the removal of out-of-date or incorrect psychological or psychiatric reports from patient files. Such reports would be handed over to the requesting patient for destruction.
2. Reports of the successful alternative therapy, accompanied by written statements by the patient confirming the improvement or cure, would be placed in the patient's file.
3. Refusal to comply by the family physician or medical clinic could be appealed to a preemption appeal authority or committee. If an appeal fails, the patient retains the right to add to his or her file the report of the successful alternative therapy and the confirming statements.

The action group believes many women will return to the family physician or medical clinic confident that they will not receive functional, psychological, or even neurotic diagnoses. The group believes descriptions of successful therapies will interest health professionals, who may adopt them in their practice or refer patients elsewhere for alternative therapy.

### Head Injuries

Head injuries, encephalitis, and encephalopathy appear to attract microbes and/or their toxins to the bruised or damaged areas of the brain (clinical observation). The excess latent viruses and toxins further aggravate patients' symptoms, disability, and behavior. Provocation and latency therapy gradually, or sometimes dramatically, improve function of the affected side of the body and mental activity. The delayed provoked aggravated symptoms can be severe for five to seven days before improvement occurs. On completion of serial dilution therapy shots, the muscle strength and coordination on the affected side improve, often to equal that of the other side. Patients with a right weak side thought they were left-handed until the recovery brought back strength to the right side.

An improvement in muscle strength from serial vaccination releases mental energy. Thoughts, ideas, and memories flood the mind, preventing sleep, until extreme tiredness occurs. The heightened mental activity extends into the next day, gradually decreasing. Serial vaccination maintains the improvement. These lucky people and their dramatic mental responses add excitement to the practice of MLV.

### Fitting, Panics, Specific Learning Disabilities, and Attention-Deficit Disorder

All patients are taking average to heavy drug dosages. A careful and detailed history is taken for evidence of viral or viruslike illnesses occurring at the onset of the illness, or during a relapse, or aggravation of symptoms. If possible, the drug dosage is reduced during the PNT and viral provocation. The provoked symptoms of a marked fixed food allergy will break through the drug dosage barrier. Panic states and compulsive actions often respond to the preliminary work-up and MLV. Specific learning disabilities/attention-deficit disorder (ADD) are managed through psychological behavior therapies and Ritalin or a similar drug. If dissatisfied with these therapies, consider a two- to three-month trial of food allergy and diet manipulation. If little or no response occurs, ask for a work-up of CRC and a selection of latent virutherapy. Some physicians, educational professionals, and many parents are concerned about long-term drug suppression of ADD. Most ADD children respond to therapy offered by the clinic. Older children confide that they do not want to go back on the drugs because their heads are clear, their physical abilities are improved, and, best of all, they have many more friends.

**IK** Jonathan, age 7, had a specific learning disability, overactivity, and was so disruptive he was removed from several schools. After a preliminary work-up, including a diet that excluded OWGGs, sugar, and honey, MLV started a marked improvement in behavior from RSV, polio, influenza, and hepatitis. After three months he was understanding what he read and was rapidly catching up with his classmates. His mother later showed me a letter from his teacher expressing amazement at the turnaround in his learning and behavior. Jonathan's mother said that he is very careful about what he eats (Galland, 1998; Hyde, 1992; Rapp, 1996).

### Multiple Sclerosis and Systemic Lupus Erythematosus

**IK** Autoimmune illness can be induced by latent viral activity (Shepherd, 1989). Multiple sclerosis and systemic lupus erythematosus (SLE) are now regarded as autoimmune illnesses, but the role of "slow" viruses and multiple latent viruses has not been ruled out. The viral role in neurological disease increases as microbiology advances. Many with neurological diseases and SLE suffer allergic, CRC, *Giardia,* and *Helicobacter* symptoms. Some patients in the early stages, and a number who have been confined to wheelchairs for short periods, appear to recover fully. The question is whether the original diagnosis of multiple sclerosis and SLE is correct.

I look for the following when selecting patients for therapy:

1. A thorough work-up has been done at a clinic or hospital. Toxic metals, in particular, mercury, cadmium, and lead, have been excluded.
2. The childhood was spent in a home with poor ecology, indoor animals, and parents who smoked.
3. The person suffered in the past from allergic symptoms and shows evidence of CRC.
4. The symptoms are similar to postviral fatigue syndrome/CFIDS.
5. The person experienced complications following vaccination or immunization shots.
6. A viral illness occurred before symptoms of either disease developed.
7. Severe measles (morbilli) or mumps occurred in childhood (this applies to patients with multiple sclerosis).
8. *An important indication:* the person suffered from recurring "flus," some of which caused temporary paralysis, numbness, mood changes, and even changes in the blood immune system laboratory results.
9. The person's employment involves working with xenochemicals, e.g., adhesives.

Multiple sclerosis patients gave exaggerated provoked symptoms during testing with latent viruses. The "shadowing effect" is frequently seen in these illnesses. Morbilli and mumps are important viruses of multiple sclerosis. MS and SLE often respond to morbilli, mumps, polio, influenza, rubella, herpes, v. zoster, CMV, and EBV. The Epstein-Barr virus is elusive at first, but six to eight months after the PW and virutherapy testing is finished, its response makes the difference between a partial recovery and an almost full recovery. If serial vaccination therapy slows down the deterioration, halts the autoimmune symptoms, and improves brain activity, a trial is justified for those patients in more advanced stages of the illnesses. Patients attending the first three to four clinics were tested in their wheelchairs. The majority now walk; others are grateful for improvements in symptoms and the slowing down of the disease process. Not all respond to therapy. My observations and experiences with the two diseases during their early stages leaves me in no doubt that the role of multiple latent viruses warrants further research, without complying with "proof medicine" requirements.

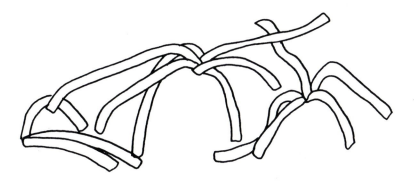

## THE HEART AND THE VASCULAR SYSTEM

OWGG proteins/glutens play games with your vascular system. They make a fool of you because the specialists' examinations, electrocardiograms (ECGs), and other medical technology tests are normal. Yet a few days later, you wake at 2:00 a.m. with a heart that wants to jump out of your chest. You may be on the job, walking somewhere, minding your business, and suddenly you feel you are going to faint and have to sit on the ground or floor. Mercifully, you remain conscious, but your heartbeat is so slow you fear it will stop. It does not, and after 5 to 10 min you get up, shaken, but thankful you are still alive.

Your angina pains begin 1 to 2 h after a lunch of whole-grain sandwiches and a thick soup with crunchy toast pieces. You may remember that you woke up 2 to 3 h after you ate an evening snack of cake or a muffin, perhaps a chocolate or two, because you know this fare helps you to sleep. You search your mind for an answer to what is happening. *Surmise:* The probable explanation is that the OWGG glutens affect the heart rate by altering the conduction of nerve impulses in the heart muscle cells of the specialized conducting system.

There is an ugly, common, dangerous aspect to OWGGs. Their glutens cause small vessel constriction or spasm of cells in the vessel walls, causing narrowing of the vessels and reduced blood flow. Those with OWGG allergies complain of cold extremities and an unexplained rise in their blood pressure. A spasm occurs in the small vessels supplying the kidneys, which complain by producing a hormone that stimulates the heart to beat more forcibly and rapidly. The body cannot tolerate a buildup of toxins in the blood system, so the kidneys must continue detoxing regardless of the blood pressure rise. As the avalanche of OWGG glutens continues to enter the body, the blood pressure increases, causing essential hypertension. The supply of blood to the kidneys and other organs is further compromised by overproduction of insulin, which stimulates the muscle cells in the vessels walls to increase their size and bulk, thereby narrowing the lumen, or passageway, and limiting blood flow. The easy way around the problem is to take drugs that lower the blood pressure, but, unfortunately, the affected vessels are not always freed of constriction and the blood takes a bypass through other vessels, with resulting drop in blood pressure. Overproduction of insulin is detected and corrected.

At the clinic, hundreds of patients with essential hypertension have recovered or lowered their blood pressure after three to four months of OWGG exclusion. Nearly all gave up their hypotensive drugs and found they could not resume eating OWGGs. Early anthropologists found that elderly people of non-OWGG-eating tribes and village communities had little or no atheroma or thickening of their arteries (Schmid, 1994). A clinic patient reported a reduction in or disappearance of angina pain, an increase in exercise tolerance, and an improvement in body warmth after three to four months of OWGG exclusion. It is suggested that the exclusion of OWGG glutens reduces the thickening in the vessel walls by absorbing the fat calcium complex accumulations, or atheroma.

OWGG-allergic patients with hypertension are encouraged to buy a home blood pressure machine and to record the fluctuations in blood pressure three to four times a day. An important reading is in the early hours of the morning, between 2:00 a.m. and 5:00 a.m. Although they continue to take smaller doses of hypotensive drugs and the readings are satisfactory during the day, they are alarmed at the high readings in the early hours of the morning. By six to eight weeks, the effects of OWGG exclusion and continuing hypertensive drug therapy leads to hypotensive light-headedness. The antihypertensive drugs are reduced or stopped. By twelve to fifteen weeks there are no raised early morning readings. When the antihypertensive drugs are stopped, the water pills (diuretics) are no longer required. Remaining water retention clears when CMV, *Helicobacter,* and *Ureaplasma* improve kidney function.

**IK**    A scientist, age 40, with hypertension over 200 refused medication. He spent four years and considerable capital searching for a cause. At the first interview, he left me a large satchel filled to the brim with old ECG tracings and medical reports from throughout the Western world. He provoked markedly to OWGGs, and after twelve weeks of exclusion, his blood pressure returned to normal. Since his recovery he attends a gym and jogs regularly. At the end of the first year of

OWGG exclusion, his reading was 105 to 110/70. He has been unable to reintroduce OWGGs. He notices some elevation of his blood pressure during the height of the grass pollen season.

**IK** A male, age 60, with hypertension had nasal problems, which he called chronic sinusitis, that were due to chronic infection and the numerous medications he was taking. The OWGG provocation markedly aggravated the chronic sinus problems for seven to ten days. There was further improvement of his nasal blocking with house dust mites and molds therapy. Three months later he was off all medications and his blood pressure was within normal range for his age. He was thrilled with the disappearance of head sensations and the improvement of his memory.

The heart and blood vessels are susceptible to active viral infections. The great swine influenza pandemic in 1918 killed thousands of people, young and old, through sudden heart failure. It is still around, and young people with influenza-related heart failure can be kept alive with heart transplants. Heart pain, increased/decreased pulse rate, and fainting sensations are often provoked by polio, influenza, rubella, mumps, Coxsackievirus, and *Chlamydia*. CMV, and to a lesser extent influenza, provokes heart pain. CMV, *Helicobacter*, and *Ureaplasma* improve kidney function, but the beneficial effect is delayed until OWGGs have been excluded for three to four months. With the improvement in kidney detoxing comes a speedier return to remembered normal health.

**IK** She had recurring flu and chronic asthma, which began to affect her lifestyle fifteen months ago. She improved on OWGG exclusion and CRC therapy. An influenza 5[7] provocation dose aggravated the influenza symptoms and her asthma, requiring admission to the hospital for oxygen therapy. An increase in fluid around the heart (pericarditis) was treated, and on discharge from the hospital a week later, her asthma had cleared, with a dramatic improvement in health. She has been unable to reintroduce OWGGs and for some years has taken influenza 5[10] at six- to eight-week intervals. She suffers from a normal number of head colds but seems to avoid catching the flu.

Exclusion of OWGGs allows the lining of the gut to recover, and the blood hemoglobin returns to normal, as there is no further loss from minute bowel ulcerations. Thyroxine and vitamin K activities are enhanced when OWGGs are excluded.

## THE EYES AND EARS

### *Eye Symptoms and Visual Disturbances*

Eye symptoms were the sixth most common complaint of a group of 350 patients experiencing chronic unexplained fatigue. With eye symptoms, where allergy stops and viruses begin is impossible to tell until the full work-up is completed. If you experienced any unexplained strange visual effects in the past, you could be in for an exciting time during provocation and neutralization. At first, I could not believe some of the descriptions from provocation. But as more and more people experienced similar visual provocations, I now believe viruses are an important cause of most unexplained changes in color intensities and visual distortions. Visual disturbances such as these have occasionally followed provocation with foods. Migraine aura is provoked and relieved by MLV. Itchiness, puffiness, haziness of vision, redness, and blue/black allergic shiners on the lower eyelids respond to MLV. *Chlamydia* is a viruslike bacterial parasite that lives in the conjunctivae surface organ cells and in the tear ducts. Antibiotics do not always eliminate *Chlamydia,* which is the main cause of recurrent or persistent irritable, itchy sore eyes, redness and puffy lower lids, and variable hazy vision. *Chlamydia, Mycoplasma pneumoniae,* adenovirus, mumps, and RSV are tested before other multiple latent viruses, whether or not they are suspected.

IK    His eyes have itched for as long as he can remember. His parents tried tying his hands at night to stop him from rubbing his eyes. By age 18, all the anti-itch SSDs had been tried. The Csds gave the most relief and were used until age 28, although periods of eye and skin itching continued despite the use of drugs. In his twenties, he developed irritable bowel syndrome and his dermatitis, present from childhood, gradually became worse. The eye specialist became concerned that the Csd therapy would cause cataracts. A conical cornea was diagnosed some years earlier, and contact lenses were worn when he could tolerate them. It was suggested that a corneal graft would be necessary for one eye. The first clinic visit provoked a five-day marked reaction to OWGGs. Itchiness of the eyes and skin was controlled with prednisone. The next visit produced another marked reaction to *Candida* and molds. After five days, the symptoms subsided. Vision appeared to be clearer and outdoor colors were brighter. At the next visit, hepatitis provocation brought about the worst skin and eye itching he could remember for months. But two days before the next visit, the itchiness was gone. The next testing session gave a marked reaction to *Chlamydia,* with pains in the neck and shoulders, chest wheezing, and intense eye itching. A week later the skin was much improved and he was able to sleep at night because all itching had stopped. The next visit, herpes and v. zoster brought on itching and hazy vision for four to five days. After this he was able to wear contact lenses with ease. By now his weight was reduced and there were improvements in memory, moods, and personality. Since then, he has experienced dramatic improvement. I have not heard whether the corneal graft operation was performed.

The whites of the eyes are moist membranes frequently affected by allergic inhalants, foods, and molds. When antibiotic eye ointments fail to relieve the itching, Csd eye preparations give relief. Long-term symptom suppression with Csds carries considerable risk of (1) changes in the eye lenses (e.g., cataracts) and (2) changes in the fluid pressure of the eyeball (e.g., glaucoma). MLV, using a selection from influenza, RSV, adenovirus, herpes, v. zoster, hepatitis, and rubella will clear the itching symptoms. Recurring small ulcers on the clear part of the eye (cornea) or a large, deep, more persistent ulcer may in time threaten the person's sight. Most of these ulcers are caused by v. zoster but may be aggravated by herpes, adenovirus, rubella, and mumps. Contact lens wearers suffer varying degrees of conjunctivitis, which may not be relieved by SSDs, so the lenses are abandoned. The preliminary work-up and MLV successfully treat intolerance of contact lenses.

The retina and visual (optic) lobe of the brain are responsible for many unusual effects during provocation. The following visual effects could be due to retina responses: a door looks twisted; others in the room have large heads or other body distortions; the floor of the room is uneven. Changes in the brightness of the colors in the room and outside are startling for some patients, with the colors changing from one to another or disappearing, the vision becoming black and white. Most alarming is a temporary blindness lasting from a few seconds up to three minutes. This provoked blindness happened to some patients in the past, so they were not overly concerned. Over eighty patients at the clinic spent their lives in a dull-colored world until MLV revealed the brightly colored real world to them. Another group wore dark glasses, not only outside, but inside buildings as well, because of a painful glare. After food allergy testing and MLV, they continue to carry their dark glasses around with them, just in case the painful glare returns.

*Surmise:* Latent viral activity in the visual areas of the brain (occipital) and spasms of blood vessels supplying the surface of the brain bring on the

aura of migraine: wavering vision, very bright white flashing lines, interference with central vision, and often inability to read type. The vision is
narrowed so that background objects are no longer seen.

IK    A middle-aged woman had "shadow" visual changes during influenza and polio provocation. Other body symptoms were provoked by
the two viruses. Her vision was enhanced; the colors around her
brightened intensely. The effect was very marked with mumps. The
improvement continues as normal vision. I was not surprised when
she told me that her mother had said, "You were very ill with mumps
at age four." Since that age she had lived in a dusky, dull-colored
world.

Eyes and vision are a common area for change-of-site responses
(CSRs). Conventional medicine treats the symptoms with suppression
medication, allowing the patient to become tolerant of the visual effects.
After some weeks or months of SSD therapy, however, a CSR transfers
symptoms to other body areas, leading to, for example, eczema, sinusitis,
bronchitis, or changes in mood and memory. Soon the patient is seeing
other specialists for the CSR symptoms in addition to the three monthly
visits to the eye specialist. People unravel their symptoms and dismiss
their specialists in reverse order, if MLV and allergy work is successful.
MLV has not caused any permanent visual effects or led to the onset of
glaucoma.

### Variable Deafness, Head Noises (Tinnitus), and Unsteadiness

We have all heard of tragedies involving sudden viral infections that
leave the victim deaf in one ear, partially sighted, or with no sense of
smell. If the deafness, tinnitus, and unsteadiness varies, there is hope that
allergy and MLV may be of help, but there is no hope for the patient who
has no fluctuation of symptoms. Active viral infections trigger one of the
following four responses: (1) a sudden loss of the senses; (2) a gradual
diminution and worsening of the senses; (3) a sudden loss of the senses,
followed by slow recovery, often with a sudden return to normal two to six
weeks later; or (4) a sudden or rapid onset of the disability, followed by
gradual recovery, but not back to normal. Some weeks or months later the
infection strikes again and there is less recovery. Over one or two years
repeated infections destroy the sensory function. It is difficult for many
patients to comprehend that latent viruses are present in the cells of their
hearing organs. Ten years ago a medical journal published an article that
described over 100 therapies for unsteadiness. Numerous therapies for

tinnitus and vertigo still exist today. Many patients attend the clinic because they are not prepared to have surgery for these symptoms. When there is fluctuation of symptoms, the majority respond to the preliminary work-up and virutherapy. What is more, they retain their recovery. Other patients associate the onset of their motion sickness with a viral infection, and they do well on MLV. They are delighted that they can at last stop taking the SSDs.

Tinnitus and vertigo, together with fluctuating and distorted hearing, are often the result of reactions to foods, xeno-SSDs, and petrochemical toxins. The mold toxins *Mucor, Aspergillus,* and *Candida* can affect the senses.

**IK**    A keen golfer recovered from Ménière's disease, a type of unsteadiness or vertigo, and was able to return to a reasonable golf handicap. He loved ham but was convinced that pork reacted on him, so he decided to exclude it from his diet in favor of his first love, golf.

Provocation neutralization with foods, molds, and especially multiple latent viruses can be dramatic, with a sudden return of hearing and steadiness and the disappearance of tinnitus. Thirty years ago, I was amazed when the exclusion of the OWGGs, in particular, wheat, cleared away an unbearable tinnitus that had made one person an invalid for the previous three years. Patients ask me, "Where is the provoking action taking place?" I reply, "It could be the specialized cells of the hearing organs and labyrinth detoxing excess latent food particles and viruses." The reduction in latent virus and the improvement in nutrition from vitamin A and zinc enable many cells to recover their function and to begin transmitting impulses to the hearing, balance, and visual areas of the brain. Most people respond to adenovirus therapy, followed by influenza and RSV. Sometimes rubella, mumps, v. zoster, polio, and hepatitis are provoked and used in the treatment with the three main viruses.

The cells of the hearing organs have some of the highest levels of vitamin A and zinc in the body. Fish oils containing vitamin A and zinc supplements reduce the risk of relapse. Heat therapies, especially saunas, are strongly recommended. Do not accept Csd drug therapy if ear symptoms are fluctuating after a sudden viral infection. Csds encourage viral activity by lowering the immune responses, whereas vitamin C discourages viral activity.

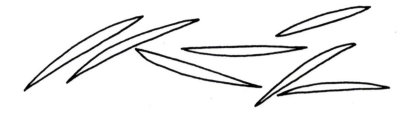

### Children's Deafness and Glue Ear

Western nations' children suffer from a sticky mucus pandemic: (1) glue mucus affecting the ears, treated by ventilation tubes or grommets; (2) bronchitis and asthma with sticky mucus, treated by inhaled Csds; (3) obstructed noses and sticky mucus, often infected, treated by Csd inhalers and antibiotics; and (4) excess mucus in the motions. These conditions have no recognized cause, so, consequently, the treatments are empirical. Sticky mucus in the middle ear of children was an unusual finding prior to the 1960s. *Surmise:* The birth control pill is a hidden cause of the sticky mucus pandemic, as I observed the pandemic developing in the early 1960s.

**IK**  I became suspicious of the pill as one of the causes of sticky mucus in 1964. Here are my findings from a clinical study of 876 families with 2,188 children between 1970 and 1983:

- **Group 1**—667 children conceived before mothers went on the pill or Depo-Provera®. Of these, 105 children had exploratory operations on their eardrums, with watery discharge in 37 and sticky mucus in 68.
- **Group 2**—1,521 children conceived by mothers who used the pill or injection for longer than nine months before stopping it and conceiving a child. Of these, 610 had operations, with 42 showing watery discharge and 568, sticky mucus.
- **Group 3**—178 families with 248 children born before the pill and injection, and 313 children born after the mothers used the pill. Of the 248 children, 28 needed operations, with 23 having watery discharge and 5, sticky mucus. The 313 had 124 operations, with 10 presenting watery discharge and 114, sticky mucus.

Children conceived before using the pill or Depo-Provera®: 1 child in 50 with sticky mucus. Children conceived after using the pill or injection: 1 child in

2.75 with sticky mucus. The survey concerned children in families in which one or more children were referred to me because of variable deafness. The findings show that use of the pill or the Depo-Provera® greatly increases the risk of sticky or glue mucus disease in children's ears. The increased incidence of sticky mucus asthma in children should be investigated along these lines because this trend shows no signs of going away. The sticky mucus appears to attract, and may be encouraged by, nose and chest viruses such as influenza, RSV, and, especially, adenovirus. Virutherapy drops with *Candida* and these three viruses improve/clear many children's ears and lungs when they present during the early stages of the disease.

Progesterone and estrogen, or progesterone alone, are synthetic xenohormones made by chemists. The xenohormones increase the stickiness of mucus in the canal of the cervix, and sperm are unable to get through this sticky mucus barrier. Women complain or notice that they develop a blocked nose/sticky nasal mucus and/or sticky chest mucus after taking the pill for weeks or months. The man-made xenohormones may affect the fertilized ovum. It is disturbing to think that man-made chemicals have penetrated to the very beginnings of a human life, the dividing ovum. It is even more worrisome to contemplate what the effect may be when xenochemicals are present after three, four, or five generations. Man-made xenohormones penetrate every tissue of a woman's body, including her ovaries. The egg that issues from the ovary, I surmise, contains natural hormones and xenohormones.

## *THE SKIN*

Not all itching, eczema, or dermatitis responds to accepted therapy; rather, they are controlled by Csds and other SSDs. Dermatologists identify chemical and contact factors through skin testing; relief occurs when these factors are eliminated. Allergists accept people after a thorough work-up by a dermatologist. The food and inhalant investigations and treatment of the CRC give good results. Virutherapy is a further dimension in the relief of itching, skin redness, burning, and other sensations occurring with skin conditions. Some patients identify the provoked symptoms as being due to a single virus. They are able to notice the difference in the type of itch, burning, or creepy-crawly sensations and the supersensitivity when touched. Many mothers report the child's eczema began immediately or some time after the child had a viral infection or was vaccinated. Skin conditions are the third most common complaint of patients. MLV using these viruses has cleared or improved skin conditions. The order of frequency is influenza, hepatitis, polio, morbilli, rubella, herpes, v. zoster, mumps, EBV, and *Chlamydia*. Relapses are successfully treated by repeating the serial vaccination.

### Hives/Urticaria

Hives/urticaria that persist after treatment by a dermatologist can respond to a thorough allergic and CRC therapy course. MLV enhances results. Relapses are a possibility, so always keep some of the drugs close at hand.

**IK**    She suffered hives/urticaria since giving up a hotel bar job six years previously. At first, antihistamines stopped the itch, but later the expensive new antihistamine drugs were needed. She consulted a dermatologist, who gave her prednisone tablets. She noticed her worst periods were during the grass pollen season. Two years ago, in desperation, she stopped drinking her favorite lager and gin. Excluding alcohol and going on several crash diets had no effect on the skin problem. They slowly made her tense and very irritable. She continued to gain weight. The first testing session at the clinic provoked a severe OWGGs response, with depression and crying. For two days after the provocation her skin "went mad." Hives and rashes came out all over her body. She stayed off work until a course of prednisone began to control the symptoms. She continued because she was determined to comply, as the friend who referred her to the clinic had undergone a similar experience. For the next ten days she had a great desire to eat toast and drink lager. But in the final two days she noticed a big change in herself. She felt a relief of tension and began to sleep. I advised her not to start the nystatin for another week. At the next visit she provoked with CRC, which further aggravated the symptoms she was getting from the nystatin. She reacted to hepatitis, which was the cause of the creepy-crawly skin sensation. Rubella was responsible for the red areas on her face and neck. After four months and no OWGGs, her weight was much reduced, the insomnia was gone, the IBS had cleared, and she was thrilled with the appearance of her skin. Her mother told me how delighted she was to have her happy, pleasant daughter once more. She contacted me some months later and said she was unable to return to eating OWGGs, but that did not worry her because she was so well and had joined the local gymnasium. "And oh," she said, "I am enjoying my new social life."

### Psoriasis

Psoriasis is treated at the clinic when conventional therapy fails. Many react to the skin preparations or are suffering toxic effects from drugs. The preliminary work-up includes special attention to provoking with the molds

*Trichophyton, Epidermophyton,* and *Cryptococcus,* despite previous successful antifungal drug therapy. Psoriasis may be of several types. The most
common is from CRC, and almost as common a cause are multiple latent
viruses. Other causes of itching are food allergies, some molds, and, at
times, chemicals. One patient was delighted with the decrease in the psoriasis areas and the loss of itching but, best of all, was an end to her moodiness
and the return of a happy home life.

### The Eczema of a Hundred Causes

**IK**  A woman with dermatitis collected a long list of possible causes and
aggravating factors suggested by the numerous physicians she had
seen over the years. She called it "the eczema of a hundred causes."
At the clinic, the preliminary work-up and MLV identified another
long list of causes, but it did not match her original list. The remains
of acne on her face and chest cleared with exclusion of OWGGs. The
itching and pain around her anus cleared with the exclusion of apples.
The strange sensations of heat and redness around her neck were due
to egg and chicken allergies. The red peeling rash on her limbs, hands,
and part of her belly, together with the itching, responded to CRC
treatment. The itching and excess mucus in her genital area finally
cleared with CMV therapy. The itching and scaling of the eyelids
disappeared with mold treatment, adenovirus, and *Chlamydia.* For
thirty years she had been unable to let people touch her, but this
cleared when *Giardia* and herpes were controlled. She described a
different type of itch that moved around the body, sometimes affecting
all her skin areas. This was due to hepatitis. The eczema became very
red and hot on her upper arms and thighs but cleared when rubella
was tested and treated. She frequently suffered crawling sensations
under the skin, and this turned out to be due to hepatitis and polio. For
the last twenty years she suffered vesicles or water blisters around the
mouth and lips, with occasional tingling and numbness. Around her
waist at belt level she always had a number of tiny, watery itchy spots.
The causes were herpes simplex 1 and 2, v. zoster, and CRC. The
improvement in her skin texture and hair she attributed to taking zinc
and the three unsaturated oils. So in the end, there were eighteen real
causes for her dermatitis. Please do not think that eczema and dermatitis conditions are easy to treat. The difficult part of the treatment is
finding the causes.

## Acne

Dermatologists and physicians use powerful new therapies and give the impression, backed up by pharmaceutical advertising, that acne "can be beaten." Acne patients coming to the clinic have tried three- to six-month antibiotics courses, hormonal treatment, and synthetic vitamin A with partial or temporary improvement. At the first visit they ask, "What is the cause of acne?" or "Why are fatigue, migraines, mood changes, depressions, vaginal discharges, and skin itching and eczema occurring months after I finish the courses?" I reply, "Acne has many causes and the delayed symptoms you are now suffering are due to a change-of-site response" (see pp. 194-197). Physicians do not accept that foods play a role in acne, but they advise against consuming sugar, chocolate, and coffee during treatments.

Most acne patients attending the clinic have marked allergies to OWGGs. The OWGGs are provoked at the first visit, and the effect on the acne or accompanying symptoms convinces them to start an exclusion, at first for three months, but often for six months, until all signs of the acne and related symptoms clear. Symptoms of CRC are nearly always present in people with food allergies to OWGGs. A skin organism, *Staphylococcus aureus,* thrives in the presence of *Candida* symptoms. Those with acne provoke strongly to *S. Aureus.* The *Candida* shots include the personalized treatment dose of *S. Aureus toxoid,* which is given once a week. During the burn-off symptoms from the food exclusion and the treatment shots, there is an increase of small blind pimples and spots over the acne areas. The areas look fiery red, feel hot, and are itchy. The marked deterioration of their facial complexion causes faint-hearted patients to stop treatment. The determined ones cover up the worst areas with makeup. Do not squeeze the boils or pimples, as most will not become pustular. Nearly all disappear in six weeks' time. A food indiscretion will cause the acne and pimples to flare within a few hours.

If skin itching and redness persist despite the food exclusion and *Candida* shots, you require virutherapy. Influenza, polio, hepatitis, rubella, morbilli, v. zoster, and herpes clear the remaining skin symptoms, or symptoms elsewhere brought on by the change-of-site response. So many people attending the clinic for CFIDS/ME, CRC, and latent viral symptoms blame the acne treatment for starting the deterioration of their health. The culprit is the antibiotic chlortetracycline.

**IK**   A woman with disfiguring acne affecting her face, breasts, and back had undergone all sorts of treatments over the past fifteen years. She had several anesthetics for chemical peel and skin-shaving procedures. The acne was still severe, with deep firm lumps under the acne scars. Complete exclusion of OWGGs began the slow improvement in her acne, and by the end of the year, the firm lumps had disappeared. She recovered with shots of *Candida, S. Aureus,* and several viruses. Her symptoms from the change-of-site response also improved. The gratifying result persisted, and eighteen months later I was introduced to her fiancé. She cannot reintroduce OWGGs to her diet, as any lapses cause a severe acne flare-up.

## MULTIPLE LATENT VIRUSES AND MUSCLES

MLV provokes dramatic muscle symptoms, such as improved grip and tone of affected muscle groups. If improvement continues, patients have a greater than 60 percent chance of recovery to previously remembered health. Muscles make up the largest tissue mass of our bodies. They are affected by the toxins of CRC and *Giardia.* Viruses cripple our body movements, enforcing long periods of bed rest, with muscle pain and wasting. Before the discovery of polio immunization, the active polio virus was believed to damage nerve cells of the spinal cord and base of the brain. Recent research shows the polio virus also affects muscle cells. Polio is not the only virus that provokes change in muscle strength. It is unusual for one virus to be responsible for all symptoms. Those of you who subscribe to journals for CFIDS/ME societies will know of the exciting new discoveries, for example, that lactic acid formed through muscle activity is a cause of the increased pain CFIDS/ME patients suffer while and after exercising. Could it be that latent viruses or other toxins interfere with the breakdown of lactic acid? Patients whose muscles are affected by polio, CMV, EBV, and other viruses constitute three different groups: (1) those who suffer a three- to four-month duration of symptoms, (2) those with a three- to six-month symptom duration, and (3) those experiencing symptoms of long duration (one year or more). The first two groups manage to continue daily activities and respond to MLV. Those in the long-duration group have tried many therapies. Their work-up should be deliberate and cautious to prevent excessive delayed symptom provocation.

The immediate provocation response is measured using a handgrip for the arms/limbs and peak flow meter for chest muscle action. Immediate and delayed provoked symptoms are (1) muscle weakness, (2) an increase in muscle strength, (3) localized knots or lumps or localized muscle spasms, (4) pain in muscles, (5) tenderness of muscles on movement, (6) pain in muscles on touching, (7) twitching or tremors of muscles, (8) a creeping and spreading contraction and then a relaxing effect of muscle groups, (9) stumbling and clumsiness, and (10) an effect on eye muscles that disturbs vision.

The polio virus provokes the majority of CFIDS/ME people with variable muscle weakness. CMV and EBV are next in importance. Muscle pain of CFIDS/ME is nearly always relieved by morbilli. Often the full benefit of polio serial vaccination does not occur until further viruses are used in the treatment. EBV, and to a lesser extent CMV, brings on muscle weakness or decreasing strength five to seven days after provoking. Both EBV and CMV make the limbs feel leaden. Muscle weakness can be tolerated for two to three days, but if it persists some patients become afraid. Once recognizing that this type of weakness has occurred in the past they are reassured. During provocation and delayed responses, viral smells are detoxed through patients' breath, sweat, and urine. After they get home, if they lie on a bed or couch for 2 to 3 h, the room may fill with the same viral smell. An important sign is passing pink-colored urine 12 to 24 h after the provoking test or a treatment shot. *Helicobacter* provocation and, sometimes, treatment shots cause patients' urine to have a cat urine smell. In the past the color and smell of the urine occurred when patients attempted to exercise but were stopped by weakness and muscle pain. Muscle pain from exercising or touch is caused by morbilli, mumps, herpes, and CMV.

Provocation testing is begun with polio to assess changes in muscle strength. Morbilli is then provoked to relieve muscle pain in the limbs. No further testing is done for one to two weeks, and then CMV is provoked because of its marked effect on muscle strength. The improvement in muscle function and strength encourages patients. The effect may be enhanced as the other viruses are provoked over the next four testing sessions. On the fourth or fifth testing session dengue and EBV are provoked.

**IK**    During a testing clinic, three women developed neck muscle weakness from provocation with poliomyelitis. Their heads fell forward and had to be supported by their hands. They could not stand up due to temporary leg weakness. A neutralizing dose restored the tone to the neck muscles, with some increased strength in the legs. One woman suddenly developed urgency. A neutralizing dose returned sufficient strength to her legs for her to go to the toilet. She feared she would be unable to get off the pan after she passed urine, so I waited outside the door with another neutralizing dose. At the same time, the third woman regained full tone in her "jelly" legs. Since that time, polio testing is limited to one person in the group. The same rule applies to asthmatics during mold, polio, RSV, ATV, and influenza provocation, and to women with urinary problems, such as urgency during provocation by *Helicobacter,* CMV, *Ureaplasma,* and *Trichomonas.*

### Viral-Provoked Muscle Symptoms and Responses

At the first clinic visit people describe their suffering from a catalog of muscle symptoms and responses (refer to the Virus-Allergy Questionnaire, pp. 300-305). The more unusual symptoms are dismissed by their physicians as affective/functional. During the worst muscle symptom periods, with marked weakness and pain in the muscles, strong feelings of fear and despair occur. MLV confirms latent viruses are responsible for and relieve many muscle symptoms, including the accompanying fear, despair, depressed mental activity, and lost motivation (mañana). If you suffer from muscle or joint symptoms, can you identify or match them with those described under muscle groups A, B, and C? If so, latent viruses and microbial toxins are probably affecting you. Patients present with considerable variation in symptoms and causes. The matching of conscious-control muscle and joint symptoms, or muscles not under conscious control, to latent viruses and microbial toxins is a recurring pattern seen at the clinic and described by patients over the past fourteen years. It is very unusual for a patient to provoke and respond to MLV without involvement of the muscles. The body has three muscle groupings that respond to MLV and certain microbial toxins:

A. Muscles controlled by consciousness or willpower; these are voluntary.
B. Muscles that get on with the work of running basic functions, such as the heart and the muscles in the gut wall; these take little notice of consciousness or willpower and are involuntary.
C. A mixed group of muscles maintaining constant strength or tone and adjusting to changes in gravity; these maintain our posture, adapt to other muscle movements, and have voluntary control, i.e., respond to consciousness and willpower.

All virus dilutions used at the clinic are capable of provoking voluntary muscles and joints and involuntary muscles. The significant and frequent provokers are the latent viruses influenza, polio, CMV, EBV, and v. zoster, and the microbial toxins *Giardia, Chlamydia,* and *Helicobacter.* Other viruses are dengue, rotavirus, rubella, Q fever, and *Ureaplasma,* and other microbial toxins include *Listeria* and *Trichomonas.*

## Muscle Groups A and C (Voluntary)

Immediate and delayed provoked responses of muscles or muscle groups convince patients that latency therapy has something to offer them. They identify the responses with same or similar events during their long illnesses. The responses reinforce their compliance with, and understanding of, latency therapy.

1. An increase of strength affecting
   a. the muscles on the front of the chest, increasing the awareness of soreness in the breasts—polio and CMV; and
   b. the muscles between the ribs and the diaphragm muscle, increasing the asthmatic's peak flow readings—polio.
2. Heightened muscle tenderness, sensitivity, and twitching is provoked and later neutralized by morbilli, polio, influenza, CMV, and hepatitis. Muscle cramping is a common symptom but is not affected by latent viruses. It is relieved by taking nutritional supplements, removing toxins such as nicotine, and detecting a food allergy—usually to the OWGGs.
3. Weakness of the muscles of the eyelids affects their movement and causes drooping—polio, influenza, *Chlamydia,* and v. zoster.
4. Contractions of muscles occur during provocation, or sudden sharp pains occur for no apparent reason, usually in the limbs, neck, and back, between the ribs (intercostal), the chest, pelvis, and diaphragm muscles—polio, influenza, CMV, v. zoster, *Chlamydia,* dengue, *Listeria,* and rotavirus.
5. Tender muscle points or painful tender points are in the neck, shoulders, and back—polio, influenza, CMV, v. zoster, *Chlamydia,* dengue, *Listeria,* and rotavirus.
6. Arms or legs become weak, together with painful areas of muscle spasm in the neck, shoulders, or buttocks—CMV, EBV, influenza, *Parvovirus, Chlamydia, Giardia,* and *Listeria.*
7. Lower leg muscles become paralyzed or suffer periods of paralysis—CMV, rubella, and *Cladosporium,* a mold. The back muscles will not support a sitting position—CMV, EBV, polio, *Chlamydia,* and *Giardia.*
8. From a tender point, a creeping muscle spasm spreads out, leaving behind painless relaxed muscles. The spasm begins around the

neck, moves to the shoulders, then proceeds down the back muscles, to the arms, and finally to the lower legs. The whole process can take up to 2 to 24 h—CMV, *Chlamydia,* and influenza.

9. CFIDS/ME patients report creeping muscle pain rather than a muscle spasm, though it, too, moves from the neck and shoulders into the limbs and clears within 2 to 24 h—morbilli, *Chlamydia,* influenza, and CMV.

10. Jerky speech delivery with variable incoordination of muscle movement, clumsiness and stumbling, and stuttering responds poorly to traditional treatment but improves with virutherapy. Speech recovers when the neutralizing doses are reached. The person being provoked is unaware of speech improvement, but others in the allergy room notice the marked changes in speech production and pitch. The patient reports an improvement in memory, making it easier to select words—polio, influenza, RSV, CMV, morbilli, and EBV.

I am able to recognize if a patient has improved from a telephone conversation or when the patient arrives for the next appointment. The change in delivery and pronunciation is obvious before the patient tells me of his or her response to treatment.

**IK**    A preteen with many of these problems and marked incoordination was an excellent patient because he wanted to play sports. During a private "man to man" talk with me he told me a secret: "I want to become captain of the school's junior tennis team." His incoordination prevented him from playing tennis, but he had learned a lot about the game. Virutherapy made his dream possible. A year later I received a card detailing the tennis team's successes and his excellent school report.

*Muscle Groups B and C (Involuntary)*

The muscle symptoms are vague, hard to define, difficult to locate, and, in the past, were dismissed as subjective/all in the head/imagined, even neurotic. Results of therapy at the clinic show regional differences or tropism of latent microbes and toxins.

1. Gall bladder and bowel pain is brought on by hepatitis, CMV, adenovirus, rotavirus, and EBV; irritable bowel symptoms by hepatitis, polio, adenovirus, mumps, CMV, rotavirus, herpes simplex 1 and 2, *Papillomavirus* (1, 2, 3, 4, and 6), *Giardia, Trichomonas,* and *Clostridium.*

2. Bladder symptoms are caused by CMV, *Chlamydia,* herpes, *Ureaplasma, Papillomavirus* 16, and the microbial toxins *Helicobacter* and *Candida,* and *Escherichia coli* and *Proteus* bacteria.
3. Changes in heart rate, e.g., tachycardia (racing pulse) or missed heartbeats are caused by influenza, CMV, polio, RSV, mumps, rubella, EBV, and Coxsackievirus.
4. Chest pains and a wildly beating heart that wants to jump out of your chest are the result of CMV, polio, mumps, RSV, rubella, and EBV.
5. Bronchitis and asthma are brought on by influenza, polio, RSV, adenovirus, morbilli, *Papillomavirus* (1-4), v. zoster, herpes, *Chlamydia, Mycoplasma pneumoniae, Pasteurella, Pertussis, Legionella,* and microbial toxins such as *Bordetella pertussis* (causes whooping cough).
6. The variety and intensity of food allergy muscle spasms and pain are reduced and improved by a combination of polio, hepatitis, rotavirus, adenovirus, mumps, CMV, and herpes.
7. Back pain and muscle spasms in the neck and chest are relieved by influenza and polio, working together, and *Listeria.* Lower back pain is relieved by polio, CMV, EBV, and dengue. Pain over the sacrum and in the pelvis is relieved by rotavirus, CMV, polio, EBV, mumps, and *Chlamydia. Giardia* and *Trichomonas* toxins further aggravate muscle spasm pain of the back (see Figure 1.1).
8. Pain in the hands and feet is provided by rubella, *Parvovirus, Mycoplasma hominis,* and *M. pneumoniae, Chlamydia,* and *Clostridium difficile.*
9. Children's ear, nose, and throat symptoms are improved by rhinovirus, influenza, RSV, and adenovirus.

### Pains In and Around Joints

Lots of people have joint symptoms from past sport injuries or accidents. Fortunately, they are treated and relieved by modern medicine. Others suffer arthritis pains from past or present infections, either active or latent, often complicated by rheumatism as people age. Symptom suppression drugs at first relieve the pain of chronic latent and age-related rheumatism. Long-term use of SSDs is liable to provide variable relief of symptoms, "a breakthrough of symptoms," or the appearance of toxic side effects. The drugs are stopped and another therapy tried. Chronic SSD therapy is better tolerated, and at a lower dose, if latent or unsuspected agents, such as *Giardia,* bacteria and bacterial toxins, petrochemical toxins, and multiple latent viruses, are detected and treated. Symptoms of pain and stiffness in the joints are called *arthralgia.* Symptoms around the joints and muscles, including their tendons, are called *fibromyalgia.* Most sufferers experience varying distress from both conditions.

Arthralgia includes sudden onset of joint pains, nagging pains in the joints, joint pains that vary or move from one joint to another, severe joint pain that prevents weight bearing, and joint stiffness. Fibromyalgia symptoms are sudden onset of pain and soreness around the joints, variable nagging pain and tenderness in the muscles and tendons, muscle jumping or twitching, heat and swelling of muscles around the joints, and tender lumps or areas (tender points) in muscles.

Arthralgia and fibromyalgia are bad enough, but when most other body muscles are painful, people are confined to bed, their symptoms mimicking those of CFIDS/ME. Arthralgia and fibromyalgia make up the sixth largest group of symptoms and the tenth most common principal complaint of 380 people questioned (a survey of clinic patients, 1992).

Arthralgia and fibromyalgia are frequent symptoms of food allergies, especially hidden or masked food allergies. Patients are provoked with six or more food extract dilutions. A small number of nonreactors do the five- or seven-day water fast, followed by reintroduction of two foods per day. Dr. M. Mandell wrote an informative book, *Lifetime Arthritis Relief System,* in 1983. His home treatment advice holds good today.

**IK** The arthritic father of a young woman who had received successful allergy viral therapy appeared at the clinic on crutches. The first day's testing provoked OWGG allergy. At the end of the second day of testing, an apple allergy was provoked and his affected joints started to swell and get very painful. He suffered crippling arthritis for three to four days and then rapidly recovered. A month later, "the apple man" was walking normally, and three months later, he was walking long distances throughout his city. He was so confident of his recovery that he purchased a house on a hill, as he had always wanted a view.

**IK** CRC treatments were introduced to the clinic in 1983. *Candida* therapy markedly improved treatment results. The introduction of MLV two years later further improved treatment results. Arthralgia and fibromyalgia respond to the preliminary work-up of anti-*Candida* drugs and latency injection therapy using *Candida* albicans, *C. tropicalis,* and *Torulopsis glabrata* (Crook 1995, 1996). Nearly all who attend the clinic were previously diagnosed and treated elsewhere for CRC. When the treatment failed, they were told they did not have *Candida*-related problems. This is not surprising because the treatments were incomplete and consisted of exclusion of sugars, a handful of nystatin pills and little or no advice about changing lifestyles. MLV has little chance of improving arthralgia and fibromyalgia without prior and ongoing control of food allergies, CRC, and *Giardia.*

Before the antibiotic era, streptococcal bacteria and their toxins caused disabilities and created misery for millions who suffered from rheumatic fever as well as heart and kidney damage. *Streptococcus* continues its damage in third-world populations, where it has developed (mutated) an antibiotic resistance and is now moving back to the industrial world (Crook, 1995, 1996; Winderlin and Sehnert, 1996). Experience at the clinic suggests the following bacteria and toxins affect muscles and joints: *Chlamydia, Mycoplasma hominis, M. pneumoniae, Clostridium difficile, Listeria,* and *Helicobacter.*

Bacteria and their toxins, originating from dental abscesses and filled teeth, affect muscles and joints, besides causing other chronic symptoms. If a tooth is under suspicion, a provocation with *Helicobacter* will bring on pain and increase tenderness, and occasionally slight swelling, one to three days later. The tooth abscess is treated, and the *Helicobacter* test is repeated two to three months later to check if the infection remains in the tooth root or socket. If so, experience suggests the tooth should be removed (see pp. 47-48).

*Giardia* toxin and infection of the gut and liver cause abdominal pains, headaches, arthralgia, and fibromyalgia, without any evidence of joint damage. *Giardia* toxin is a common cause of variable, often excruciating, chronic hip pains, persistent knee pain, and lower back pain. *Giardia* provokes symptoms in affected joints and muscles two to three days later. A course of the anti-*Giardia* drug metronidazole will bring on these prolonged delayed symptoms, alarming the patient, who stops the drug just when it should be continued. *Giardia* resistance to the drug is widespread, and the treatment test results may be disappointing.

**IK**    Among the first three or four patients provoked with *Giardia* was a confident skeptical patient with joint, hip, and muscle pain. He was sure there was no problem because he experienced no immediate provoked symptoms. He telephoned on the third day to announce nothing had happened and then inferred that the testing session was a waste of time and money. It was quite a different personality who telephoned on the fifth day to say he could hardly get out of bed. He was unable to go to work because of the severe joint and muscle pains. His confidence in earlier negative laboratory tests and colon examination for *Giardia* was shattered. Four months after starting latency therapy he was back on the golf course after a three-year absence.

Petrochemical toxicity is another cause of arthralgia and fibromyalgia.

**IK**    A woman in her forties suffered from sick building syndrome; her main complaint was a strange stiffness in her joints, which disappeared a few days after she was on holiday. She eventually left her job when her joint symptoms became disabling. Within three weeks of leaving the job, however, daily saunas returned the joints to normal.

Viruses present in joint tissues, such as Rubella, have long been known to persist years after the active or acute infection. Other viruses besides rubella are influenza, polio, hepatitis, herpes, *Parvovirus,* dengue, EBV, and v. zoster. Suspect a viral cause of joint and muscle pains when influenza goes through a community and arthralgia and fibromyalgia are aggravated, without the symptoms of influenza.

Follow this plan if you suspect latent viruses are a cause of joint and muscle pains.

1. If the medical work-up, including examination, X rays, and blood tests, is normal, and your physician reports that you have no clinical problems, request an allergy work-up.
2. If your physician refuses, seek an allergist and schedule an allergy investigation. Ask the allergist to check out CRC, *Giardia,* and *Helicobacter.*
3. Contact your mother, or relatives who knew you as a child. They may remember suspicious viral illnesses or vaccination reactions you suffered.
4. Consider multiple latent virutherapy if relief is not adequate, and complete any of the preliminary work-up that was not performed.
5. Complete the viral work-up by requesting provocation testing of dengue, *Chlamydia, Mycoplasma hominis,* and *M. pneumoniae, Parvovirus,* and Lyme disease.
6 Do not accept therapy with nonsteroid anti-inflammatory drugs (NSAIDs) and/or antianxiety or antidepressant drugs. They interfere with testing, provocation, and MLV by lowering sensitivity and the immunities. Those who have been on one or more years of treatment with these drugs must expect slower provocation and virutherapy responses.

### Tender Points

IK What are tender points? They are localized tender firm areas in the muscles that usually respond to heat, physiotherapy, and massage. One explanation for their existence is the muscle spasm and pain referred by a nipped, inflamed nerve from a past bony injury.

Consider the following questions:

1. Do your tender points recur in the same part of the muscle, or elsewhere, days or weeks after therapy?
2. Do they recur weeks or months after a corticosteroid injection into the points?
3. Following the symptom suppression injection, do new tender points arise elsewhere in the muscles?
4. Do the tender points increase or decrease in number in a given area with increased intensity of pain and tenderness?

MLV has provoked and then relieved tender points, often with characteristic detoxing body smells. During the serial vaccination with the provoking virus or viruses, people report they no longer need physiotherapy or massage. Occasionally, the provocation brings on an extended spasm and relaxation sequence that spreads to other body muscles, sometimes into the limbs. Following a marked provocation, tender points clear up or disappear; later they may reoccur at longer intervals. A possible explanation is that virutherapy decreases the load of latent virus in the muscle cells. The old injuries continue the referred pain, but without tender point formation. Some lucky people get relief of tender points from a single virus, such as rubella, polio, CMV, dengue, or EBV, but usually three or four viruses make up the treatment (see Figure 1.1).

### Chronic Back Pain

MLV relieves neck, middle back, and lower back pain. Undue attention is given to vertebral and disk lesions, with hardly a mention of latent viruses as a cause. Many patients had good results from virutherapy, after months, sometimes years, of treatment directed at the bone and disk lesions. Most showed minimal X ray bone changes for the extent of their disabilities. Several were suspected of malingering. I have not yet detected a malingerer. The clinical picture highlights the principal viruses:

1. The neck muscles respond to influenza, polio, and the bacterium *Listeria.*
2. The muscles at the level of the chest respond to influenza, polio, CMV, *Chlamydia,* and dengue.
3. The muscles at the lumbar level respond to polio, CMV, EBV, and *Giardia.*
4. The muscles at the level of the lower back or sacrum area respond to CMV, rotavirus, *Ureaplasma,* polio, EBV, mumps, *Chlamydia, Helicobacter,* and *Trichomonas.*

Many relieved by virutherapy remarked on the loss of tenderness in the pelvic joints and deep in the pelvis. A patient was relieved of sacral pain of several years' duration on excluding the potato family of vegetables.

**IK**   John's back pain restricted his lifestyle for two to three years. He tried extensive work-ups and approved therapies. He is sure MLV boosted the improvement of his back almost to normal. When Jane "pulled her back" while gardening, she started physiotherapy and manipulation. John persuaded her to try virutherapy, as some of her back problems remained after two to three weeks of her chosen therapy. Polio and influenza relieved her symptoms within thirty-six hours, and CMV provided relief beginning on the fifth day.

Men, ages 68 to 77, used polio and influenza shots, on average, six to ten times a year for the past nine years to get relief from nagging middle back pain.

MLV for the sudden onset of unexplained back pain needs further investigation. A quick end to sudden onset, acute back pain suggests a muscle spasm has been relieved. *Surmise:* MLV has little or no effect on bone and ligament lesions, but CMV helps by reducing the waterlogging (edema) of swollen injured tissues, such as the nerve coverings (neurolemma). Saunas and local applications of heat, and sometimes cold, relieve chronic back pain because they influence the inflammatory process and, I suggest, reduce the recently increased load of latent viruses.

Repetitive stress injury and temporomandibular joint pain syndrome have responded to the preliminary work-up and CMV, EBV virutherapy, much to the surprise of patients and myself. Sometimes the allergies to food and the effects of CRC, *Giardia,* and *Cladosporium* are important. I observed overall improvement in health and immune responses, together with a reduction in excess body fluid (edema) that is necessary for long-term improvement. Back pain, repetitive stress injury (RSI), temporomandibular joint pain syndrome (TMJ), and other fibromyalgia conditions are a huge financial burden for the insurance industry. The same conditions with evidence of injury may have an added latent component. If latency therapy provides improvement, the remaining symptoms are probably due to the structural injury. I have yet to read an article in a medical journal that clearly suggests, and recommends, allergy and latency investigation and therapy for these industrial disabilities.

RSI and CFIDS/ME are on the increase. One patient commented, "My RSI arms and hands seem to have that chronic fatigue syndrome." The widely differing theories and therapies of RSI are directed toward the affected limbs, with advice on improving work conditions.

I was surprised, even amazed, when several patients with RSI experienced changes in their jaws and temporomandibular joints when provoked with EBV. Painful jaw and chewing problems occur before, during, or after a flare-up of RSI. RSI patients experience fleeting fibromyalgia, pain in the lower leg muscles, and a variety of latent symptoms described in this section. Most RSI patients record allergic symptoms such as IBS, asthma, chronic sinusitis, and migraine on the clinic questionnaire. *Surmise:* Many RSI patients have associated fibromyalgia, allergy, and latency symptoms. When the whole problem is treated, recovery and relief often occur. Patients who gain little or no relief from the narrow "scientific medicine" concept of RSI therapies should be offered allergy and latency work-ups.

### Dengue Fever and Muscle and Joint Aches

Clinic patients who lived in or visited tropical countries should recollect whether they ever caught a fever after being bitten by mosquitoes. Did they suffer sweating, skin itching, depression, and muscle pains? For some, the symptoms may have been mild, for others, severe. The symptoms may have been dismissed as a bad case of influenza or infection of the gut. Six years ago I was frustrated to find a number of patients who reached a plateau of improvement but progressed no further. I studied the symptoms of the chronic stage of a number of tropical viral infections. The description of chronic dengue fever seemed to match the symptoms of my patients. Dengue belongs to the group of viruses known as the arboviruses, *ar* for arthropod (insect), *bo* for borne, plus virus. They are carried between man and animals by an insect, often the mosquito or tick. This group of viruses deserves more research, as its persistent and fluctuating latent symptoms are similar to those of CFIDS/ME. Some arboviruses can be fatal.

The provoked symptoms of dengue appear on the fourth to seventh day. Imagine the surprise of those tested when they awaken in the middle of the night, swatting their arms and legs, as if they were being bitten by mosquitoes. Could it be that some of the dengue latent virus deposited, or injected, by the mosquitoes is still present in the damaged cells beneath the skin? Dengue virutherapy clears or improves arthralgia and fibromyalgia and jump-starts perspiration. Popular, inexpensive air travel has spread dengue to many countries that were previously free of it. I consider no work-up for CFIDS/ME to be complete without testing for dengue fever and *Parvovirus.* Arboviruses known to cause infections locally or in neighboring countries are added to the testing list. A patient who had lived in an eastern U.S. town developed headache and fatigue some years after returning to New Zealand. Both the patient and I were surprised when he provoked to eastern equine encephalomyelitis virus. A patient who had contracted active malaria while in tropical countries suffered fluctuating symptoms after returning to New Zealand. Malaria concentrate is not available for use in treatment.

*Mycoplasma hominis* and *M. pneumoniae* are microbes between a virus and a bacterium. They provoke chest symptoms, arthritis pains, and swelling that are distinct from those provoked by *Giardia,* dengue, and *Helicobacter.* Some people had a dramatic clearance of joint pain and swelling. *M. hominis* and *M. pneumoniae* are worth provoking when the patient suffers from problem joint pains. What is in a name? The *Mycoplasma* species are not fussy about where they settle. Sometimes one will provoke the lungs without the joints and the *Mycoplasma* named for the lungs will instead provoke the joints. One or both *Mycoplasma* species will provoke bacteria that prefer to live in the bladder and urethra *(Ureaplasma).* Naming organisms according to their preferred territory of the body is convenient, not scientific.

The regrowth of forests in eastern America has encouraged a return of deer, many of which are protected and will approach houses, especially vegetable gardens, without fear. The deer bring with them ticks, and their parasitic bacteria, which enter the victim's body through the tick bite. Lyme disease is on the rise. Similar tick and bacterial diseases occur on the other continents. The symptoms of Lyme disease mimic those of CFIDS/ME. Although susceptible to antibiotics, eradication takes time, or a chronic condition results. Perhaps latency therapy using the bacterial extract dilutions could speed recovery.

### *Osteoarthritis*

It has long been known that allergies to foods and molds aggravate joint pains and restrict movements of sufferers with osteoarthritis. Recent medical findings report that CRC, *Giardia,* and some bacteria toxins, such as *Mycoplasma hominis* and *M. pneumoniae,* are additional causes. If you are over sixty, and have come down with influenza, you need no convincing that viruses aggravate. So it is not surprising that MLV has reduced the symptoms of osteoarthritis, especially in the hip joints. Many get considerable relief of hip pains from serial vaccination using *Giardia.* Be careful during the work-up not to aggravate symptoms by heavy lifting and too much walking because you are experiencing an improvement. Should you suffer from the type of rheumatoid arthritis that does not have the rheuma-toid RH (monkey) factor in the blood, consider the preliminary work-up and include *M. hominis* and *M. pneumoniae, Parvovirus,* rubella, influen-za, v. zoster, *Clostridium,* and *Legionella* in the MLV. Rheumatoid disease of the spine may be aggravated by *Clostridium* bacteria that are normally present in our intestines. Provocation with *Clostridium* dilution $5^{15}$ pro-voked marked symptoms for three to four days, then provided consider-able relief of the previously treated chronic rheumatoid arthritis of the hands and feet. Serial dilutions have maintained the improvement. I cannot offer an explanation.

The benefit you obtain from the preliminary work-up and virutherapy is boosted by other supporting treatments, such as heat therapies, saunas, baths, heat pads, and short-wave therapy. Practice good home ecology, avoid known allergic foods and substances, keep away from petrochemi-cals, and continue adequate exercise and limb movements. SSD treatments encourage people to hang on to their faulty lifestyles. The easy option is to take the powerful nonsteroid anti-inflammatory drugs for the joint, tendon, and muscle problems of osteoarthritis or methotrexate and gold therapy of rheumatoid arthritis. Sometime in the future, however, they may let you down, and you will be left with long-term side effects of Csds and NSAIDs, lowered immunity levels, and several change-of-site responses.

Any viral antibodies detected in your blood may be no more than "viral ghosts" from the past. Blood tests do not predict the latent viruses affect-ing you in the present. Viral provocation and neutralization can give you the answers.

### Deep Bone Pain

Deep bone pain cause sufferers to worry that they may have leukemia or a bone tumor. Most suffered with deep bone pain for years and gave up complaining because they were told it is a functional condition with no known treatment. The pain starts deep in one bone and then moves into other bones, affecting the long bones of the limbs, sometimes the shoul-ders, and the pelvic bones. The pain prevents a good night's sleep because drugs give little relief. After provocation and neutralization by dengue or EBV, people report the pains improve or disappear. Additional help in pain relief comes from MLV with hepatitis, herpes, v. zoster, and CMV. Some people report other sensations deep in their bones, which they describe as irritating rather than painful. I have no idea why deep bone sensations are provoked by MLV.

## URINARY TRACT SYMPTOMS

Not long after I started virutherapy, I was asked by women patients if latent viruses could be the cause of their untreatable, recurring "second curse" (all had undergone work-up and treatment by gynecologists and urologists). What they meant was *urinary tract dysfunction* and *bladder dysfunction.* The symptoms are: (1) frequency, (2) burning sensations in the urethra while passing urine, (3) constant awareness of the bladder, (4) stress leakage (incontinence), (5) pains in the loins coming from the kidneys, and (6) water retention in the body (edema) that fluctuates. It is not surprising that nearly all affected are women (bladder infection in men is very unusual because of the anatomy of the genitourinary organs).

Physicians see more infections in the urinary tract than in any other part of the body (venereal infections are not included in the discussion). The three main patterns among women who suffer from urinary tract infection are as follows: (1) most have one or two infections a year, (2) 20 percent have up to ten infections per year, and (3) a small number of unfortunates have continuous infection of the urine that is often symptomless. To give some idea of the long-term problems, 40 percent of elderly people in institutions have varying degrees of urinary tract infections. The most common infection of the urinary tract is caused by a bacterium, *Escherichia coli.* Conventional treatment of *E. coli* with antibiotics does not always clear the problem. If the preliminary work-up and MLV do not clear away the *E. coli* symptoms, then serial dilution provocation of *E. coli* is started.

Useful information about "bladder troubles" is hard to come by; see Dr. Charles Shepherd's description in his book *Living with ME* (1989). Antibiotic treatment of urinary problems is disappointing because the infections tend to recur. In addition, some "bladder infections" are not caused by bacteria so antibiotics do not help. A urinary tract infection is just as likely as influenza to cause a relapse or deterioration of symptoms elsewhere. Moods, memory, muscle weakness, and chronic fatigue relapses can follow a single urinary tract infection. The preliminary work-up must be thorough, as a hidden food allergy, such as to OWGGs or citrus, cancels out any benefits from MLV. CRC, CMV, *Helicobacter, Chlamydia, Giardia,* and *Ureaplasma* are provoked before multiple latent viruses. Patients' responses to, and comments about, provocation testing and serial dilution therapy suggest that these microorganisms frequently are not considered when treating urinary tract and bladder dysfunction:

1. Cytomegalovirus.
2. *Helicobacter* is not eradicated by the triple therapy of two antibiotics and bismuth powders. At the end of the treatment, negative cultures for *Helicobacter* are unreliable. *Helicobacter* provocation detects latent toxin in the brain (sleepiness, fatigue, and coldness), and its presence in the gut and urinary tract (indigestion and burning sensations in the gut, a cat pee smell on the breath and in the urine).
3. *Chlamydia* is considered an active venereal disease that responds to antibiotic treatment. Other *Chlamydia* infections occur in the eyes, nose, chest, and prostate, together with spasms and pain in the muscles of the shoulders, neck, inner thigh, and lower leg (see related discussions in the sections The Eyes and Ears, pp. 72-77, and Nose and Chest Conditions, pp. 37-44). During provocation, a few people experience mental changes such as feeling happy, an overall feeling of well-being, and improved memory and performance. *Chlamydia* serial vaccination shots, on occasion, gave amazing relief of urinary tract problems.
4. CRC and *Torulopsis.*
5. *Ureaplasma* and *Mycoplasma* are bacteria belonging to the family Mycoplasmataceae. *Ureaplasma* splits urea to form the ammonia smell accompanying chronic and intermittent bladder dysfunctions. *Mycoplasma* species represent the smallest bacteria. They do not have a cell wall or membrane and are able to enter living cells to become latentees (see *Mycoplasma pneumoniae* and *M. hominis* on p. 42). *Ureaplasma* provocation has immediate symptoms and marked delayed symptoms, appearing 12 h after provocation and lasting one to two days. The disappearance of the ammonia smell signals the end of the provocation. Women tell me that latency therapy with *Ureaplasma* gives relief without recurrences, in contrast to past antibiotic treatments. All feelings of unease disappear, and they experience a sensation of relaxation in the bladder and genital area not present with previous therapies. Children respond well to *Ureaplasma* provocation. The bacterium appears to be one of several causes of bed-wetting, urgency, frequency, and irritation in the genital area of young girls. *Mycoplasma hominis* and *M. pneumoniae* provocation has caused prostate and urethral unease and pain in men with and without enlarged prostates. *Ureaplasma* provocation and MLV should be offered to all people with chronic bladder and urethra problems.

**IK** 6. While being provoked or using serial vaccination treatment with human *Papillomavirus* 1 through 4 for warts, patients experience pain, unease, and irritation in the prostate and urethra, or the female genital area. *Papillomavirus* 16 is one of the causes of cancer of the cervix. That the same virus is a cause of cancer of the prostate has been discussed in the medical literature. So far blood antibody tests and PCRT of prostate cancer biopsies have not shown *Papillomavirus* to be present (Englehard, 1994). Another microbe, the protozoan *Trichomonas*, will provoke genital, bladder, prostate, and urethra symptoms in some people. Delayed symptoms are extreme fatigue, similar to CFIDS/ME, and, at first, diarrhea, followed by intermittent diarrhea and constipation, with foul flatulence. Stubborn irritable bowel syndrome has greatly improved with *Trichomonas* serial vaccinations.

If the response to treatment is slow or disappointing, despite provocation with the previous organisms, it could be due to previous, or current, cannabis use (see Cannabis/Marijuana, pp. 56-57).

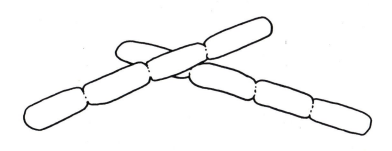

### Cytomegalovirus (CMV)

You should know how important CMV virutherapy is for women with urinary tract dysfunction, or who suffer from latent glandular fever. Some have asked, "Why glandular fever? Isn't it caused by the Epstein-Barr Virus?" I reply, "Correct, but CMV is like EBV; they both belong to the herpes virus family." This wide-ranging virus is better understood and identified from its symptoms and effects on many parts of the body. You could say, "Where EBV goes, you are sure to find CMV lurking, waiting to cause symptoms when there is an EBV relapse." CMV infects and kills cells lining the urinary tract, causing the cells *(cyto)* to swell and join together to form large *(megalo)* cells that soon burst and die, releasing a load of infective viruses. If these cells are found in your urine test, it means you have active, or possibly latent, CMV.

The following are important facts about CMV Virutherapy:

1. It reduces inflammation, swelling, discomfort, and sensitivity in the bladder and genital areas. The accompanying pains in the loins disappear.
2. CMV and *Helicobacter* virutherapy, together with CRC and *Giardia* treatments, clears many chronic urinary tract infections.
3. Unexplained waterlogging of the body (edema), especially of the breasts, is improved. Large quantities of urine are passed for 12 to 24 h after provocation, resulting in rapid weight loss. Long-term treatment allows many women to reduce or stop the use of water pills (diuretics).
4. Besides losing excess body fluid, men notice improvement of loin and lumbar pains, with disappearance of uncomfortable erections, painful ejaculations, and annoying dull pain after intercourse. CMV provocation, at times, stimulates pain and sensations in the prostate area. I surmise that it may have a role in prostate enlargement.
5. CMV is one of three viruses that improves muscle strength. CMV improves the muscles of the legs, hips, and the lumbar and sacral regions of the lower back. A few patients experience a remarkable recovery of strength in the shoulders and arms from serial CMV shots. CMV shots improve bladder control and possibly help to restore bladder holding capacity.
6. CMV virutherapy improves nasal symptoms, chest pains, and chest tightness. Asthmatics who are using inhaled corticosteroid preparations obtain improvement in the nose and chest. Liver and gall bladder pains are relieved by CMV virutherapy.

**IK**    A woman with persistent liver symptoms and abnormal liver test results consented to a liver biopsy, mistakenly believing that somehow the findings of the biopsy would provide a treatment. CMV was present in the liver biopsy, but no treatment was available. She continued to have the liver pain and, at times, severe pain in the biopsy wound. She attended the clinic, and after the preliminary work-up, CMV was the last virus tested. To her amazement, CMV $5^{18}$, a very high dilution, relieved both the biopsy and liver pain. Serial vaccination with three or four other viruses and CMV improved her health and relieved the pain. The liver function tests are almost normal. She complained to me, "Why didn't they provoke me like you have? It would have saved me all the expense and suffering. I was mad when they finally told me there was no treatment after the operation." I replied, "Scientific medicine does not use anecdotal tests and treatments, despite their obvious clinical benefits."

7. Difficult-to-treat heart symptoms often turn out to be due to CMV. These include heart thumping that wakes you with the feeling that your heart will jump out of your chest; a racing of the heart (tachycardia), so that you become faint and have to sit down; a slowing of the pulse rate that causes you to wonder when the next heartbeat will occur. All these symptoms are present without chest pain. Angina pains reduced then cleared following a year of serial CMV vaccination shots.

8. CMV virutherapy brings about improvement of depression, moods, and insomnia. A surprising benefit is enhanced mental activity and memory.

9. Successful CMV virutherapy assists in the treatment of EBV (glandular fever). Experience shows it is difficult to treat glandular fever unless the other three herpes viruses, Herpes simplex 1, 2, and v. zoster and CMV are provoked and virutherapy is underway. CMV virutherapy is improved if rotavirus provokes symptoms and is added to the serial vaccination shots.

10. Low-dose thyroxine therapy aids the effects of CMV virutherapy, increasing the fluid loss and improving moods and memory. Do not let normal thyroid laboratory tests stop you from taking small doses of thyroxine if your allergist suggests a six- to eight-week trial. Patients attending the clinic begin with one-quarter of the 0.05 milligram (mg) thyroxine tablet and may find it is adequate. If not, the dose is slowly increased over the next four to six weeks to half a tablet twice a day.

**IK**    Some years ago a large, tall, overweight woman provoked to CMV. I prescribed a potassium salt substitute and low-dose thyroxine, with written instructions on how to use it, starting at one-quarter of a 0.05 mg tablet daily. She was persuaded by a knowledgeable health worker friend to take two of the tablets a day because this was the minimum dose the doctors at the hospital prescribed. Five days later, when the prolonged provoked symptoms began, she contacted me with a sorry tale. The good news: for the first three days after testing she passed more urine than usual, but on the fourth and fifth days she kept close to the toilet by day and by night. The fluid loss was amazing; she had lost thirteen pounds. Her breasts returned to an acceptable size for the first time in ten years and there was a marked reduction in her abdomen and buttocks. Best of all, the bags under her eyes and the fullness around her neck decreased. The bad news: she was "all revved up" and developed loin and throat pain. After a talk about doing the virutherapy treatments in a gradual and progressive manner, and the dangers of thyroxine, she promised to comply. An OWGGs food allergy was detected during the preliminary work-up, but there was little weight loss in spite of a complete exclusion. Following the dramatic CMV provocation, she began to lose more weight. Six months after the last testing at the clinic she visited us to show off her new slim figure and lovely complexion.

### *CMV and* Helicobacter

Some women call these two "the urinary twins"; other women and men call them the "sexy twins." CMV gets along fine with *Helicobacter, Chlamydia, Ureaplasma,* and human *Papillomavirus,* to our discomfort in the genitourinary areas.

**IK**   *Helicobacter* is a bacterium that is very good at evading antibiotics and becoming resistant to them. The following are some important findings about *Helicobacter:*

1. *Helicobacter* provocation gives many symptoms similar to those of CMV. A burning sensation accompanies the pain and symptoms of *Helicobacter.*
2. *Helicobacter* provokes burning symptoms from the stomach, usually indigestion, and sometimes from the intestines and colon.
3. Immediate provocation brings on intense tiredness, lethargy, even sleep, and the characteristic cat urine smell. For a few people, it was the principal cause of their CFIDS/ME. *Helicobacter* fatigue does not relapse after the successful serial vaccination course is completed.
4. *Helicobacter* provokes pain and sensitivity in teeth with inflamed tooth ligaments or root abscesses. *Helicobacter* and its close relative *Campylobacter* are present in most people's mouths. *Helicobacter* provocation of nose and chest symptoms occurs, even though culture swabs of the area are negative.
5. Serial vaccination shots stimulate kidney function and, as previously described, aid in the loss of body fluid.
6. A strong characteristic smell pervades the urine, motions, sweat, and breath for two to three days after provocation, and sometimes after shots. The smell is similar to that of cat urine and can be so strong that it has alarmed people. It is the same smell they noticed on their breath and clothes months or years previously.

## The Sexy Combination

**IK**  Imagine my surprise when I first began using *Helicobacter* with CMV provocation and virutherapy. Letters and phone calls told of renewed sexual interest and activity. That year, about 100 women felt loving again and wanted intimacy. About sixty men regained their libidos and erectile-ability. There are happy endings for those using *Helicobacter* and CMV "shots." Later additions are mumps and *Ureaplasma.* Mumps may provoke ovary and testis tenderness or discomfort, prostate gland secretion, and erections during sleep (see *Papillomavirus,* p. 174). This modern-day love potion will not work its magic for those who (1) disregard an OWGG allergy or (2) have not detoxed cannabis. There must be total OWGG exclusion, and no cheating—please!

## No Desire for Lovemaking

Many times women have said to me, "If only I had been treated for CRC and given virutherapy instead of that silly psychological stuff." But the preliminary work-up and CRC, including *Giardia* and *Chlamydia,* do not restore former levels of sexual drive and response in all. I was surprised how excluding OWGGs relieved much of the unexplained muscle tension, restoring relaxed lovemaking and improving relationships. CRC treatment and MLV reduce or eliminate distorted mental attitudes about sexual feelings, decrease the frequency of unexplained periods of sexual drive, or provide a remedy for a lack of sexual drive. The end result of the work-up is disappearance of jealous or possessive feelings. It also eased arousal and orgasm and restored loving feelings in relationships. Read what Drs. Truss and Crook discovered about CRC and sex problems (Crook, 1995). One woman said, "MLV dotted the i's and crossed the t's of CRC treatment for sexual problems."

RSV, polio, morbilli, herpes, rotavirus, hepatitis, mumps, *Papillomavirus,* and the important CMV have all helped to return normal sexual drive. A number of men told me serial vaccination with hepatitis cleared their main complaint—it stopped unwanted and sadistic macho thoughts that came upon them during sexual contemplation or arousal. They could not understand why these thoughts came into their consciousness and had "put them in the back of their mind." Hepatitis and herpes made these thoughts seem like real events. Hepatitis and herpes play cruel tricks on some women, making their skin extremely sensitive so that they cannot tolerate fondling. They plead "get it over quickly." The same women hate being in crowds because they must have space around them. So it is not surprising that these women want single, not double, beds. MLV can clear away these cruel symptoms.

**IK**    A woman experienced reasonable relief from the CFIDS/ME. She attended the clinic for the remaining symptoms of severe headaches and a constant background head pain. She later told me the severe headaches were brought on by lovemaking, or whenever she contemplated making love. Previous hormone treatments had failed. The preliminary work-up, in particular, CRC, markedly decreased the severity of the headaches, but they recurred severely when she made love or even considered making love. She was surprised when additional MLV therapy cleared the remaining symptoms of her CFIDS/ME, the constant head pain, and the headaches associated with lovemaking.

### Genital Herpes and Warts

**IK**    Herpes, from *herpo* (Greek), meaning to creep, is an appropriate name for a virus that creeps along nerves, leaving vesicles or watery blisters that spread along the skin covering the area of the nerve's sensations. Herpes simplex 1 affects the body above the hips and sometimes causes genital herpes vesicles. Herpes simplex 2 is confined to the skin areas below the hips and includes genital herpes. Genital herpes attacks of vesicles and pain are treated with an antiviral drug, acyclovir. The problem is its cost. I obtain provocation results that rapidly clear genital herpes vesicles and prevent recurrences, as long as serial vaccination with herpes simplex 1 and 2 and v. zoster is continued at intervals of three to four weeks. Many are afraid that provoking with the herpes viruses will flare their genital herpes. The opposite occurs. Women appreciate the return of painless passage of urine and pleasant intercourse. Patients with a long history of venereal herpes are advised to do the full preliminary work-up and MLV to restore normal immunities. There is no quick-fix single-virus treatment for venereal herpes. A return to old habits and lifestyles brings on recurrences that become increasingly difficult to treat. Genital warts and venereal acuminata are provoked with *Papillomavirus* 6 and treated following the preliminary work-up and MLV. After four to six weekly shots the number and size of warts decreases. Thereafter, shots at two-week intervals are continued for four to six months until most, if not all, of the warts have cleared. Relapses occur if old lifestyles are resumed because overall immunities are again depressed.

## SLEEPING DISORDERS

I am impressed by the frequency of sleeping disorders in allergic, petrochemical, CRC, and multiple latent virus sufferers. I am alarmed at the quantities of hypnotic sleeping tablets or stimulants (coffee and caffeine) they use. A few have days or weeks of insomnia, then periods of extreme sleepiness. Health books on allergies and nutrition describe how common sleeping disorders are; yet books on sleeping disorders pay little attention to allergies and latent viruses. During provocation and neutralization, it is not unusual for someone to fall asleep, or to become so sleepy that he or she can barely describe the provoked symptoms. *Helicobacter* caused several people to curl up in a testing room chair and sleep there for 2 to 3 h. CRC, house dust, and molds provocations may induce sleepiness. The following latent viruses are important causes of sleeping disorders: EBV, CMV, herpes, influenza, morbilli, hepatitis, and v. zoster. (Latent viruses that elate and keep people awake are: RSV, polio, rubella, rotavirus, herpesvirus 6, and *Chlamydia.*) Sleepiness occurs toward the end of a sauna, and it is not unusual for patients to sleep for 2 to 3 h on returning home. Detoxing or excretion of petrochemicals, mold toxins, and latent viruses occurs during sleep. Have you ever woken drenched in perspiration after a questionable meal or exposure to petrochemicals? Do not arrange to attend any social engagements after attending the clinic, as delayed sleep may occur 6 to 8 h later.

IK    A confident woman took this warning lightly and arranged a dinner party for twelve on the night of her visit to the clinic. Her friends served the meal and had a great party while she slept. At 2:00 a.m. she received her guests in the bedroom as they were leaving. She had no hard feelings as she later made a great recovery.

Who has not experienced severe influenza with two to three days of sleeping and sweating? It is not surprising that latent viruses are a cause of sleeping problems. In time, I believe petrochemicals, including xeno-SSDs, mold toxins, and food and inhalant allergies, will be recognized as causes of sleeping disorders. Obtaining confirming "scientific" laboratory tests, however, will be a real problem. After ten years or more of interrupted sleep from skin itching and joint aches, irritable bowel, bladder, and vagina, patients, and I, are amazed how quickly the preliminary work-up and MLV restore sleep. The investigation of insomnia should be thorough to identify all principal factors. It is the removal of these factors, including xeno-SSDs, no matter in what order, that restores normal sleep patterns.

Sometimes it takes two to three months for all factors to be identified and removed.

**IK**    A woman with a skin itch, but no skin eczema, except where she scratched, had not slept normally for twenty-five years. Hepatitis was the main source of the itch, and the "shots" quickly cleared the skin itch. She promptly started sleeping normally, with no need for sleeping tablets, despite having used them every night for twenty-five years or more.

Do not throw out your sleeping tablets; they could be useful if insomnia is provoked during treatment or you suffer a relapse. It is not unusual for successfully treated people to tell me of the relief of their insomnia and the thrill of being able to sleep through the night and wake up refreshed.

### Sleep Apnea

Male patients with sleep apnea scare their sleeping partners. Deep sleep, especially after physical exertion or drinking alcohol, brings on irregular breathing and snoring. Soon the breathing stops, followed by choking noises, a jerking of the body, a move to a new sleeping position, some deep snoring breaths, and back to the cycle's beginning. Men with sleep apnea problems wake tired and underperform during the day.

Apnea has many causes, so if your partner thinks you have sleep apnea see a physician or surgeon who specializes in the condition. Before agreeing to surgery on your soft palate, throat, or nose, try the following:

1. Sleep with the head of the bed raised on 25 to 30 cm blocks (10 to 12 inches [in]). Do not use extra pillows because the increased bending of the neck could aggravate the sleep apnea.
2. Do not drink alcohol after 4:00 p.m. Take a magnesium supplement just before retiring.
3. Do not become too exhausted from physical exercise during the day.
4. Weight reduction is very important. Are you sure you do not have an OWGG food allergy? The back of the tongue has little or no muscle; it is padded with fat. Being overweight adds fat to the back of the tongue, which enlarges it and narrows the width of the airway.
5. Successful dust and food allergy therapy clears blocked noses and improves chest function. If there is an OWGG food allergy, total exclusion decreases the body weight. Cleaning the bedroom, cleaning the walls and curtains, and removing old carpet to reduce dust and molds helps most patients with inhalant allergies.

6. Muscle tone during sleep is improved with MLV, polio, influenza, CMV, RSV, EBV, *Chlamydia,* and CRC.

If sleep apnea is not improved by these treatments, you should go to an apnea clinic for a medical and surgical assessment.

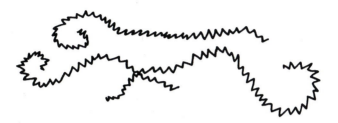

### THE VIRUS-ALLERGY LINK
### AND CHILDREN'S RESPONSES TO MLV

The following checklist may help you understand the role MLV plays in helping children's conditions—but first an explanation. The responses to MLV and the symptoms from testing or provoking vary so much in children that I am unable to do more than generalize. Rashes, behavior, and food problems sum up most children's complaints seen at the clinic. Add to these the "sticky mucus diseases" that appeared during the early 1960s, becoming persistent in the 1970s and lasting into the present: glue ear, sinusitis, asthma, bronchitis, and bowel conditions with increased mucus.

1. Have no fears about the treatments. Be prepared to drastically change lifestyles, eating habits, and the home and/or school ecology.
2. The preliminary work-up is simpler than for the adult. More attention is paid to food allergies, house dust mites, and CRC. Two to three other microbes and between four to eight viruses are provoked.
3. You and your partner may have to change your lifestyle during the treatment period.
4. No "shots" are given to children under the age of fourteen. All treatments are delivered under the tongue as drops (see pp. 198-203).
5. On average, two to four trips to the clinic are adequate because recovery is faster in children.
6. The 3 to 4 h testing sessions at first seem excessively long, but they pass quickly when drawing, writing, and reading activities are encouraged. (No felt pens please.)

7. Children are able to stop their inhaled Csd treatments for obstructive nose, bronchitis, and asthma much sooner than adults.

8. Overactive children and those with hyperactivity and memory loss (attention-deficit disorder [ADD]) respond well to therapy, and many are able to stop taking their drugs, providing they comply with lifestyle changes.

9. Be sure to record in the symptom questionnaire any viral illnesses that affected the child more than other children in the neighborhood. Describe any immediate or delayed vaccination reactions (up to eight weeks), as the same viruses may be responsible for present symptoms.

10. Parents learn to examine babies' mouths and children's throats for teething, coated tongues, or inflamed throats. Ask your family physician for recommended health books on childhood nutrition. The following supplements are necessary for your child to respond to allergy treatment and virutherapy: preparations of zinc, calcium, and magnesium; a selection of unsaturated vegetable oils (olive, sunflower, safflower, flax) and a fish oil (salmon, cod liver); vitamins A, B, and C; and a saturated fat, preferably butter (do not use margarine), unless you have a dairy allergy. Parents are encouraged to use simple allergy provocation tests to identify minor food allergies or intolerances (Crook, 1996; Rapp, 1992).

11. Help your school-age child by interviewing the teacher two or four times during the term, regarding progress in behavior and learning. Improved classroom and activity reports are important signs of successful therapy. Most allergists like to receive copies of school reports, especially if they are posted by the child.

It continues to surprise parents, and me, how previously "hard to manage" children can make a real effort to comply, without much complaint, once they experience the good effects and improvement of virutherapy.

One little fellow of five told me, after his nose was cleared and his behavior had improved, "I like Mum's beaut [excellent] cooking now; it used to taste like chewed up lavvy [toilet] paper."

I could write another book on children's latency symptoms, treatments, and responses. The summaries that follow are of the main symptom patterns remaining after inhalant and food allergy therapy.

### Infants and Toddlers

Infants seen at the clinic have cradle cap, nappy or diaper rash, a variety of other skin rashes, and restless or sleepy behavior. They have generally had one or more antibiotic courses. Infants and toddlers are provoked in the same manner as children up to age fourteen, with sublingual or "under the tongue" drops. The first visit involves testing for three or four principal foods, house dust, mites, molds, and *Candida.* The second visit includes tests for influenza, rhinovirus, and RSV; if a whoop is present, for pertussis (whooping cough); if green nasal mucus, for *Pseudomonas aeruginosa;* if recurring colic/mucus with motions, for rotavirus and adenovirus. A third visit may be necessary, if urinary tract infection is disrupting potty training, for testing with *Giardia, Helicobacter,* CMV, hepatitis, and *Chlamydia.*

The neutralizing of provoked symptoms is usually obvious to the mother and the physician. The treatment drops contain viral and bacterial doses, on average, between $5^5$ to $5^8$ and, for *Candida,* $5^{12}$ to $5^{15}$. Infants and toddlers recover as soon as (1) sugars, honeys, and any allergic foods are excluded, (2) nystatin tablets are divided into eighths, and even sixteenths, and given with food two or three times a day, and (3) sublingual treatment drops are begun. For best results, home cook all foods. It is not practical to exclude all supermarket foods that contain small amounts of sugar, preservatives, dyes, and additives. With treatment under way, and the child's health improving, it is easy to recognize and test any food that seems to upset the child.

### Children Four to Nine Years

#### The Sugar Problem

**IK** "How can I stop my child from eating sugar? You should see the tantrums and the bad moods that follow when I take away the sugar." My reply to this common complaint is, "Some parents give up the battle and dole out the sugar, but sugar encourages many of the organisms we are talking about." It saddens me when I tell the parents there is no point in bringing the child back for treatment because they cannot control the sugar problem. In the past, I treated groups of children who continued eating sugar. I eventually convinced the parents of the need for two to three months of sugar control for an improvement in behavior and health. The sugar controversy grinds on. Who to believe? Forget the "proof medicine scientific trials" and the "sugar is a food" of the media. Provoke your child with sugar, dyed candy, and chocolate. Believe your own observations, not the contrived media messages.

Many children suffer a severe relapse following a birthday party. For seven to ten days following the party, it is difficult to get any beneficial response from sublingual viral treatment drops. Mothers can manage the eating at birthday parties by careful presentation of foods on the table, covering half of the table's surface with savories, meats, cheeses, and nuts, and placing the traditional sugar, fruit, and cake dishes on the other end of the table. Mothers report that most of the "junior" guests start with foods on the first half of the table, dipping into the sweet foods only after the other dishes have disappeared. If your child is the birthday host, you have the opportunity to control children's sugar intake further by making the traditional dessert dishes with nonallergic ingredients, natural sweeteners, and a minimum of cane sugar. Fast foods are not a suitable substitute for the savory half of the table because they contain excessive amounts of xenochemicals and sugar.

A common sense exclusion of obvious food additives will help in the child's treatment. Although hard work, if you are familiar with the Feingold Diet, follow the instructions for avoiding man-made food additives. I ask mothers of sugar-addicted children to check for detoxing food colorings on their pillowcases. If the children drink large quantities of soda, it is not unusual for the coloring on the pillowcase to match the soda. Provocation with mumps sublingual drops causes a pain in the pit of the stomach and/or overactivity (ADD) in sugarholic children. Mothers are impressed by the provocation and make a real effort to control sugar in the home. Active mumps infection with destruction of many, or all, of the insulin-producing cells of the pancreas is a frequent cause of teenage diabetes (type I) (see Carbohydrate Control and Diabetes I and II, pp. 52-53).

## Fussy Eating and Main Meal Reversal

I hesitate to write about the complicated subject of fussy eating. A great number of books and articles written by psychologists and pediatricians highlight the social and ethnic factors, in addition to medical causes, behind fussy eating. Nowhere in this literature have I found reference to latent viruses. At the first clinic visit, parents admit that they do not know what to do: "How much notice should be taken, or should it be disregarded?" If fussy eating is starting to concern you, and the child's health is sub par, suspect a food allergy and do simple food family exclusions, beginning with the OWGGs (see p. 170). Always suspect a food that is consistently spat out or thrown on the floor or is a favorite food that provokes delayed mood or behavioral changes. Consult an allergist for a food work-up and a trial of CRC, *Giardia,* and *Helicobacter* therapy. Successful *Giardia* and *Helicobacter* antibiotic therapy should be followed by *Giardia* and *Helicobacter* treatment drops to lessen the frequency and severity of relapses. The gut viruses, adenovirus, hepatitis, polio, rotavirus, and mumps, at times, restore children's appetites and relieve bowel symptoms. Nasal blockage prevents the finer tastes and smells of food from reaching the smell area of the nose. These children will choose foods whose taste is detected by the tongue—salty, acidic, or sugar sweet foods.

An unsuspected cause of fussy eating is main meal reversal, possibly an inherited behavior. Children eat a substantial breakfast but will only pick at the evening meal. If your child's appetite is strong in the morning, you will need to take time and patience to train them to the accepted adult meal pattern of modern life. They may not change, however, until age eight or nine. A few adults attending the clinic are unable to eat a substantial meal in the evening, despite their best endeavors. They have no appetite, and if they eat an average amount of the food, they feel nauseated; some even vomit. Check out main meal reversal before seeking professional advice on fussy eating.

### Sinusitis, Bronchitis, and Asthma

An allergic factor is nearly always present with these conditions. Parents begin a basic work-up of improving home ecology, trying food exclusion diets, eliminating sugars, putting pets outside the house, and removing old bedroom carpets. The resulting improvement encourages parents to continue these measures, and, in time, children become aware that certain activities or foods make them sick. Further help comes from an allergist who detects other hidden food and inhalant allergies, CRC, *Giardia,* or worms. If the overall improvement in the nose and chest is disappointing, start latency treatment in the form of sublingual drops of CRC and influenza, RSV, and ATV, followed by provocation of polio, morbilli, and *Mycoplasma pneumoniae* (for an explanation of the effect on the lungs see pp. 42-44). If the child's cough is not the allergic food "bark," it will probably respond to morbilli, *Chlamydia,* and *M. pneumoniae* added to the treatment drops. When a whoop, or suspicion of it, is present at the end of coughing, pertussis (whooping cough) $5^4$ to $5^6$ is remarkably effective. Testing with pertussis at the clinic brings on the typical cough and whoop. *Pseudomonas aeruginosa* provocation and serial vaccination is particularly useful in getting rid of the green nasal pus. Foods taste better with an open nose. Children respond rapidly, and the majority are able to dispense with their Csd inhalers. Their confidence in themselves is restored, often with remarkable improvement in schoolwork and sports activities. Parents are advised to keep a supply of asthma medication in the home, as temporary relapses can occur.

### Headaches, Sore Muscles, and Abdominal Pain

Some children may suffer from these three symptoms together or in sequence (change-of-site response). As the headache is treated and improves, the pains switch to the abdomen or muscles. Having shown no response to conventional treatment, these symptoms may have common or separate causes. Latent virus provocation and therapy for headache is influenza, RSV, and polio; for the sore, painful muscles, morbilli; for muscle weakness, polio, CMV, and *Chlamydia;* for abdominal pain and bloating, hepatitis, polio, CMV, rotavirus, and adenovirus. CMV and EBV frequently provoke abdominal pain that could be coming from inflamed lymph glands draining the intestines. MLV can bring about a dramatic recovery within four to six weeks for children age eight through sixteen. Active glandular fever with a positive blood test may respond, on average, to PW, MLV, and EBV $5^{15}$ to $5^{20}$, CMV $5^{12}$ to $5^{18}$ virutherapy.

### Bed-Wetting and Sleeping Problems

Disturbed sleeping, behavioral problems, overactivity, or hyperactivity/ ADD may be intermittent or continuous (change-of-site response). Seek pediatric and psychological advice before starting allergy treatment and MLV. Conventional medical therapies favor SSDs, but if parents are unhappy about the use of Csd skin creams for years to come, it is best to seek an allergist's opinion. Most successful treatments of bed-wetting (enuresis) are a combination of the three therapies. Ask for deworming pills before starting the food allergy investigation. If you still suspect worms, ask for provocation with roundworm extract. Crops of skin warts suggest poor immunity and nutrition. After six to eight weeks' attention to good meals and nutrition, there may be no improvement. Do serial dilution and provocation with *Papillomavirus* 4 and 6, and add to a treatment dropper bottle.

Grass pollens and OWGGs are common causes of insomnia and disturbed sleep. Other foods known to cause disturbed sleep are citrus, apples, and pears. Sugar, honey, and foods with a high content of mold or yeast should be excluded. Following the allergy work-up, CRC, *Giardia, Helicobacter, Chlamydia,* CMV, and *Ureaplasma* are provoked, and the significant microbe treatment doses are added to the dropper bottle. Skin itching and crawling sensations under the skin keep children from sleeping and make them tired and irritable during the day. Suspect hepatitis, herpes, rubella, and v. zoster. It is not generally known that polio and hepatitis may cause children's nightmares. Children in the four-to-nine age group require at least three to five visits and two to three treatment dropper bottles. Progress is often interrupted by relapses. Parents should give the treatment a six-month trial. It is rewarding for parents, and me, to see the gradual change for the better in personality, learning ability, and physical performance. One mother's comment comes back to me every time I treat a new child with these problems: "I've got my lovely boy back after that terrible vaccination reaction."

**IK**   Ronald, age 8½, wet the bed most nights. Medical and surgical investigations were normal. Previous treatments gave relief for two to six weeks. An allergy to soy and citrus foods was uncovered. The exclusion of sugar, honey, and allergic foods, and treatment drops for CRC, *Helicobacter, Ureaplasma,* and CMV, together with psychological therapy, resulted in an occasional wet bed. As the boy's self-confidence returned, the treatments were phased out over the next six months. Ronald sent me his excellent school and sports reports for the next two years.

## Memory Loss

**IK**   Chronic fatigue immune dysfunction syndrome can descend on a child and wreak havoc with his or her development. A previously normal child who is doing well at school develops a loss of memory for immediate and/or past events following a severe cold or viruslike illness, possibly influenza, and sometimes following vaccination or a vaccination reaction. Schooling and social events turn into ordeals, and the child becomes depressed and loses confidence. The children I see all had psychological treatment with no lasting improvement. They were forced to give up schooling because they could not recollect what they are told and, if given written instructions, may be able to read them but could not remember. This is not attention-deficit disorder. Several children with memory loss, depression, muscle pain, and weakness suffered terrible mental and personal anguish at the hands of psychiatrists, psychologists, and teachers. The professionals were influenced by the medical diagnosis dogma, "CFIDS/ME is functional." Teachers with the "snap out of it; pull yourself together" mind-set forced parents to withdraw the children from school. When the children recover, the parents change schools if the teachers refuse to change their attitude toward CFIDS. Important viruses used in the treatment of marked memory loss are RSV, polio, influenza, morbilli, hepatitis, rubella, v. zoster, rotavirus, and EBV.

## Behavior and Attention-Deficit Disorder

Sudden behavioral changes are a feature of provoking with sublingual (under the tongue) drops. Fortunately, nearly all alarming provoked behavior is quickly neutralized. The problem is delayed behavioral changes that occur 3 to 5 h later, when the family returns home. Parents can put up with provoked behavior because they are now convinced that a cause or causes exist and they understand what is happening. The same aggressive behavior and personality changes so often seen in the schoolroom or on the playground are provoked during testing sessions. Aggressive behavior in older children becomes dangerous during team sports or playground games, and they have little or no recollection of their behavior. Important provoking viruses are hepatitis, polio, RSV, influenza, CMV, and EBV.

**IK**    A girl, age 9, started kicking the furniture of the allergy room and her mother's legs during provocation with polio drops $5^5$. Her behavior deteriorated further on $5^7$ (25 times more dilute), but it cleared on $5^9$ (625 times more dilute). The mother then remembered a temporary behavioral change occurred some weeks after the polio oral vaccination. The removal of poultry from her diet and the use of drops with CRC, polio, RSV, and adenovirus restored her previous sensible, happy schoolgirl behavior, and she later brought home very good reports.

Children with violent behavior problems suffer from fearful dreams and nightmares. They will not tell you about the nightmares until their behavior is improving because they cannot remember them or think that nightmares are a normal occurrence. When medication fails to clear nightmares, children exhibit complex behavioral problems. MLV, combined with psychological and nutritional therapies, can reverse the behavioral patterns. An important observation is that violent behavior in children responds to hepatitis therapy in a manner similar to violent behavior in adults. Symptom suppression drugs are preferred by many families, but this allows children to continue their faulty lifestyles and food habits. Every so often violent behavior breaks out from under the control of the SSDs. Nearly all parents who bring their children to the clinic have experience with SSDs. Children brought up on the SSD Ritalin (and other caffeine-derived drugs) are at risk of acquiring prison records by their early twenties (Rapp, 1996).

Families attending the clinic who change their children's diet and lifestyle were rewarded by a return to normal behavior without drug therapy. Children with violent behavior and ADD attending the clinic had a high incidence of past head injuries, viral or bacterial meningitis, and undiagnosed encephalitis. The recovery of normal function following provocation and treatment is more marked than the improvements noticed in adults.

**IK**   A boy, age 11, became autistic as an infant, following a triple vaccine shot that included pertussis (whopping cough). He provoked strongly to pertussis $5^{15}$ and improved on its latency therapy. OWGGs exclusion and MLV with polio, rubella, CMV, and EBV combined to improve the strength of his limbs, coordination, and behavioral tics. The latency therapy revealed an excellent memory and quick recall, advanced writing expression, but, unfortunately, little improvement in speech.

*Tonsils and Adenoids (T&A)*

The modern approach to T&A infection and enlargement offers alternatives not available forty to fifty years ago when removal was encouraged by public health authorities. Your family physician and otolaryngologist (ear, nose, and throat) surgeon advise an operation for your child's infected and blocked nose, chronic infected and painful throat, and variable deafness, with the glue ear mucus. The reasons and risks for the operation are explained. Parents may hesitate because, nowadays, so many children grow out of the condition. Request a referral to an allergist who uses the provocation neutralization technique. The allergist gives you advice on lifestyle, food, and home ecology. The allergist tests for allergic foods, dusts, and CRC and suggests medication and nutritional supplements. You are advised to inspect the tonsils for appearance and size twice a week. A response to the preliminary work-up should be obvious in six to eight weeks. If not, ask for a trial of MLV. The important virus, to give its original full name, is adenotonsilvirus, now called adenovirus. At the first virutherapy visit, adenovirus, influenza, and respiratory syncytial virus are tested and, if significant, added to the dropper bottle of *Candida*. Occasionally a second visit is required to test glandular fever (EBV), other viruses and bacteria, and whether there were reactions to vaccinations or severe childhood infections in the past. A separate EBV treatment drop bottle is made up because drops are given every two to three weeks. Adenovirus and EBV boost the effects of other viruses by reducing the tonsil and adenoid bulk and the size of enlarged tender glands in the neck. EBV relieves the sore throat on the back wall of the gullet. The EBV sore throat is constantly being misdiagnosed as low-grade tonsillitis. Many useless symptom suppression T&A operations are performed with little or no improvement of the sore throat.

If there is no response to the allergy and virus work-up after three to four months, and the infections continue, consider the operation option. The delay in treatment will not be a waste of time. I have repeatedly observed that children who received the work-up and nutritional therapy experienced improved immunities, but although surgery was still needed, they suffered far less postoperative pain, the recovery period was reduced, and there was obvious benefit from the surgery.

## THE VIRUS-ALLERGY SCORECARD FOR UNTREATABLE ALL-IN-THE-MIND SYMPTOMS

### Instructions

- Score one point for each symptom you identify with in the symptom group.
- Do not score symptoms with known causes or those treated in the past and relieved.
- Many scorecard symptoms were diagnosed as psychological. The results of virus-allergy link therapy suggest otherwise.

### How to Score

The probability of the virus-allergy link information improving your symptoms is:

- Score under 8, low or not applicable.
- Score 8 to 12, moderate to good.
- Score over 12, good to very good.

## The Virus-Allergy Scorecard

| Symptom Group | Points |
|---|---|
| Do you suffer recurring flu or fluctuating virus-like symptoms (1)? With little or no relief from antibiotic courses (1)? | |
| Within the last year, have you passed a thorough medical work-up (1)? Do you feel like a puppet manipulated by viruses and toxins (1)? | |
| Do you suffer fluctuating unexplained fatigue (1) and/or lack of motivation (1)? Are you diagnosed as neurotic, your symptoms all in the head (1)? Are you taking symptom suppression drugs, e.g., antidepressants, NSAIDS, etc. (1)? | |
| Do you suffer "no cause" depressions, cry a lot, and/or have morbid thoughts (1)? Fluctuating swelling and soreness of lymph glands (1)? Sore throats and "heavy as lead" arms and legs (1)? | |
| Do you have strange head symptoms (1)? Suffered a mild to moderate (1) or severe (2) head injury? Scary or strange dreams (1)? Memory loss or reading problems (1)? Attention-deficit disorder or dyslexia (1)? | |
| Do you get argumentative, aggressive (1)? Or retreat into yourself for no reason, antisocial behavior (1)? | |
| Do you relieve your stress or neurotic symptoms by smoking nicotine (1)? By drinking alcohol (1)? By drugs such as cannabis, cocaine, etc. (1)? | |
| Did you suffer postvaccination reactions (1)? Unexplained viral infections causing brain symptoms or a severe illness with one of the childhood viral fevers (1)? Glandular fever, cytomegalovirus, hepatitis, dengue infections (1)? | |
| Do you suddenly become cold, with "icy" extremities, for no apparent reasons (1)? Have sleepy periods you cannot fight off (1)? Reversal of sleeping patterns, sleep disorders (1)? | |
| Do you suffer irregular heart rates, pounding, "heart" pains (1)? Water retention problems (1)? | |
| Do you suffer recurring symptoms and infections of the vagina, prostate (1)? Bladder, kidney, urinary tract symptoms/infections (1)? Endometriosis, pelvic inflammatory disease (1)? | |
| Do "virus infections" aggravate chronic sinus and asthma (1)? Cause migraines, head pains, or aggravate a constant background head pain (1)? | |
| Do your peak flow readings vary for no apparent reason or not correlate with your physical activity (1)? Do the muscles between your ribs ache and prevent you from taking a deep breath (1)? | |

| | |
|---|---|
| Is your skin itchy, constantly red, supersensitive, or do you perspire excessively (1)? Do you have fluctuating "pins and needles" or numb sensations (1)? | |
| Do you have fluctuating muscle strength in your limbs or back (1)? Fluctuating joint pain (1)? RSIs/tender points; neck, back, and shoulder pain (1)? | |
| Have you variable visual effects and/or unsteadiness (1)? No-cause itching, burning eyes (1)? Chronic pain in or around an eye (1)? Does your child suffer from glue ear (1)? | |
| No causes found, no effective therapies for IBS, celiac disease, CRC (1)? Chronic diarrhea, frequent or foul motions, burning indigestion (1)? Fluctuating liver/gall bladder, "Hepatitis-like" symptoms (1)? | |
| Did home exclusion of certain foods and beverages or an exclusion diet give little or no relief (1)? | |
| **TOTAL** | |

Chapter 3

# Getting Acquainted
# with the Preliminary Work-Up
# and Multiple Latent Virutherapy

## LATENT VIRUSES AND THE LINK WITH ALLERGY

### Active and Latent Viruses: What Are They?

**IK** "What is a hidden virus, doctor?" It is the first question people ask me on arriving at the clinic. They want to know why they have vague, changing, undiagnosed symptoms that are given the labels of psycho-somatic, affective, or dysfunctional. A hidden virus is a latent virus, stealth virus in medical jargon. The dictionary defines latent as present, but not showing. Hidden viruses gradually bring about a wide range of vague symptoms in people who constantly, or at times, suffer periods of unex-plained tiredness from fatigue and/or faulty memory. Their motivation disappears; they cannot concentrate on work, beginning or finishing a job, or any mental activity. Occasionally, the onset is sudden. Some call it, "the tiredness or mañana illness." Mañana in Spanish means tomorrow but is another way of saying, "You are unable to get up and get going," or "You have lost your motivation." Patients with hidden viruses frustrate their physicians because no causes for their symptoms are found from clinical examinations, laboratory tests, and medical technologies.

"Why are hidden viruses different from other viruses? I know when I have a viral head cold or influenza." I explain, "The viruses we all know, such as mumps, measles, chicken pox, and shingles, are active viruses. Our family physicians recognize the active viral infections and send us for blood tests to confirm the diagnoses. The blood tests report the presence of antibodies to the active viruses, indicating the body's blood immunity is dealing with the active infection."

Put another way, common human viruses are *active* and *latent*. Latent means hidden activity, whereas an active virus is one causing recognized viral infections. A latent virus causes ill-defined symptoms that are usually dismissed as subjective or functional. Laboratory testing detects no antibodies for latent viruses. If you get run-down or your immunities are depressed, latent viruses could be the cause of your tiredness and functional symptoms. It is not known why latent viruses do not leave any antibody marker or memory in our blood immune system, called the natural immune system (NIS). There are no inexpensive latent laboratory tests available. The PCRT sometimes detects latent virus DNA in blood and biopsies of body tissues. A clinical allergy test called provocation and neutralization is modified to detect latent viruses and to provide a starting treatment dose. I am often asked, "What sort of a virus is the HIV, the AIDS, virus?" I reply, "At present researchers consider it an active virus because it stimulates blood antibodies." The HIV virus test is positive if antibodies are present. Researchers suspect there is a latent form of HIV, as many with obvious AIDS have negative antibody tests for HIV but positive PCRTs. If a concentrate of HIV proteins were available, serial dilution provocation with HIV might be a way of confirming the presence of HIV in a latent form.

### Are Latent Viruses Living in My Body?

Latent viruses invade our bodies by stealth during a viral infection or vaccination. They slip past our bloodstream's immune system to enter our organ cells. The various viruses are attracted to preferred organs; for example, respiratory syncytial virus prefers the lung and brain (tropism). Medical science has developed harmless weakened living viruses that protect us against the same active viral infection. Vaccination stimulates blood antibodies and *(surmise)* places latent viruses in organ cells. The provocation neutralization test (PNT) will not detect latent viruses unless there is an excess in organ cells. Should you suffer a serious loss of health or fitness and the latent viruses are no longer controlled, they spread and enter more body organ cells to bring on fatigue and neurotic symptoms. Provocation neutralization testing will then detect excess latent viruses.

Do not worry about latent viruses in your tissues. Keep healthy and fit and your bodily defenses, the blood natural immune system, and individual organ cell immunities will protect you from active viral infections and a dangerous buildup of latent viruses. Persisting unexplained functional mind and memory symptoms and fatigue continue during prolonged SSD courses. Multiple latent virus symptoms do not figure in clinical textbook descriptions of symptoms and causes of illnesses. You may think—or ask—"What is this latency immune system? Why do we need it? Isn't the blood immune system adequate?" I reply, "Wait until you read the section One or Several Immune Systems?" (see pp. 145-147).

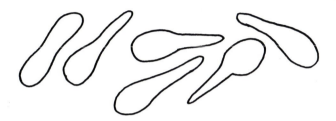

### *Why Suspect Latent Viruses?*

Patients' views and opinions are important to me. Read what these people told me at their first visit to the clinic. Provocation neutralization testing detected latent viruses in all of them, and the treatment doses helped them to return to normal health.

- Conventional and alternative therapies improved my health, but I am not yet back to the health I remember when I was well months ago. No more treatment is offered. The possibility of viruses causing my symptoms was discussed with a physician, but, sadly, he could offer no explanation or therapy. My symptoms continue.
- I read a lot of books and pamphlets at the Chronic Fatigue Association. The information did not help me to understand my strange and untreatable illness. It was suggested that a chronic type of virus could be stirring up the variable intensity of my symptoms. The paperbacks on chronic fatigue suggested rest and psychological help. That was all. I could not afford the expensive treatments they recommended.
- The onset of my illness was sudden, as if an infection had occurred, but all the laboratory tests were normal. It has continued this way over the months, but I am no better.
- I had an illness like glandular fever that I seemed to recover from after I had several antibiotic courses. Some months later my health deteriorated. My symptoms were diagnosed as functional or psychological because a complete and thorough hospital examination was normal.
- My mother remembers a severe, viruslike illness I had as a child. She thinks the physician who attended me diagnosed it as one of the childhood fevers. My health remained poor following this illness, and I have

always been less active and weaker than my friends. Over the past six months I became very tired and developed psychological-like symptoms. All the tests are normal, but I'm sure *that virus* is still in me.

- I had a severe vaccination reaction and/or I had a strange illness several weeks after the vaccination. I now think the vaccination was responsible for my present tiredness and symptoms. I improved for two to three months after an allergic work-up for inhalants and foods. The diet was difficult, and I gave up. The symptoms returned.
- In spite of the allergy work-up, the symptoms started to return again, but not as bad as when I started the work-up.
- I had an allergy work-up and was treated for *Candida*-related complex. I took nystatin drugs. Sugar and honey were restricted. Symptoms were aggravated for three to five days and then I improved a lot. The nystatin tablets were no longer helping me six weeks later. I increased the dose (and the expense), but it has not made any improvement. All through the treatment I continued the allergy advice and shots.
- **IK**   I attended an allergist who gave me serial titration and provocation neutralization testing and therapy. In addition, I took nutritional supplements and started a rotary diet. Later, therapy was given for CRC symptoms. *Giardia* was diagnosed and treated. I had a good response, but I still get relapses lasting a few days or one to two weeks. They usually occur when I have a head cold or the flu. I reckon I am 70 percent improved, but not back to the health I remember.

I selected this mixed bag of patients who were sure their fatigue and functional symptoms had a viral cause. Many and varied are the original causes of their illness: a severe skin burn; an anaesthetic; a severe or prolonged exposure to antibiotics; severe side effects from drugs or antibiotics, an anaphylactic attack, a trip to the tropics or the East, a mosquito, wasp, or animal bite; working in a "sick" building or in a toxic trade; and recreational drug use. Marijuana/cannabis appears to markedly increase susceptibility to multiple latent viruses.

### The Strange Symptoms of Latent Virus Overload

This book describes a wide range of bizarre and functional symptoms with which you may identify. You will be convinced they are for real when latent virutherapy provokes or aggravates and then relieves them. Latent viruses add to or change symptoms of nonviral and allergic illnesses. They alter the effects of drugs, in particular, symptom suppression drugs.

**IK**   A woman in her early thirties is now coping very well on allergy, CRC, and MLV. Many of her bizarre and strange symptoms, diagnosed over the years as functional, are improving. In the past she had little or no help from her family physician. She no longer mentioned the symptoms to the physician because they were considered to be "all in her head." She lost confidence in the medical profession because she believed the earlier treatments were arranged or pre-empted before she put a foot in the family physician's room. She no longer wanted to talk about her symptoms with close friends and relatives for fear of being branded "neurotic." Whenever the symptoms were present she felt guilty. She called these unreal, "not to be talked about" symptoms, her "functional fantasy." She was most surprised when several of her fantasy "sickies" were brought on or provoked by multiple latent virus testing. After two further testing sessions she summed up the courage to speak to me. It was a great relief to her when I agreed the strange and bizarre symptoms could be provoked by latent viruses. Two months later, after more testing sessions and three serial vaccination courses, one of which was hepatitis, all her fantasy symptoms disappeared. She was still afraid that the symptoms would relapse. Some three years later she sleeps at night, without fear of being woken up by terrifying dreams, which were brought on by latent hepatitis. Her fantasy symptoms have not recurred.

### Where Is the Link with Hidden Latent Viruses and Allergy?

Multiple latent virutherapy is a new concept of diagnosis and treatment for many conditions, including those with vague neurotic symptoms. Latent virutherapy by itself appears to treat some of the active virus symptoms, but when combined with allergy therapy, it becomes an important tool in the patient's recovery. The virus link with allergy, CRC, and some medical therapies is valid when the patient returns to previously remembered health and again is active and happy. So obvious is the benefit of The Virus Allergy Link that medical treatments are reduced, modified, and often stopped.

Many patients had benefits from other medical treatments before attending the clinic, but the improvement was not sufficient to return them to remembered health. Some who recovered remembered health later suffered relapses, usually from an influenza infection. Relapses are always a threat, but the latent virutherapy-allergy linkage markedly reduces, and often eliminates, the risk of these influenza relapses. The improvement in memory and well-being that the linkage brings is far superior to either virutherapy or allergy therapy alone. Come to think of it, a considerable number of people condemned to the "diagnostic rubbish or trash bin" when the SSDs failed are freed by these therapies.

The following are latent virutherapy-allergy links:

1. *The sinusitis link:* Conventional allergy work and antibiotics are disappointing until latent virutherapy is linked up using influenza, respiratory syncytial virus, and adenovirus.
2. *The asthma link:* Allergy therapy improves the airways of the lung and raises peak flow readings. MLV improves the air sacs' (alveoli) exchange of oxygen, carbon dioxide, and toxin excretion in the breath (pp. 42-43). People with asthma find their energy markedly improves, and they become warmer and look a better color. Most are able to stop their inhalers and other SSDs.
3. *The irritable bowel syndrome link:* Food allergies are present, but improvement varies with therapy and elimination of suspected foods. Latent virutherapy enhances the response when polio, hepatitis, mumps, adenovirus, rotavirus, and CMV are used. The symptoms from accidentally eating an allergic food are decreased, and several previously allergic minor foods can now be eaten without symptoms.
4. *The skin link:* Few chronic skin conditions will completely clear and remain clear of rash and itch with allergy therapy using dusts, molds, and foods. Latent viruses link up to allergy, and the two do a much better job of clearing the skin of symptoms and future relapses, using influenza, hepatitis, polio, morbilli, rubella, herpes, v. zoster, and EBV.

You will recognize more latent virutherapy-allergy links as you read about various diseases and conditions in Chapters 2 and 5. It is not known why the linkage of allergy and latent virutherapy produces such gratifying and enhanced results.

## CONSULTATIONS AND DIAGNOSIS

### How Long Are Consultations or Office Visits?

No symptom suppression drugs or treatments are prescribed for your symptoms because examination and laboratory investigations fail to find any causes. Allergy and virutherapy methods will probably find causes for your functional all-in-the-head symptoms. Do not expect a ten-, fifteen-, or twenty-minute visit. Be patient and expect visits to the testing room to last three to four hours. The checkup is not going to be easy for you, the nurses, or the physicians. But you will not be bored stiff, as there is plenty to read and learn while the testing continues. You discover new explanations for those strange undiagnosed symptoms that come upon you from time to time, or that keep you company day in and day out, messing up your life. Your past illnesses, injuries, and operations are described in the clinic questionnaire (see Appendix II). Tell the health professional any pertinent details regarding the questions you answered. Ask how answers that interested the health professional might affect your work-up and therapy. Past infections by viruses, bacteria, or unknown causes could be provoking your fluctuating symptoms. At least 80 percent of patients recall some past minor or severe head injury (see Head Injuries, p. 66). If you suspect, or vaguely remember, a head injury, for example, from a fall off a bike or out of a tree, it is possible your parents may recall the details. *Past injuries are very important,* as latent viruses seem to be attracted to damaged or bruised organ cells, especially brain neurons. Engage in conversation, as other patients in the testing room will be keen to discuss food preparations, recipes, and life-style changes.

**IK**  Charles, age 48, suffered from uncontrollable right-side migraine headaches that were accompanied by a nagging deep head pain. He had been frustrated at sports by the weakness on the left side of his body. Influenza, polio, and morbilli virutherapy resolved the right-side head pains and increased the power of the left arm and leg, almost equal to that of the right. He knew of a right-side head injury from a motorbike accident that he had suffered at age 16. His older sister recalled a fall off a horse when he was age 5.

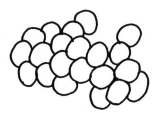

**Waiting for the Diagnosis (The Frustrating Consultation)**

Patients call it the frustrating consultation or office visit. Have you experienced the following at your family physicians' office? The physician sums up the examination, laboratory tests, and any medical technology reports. The interview proceeds as follows: "Mary, the tests and examinations are normal; the drugs and antibiotics have not helped you. It is possible you have a virus infection that will not go away. You will have to live with it till it clears." Mary asks, "What is the name of the virus and can you treat it?" Her physician replies, "The tests did not detect any viruses. There is no treatment for this sort of virus. I want to see you again in three months for a review."

Hundreds of people attending the allergy and virutherapy clinic experienced such consultations with their family physicians. Sadly, their viral symptoms did not go away as predicted. They tell me how they dreaded that crucial visit and felt let down because of the expense of the medical technology and specialist visits. It is comforting to know that you have no serious or dangerous condition, but many have lingering doubts in spite of their physicians' reassurances. They want to know *why* their fatigue, difficulty getting started or motivated, moods, and variable and unreliable memory were not matched to causes. There is no explanation given for their increasing pains, tenderness of muscles, changes in the way their organs are working, skin sensations, dermatitis, chest symptoms, and many other, often bizarre, symptoms.

Stress is suggested as a cause of their symptoms. To understand how stress is affecting them, they consult psychologists and psychiatrists. But after a period of failed treatments, they resent the suggestion that their personality is at fault, and being labeled as neurotic. They are sure, in their own mind and body, that the symptoms they are experiencing are *real,* not imagined or due to faulty brain activity. A trial of antidepressant drugs often improves symptoms. Unfortunately, antidepressant drugs interfere with latent virus testing and therapy. The drugs are reduced to minimal levels or stopped by about the third or fourth visit to the clinic, at which stage most patients have stopped their antidepressants.

Health books on allergy and CRC led many to consult allergists or physicians who specialize in these areas. They obtain little long-term benefit from the advice of allergists who use skin prick or scratch tests and SSDs, antihistamines, corticosteroids (Csds) and nonsteroid anti-inflammatory drugs (NSAIDs) for joint and fibromyalgia complaints. Another cause of failure is the allergist who restricts a diagnosis of food allergy to prick or scratch tests and blood immunoglobulins (RAST, ELISA food tests) (see p. 146). Many abandon conventional treatment to seek relief from alternative health professionals. Dieting and nutritional supplements at first improved many of their symptoms, but as the months went by, the old symptoms began to reappear. Many call this frustrating, expensive saga "the million-dollar work-up."

*The Million-Dollar Work-Up*

- "I've carried out all suggestions and therapies of the physicians and had surgery from the surgeons I consulted over the last three years. I spent a lot of time and money on psychological therapies. I don't think there is any improvement from all these treatments, and the relapses continue."
- "I had numerous examinations and received treatments that turned out to be ineffective. I had numerous blood tests and screening. All they tell me is that I do not have cancer, or any known progressive illness, and I should consider myself healthy. I know, however, there is something wrong going on inside me."

Symptom suppression medication depends on the patients' immunities improving while the symptoms are suppressed. But recovery during symptom suppression does not always occur, and when the course is finished, the symptoms of the illness reappear, sometimes with additional ones due to the toxic effect of the drug course. Attempts to suppress the symptoms for a further period, by increasing the dosage of the drug, usually fail. When it is obvious that the medical therapy has failed, the patient may be referred to symptom suppression surgery. Those with financial resources seek relief from alternative health operators. Eventually, the financial resources are exhausted and the patients complain of the frustrating useless therapies as "the million-dollar work-up."

### *Are You Losing Confidence in Your Physician?*

Why are you losing confidence in conventional medicine? Your physician was unable to *restore* your *remembered health* and *vigor*. Should you now visit another physician? You hesitate, as you do not want to go through another expensive duplication of laboratory and modern technology testing. Patients sum up their situation this way: They suspect their symptoms and illnesses are being fitted to the available laboratory and diagnostic technology. If their symptoms do not fit an accepted illness, they are given a diagnosis of functional, psychological, even neurotic/psychiatric problems and handed a referral to a psychiatrist. When the results of the investigation are given to them, they realize the laboratory tests and other technology were not related to their symptoms (inappropriate). Their physicians seem to be looking for one cause, whereas the patients have a gut feeling that their symptoms are the result of several causes.

Prior to visiting the clinic, patients experienced symptom suppression drugs and antidepressants, with little, if any, benefit as the months went by. Side effects became more of a burden; drugs and dosage were changed, often at considerable expense, but, sadly, they gained little or no improvement in their problems. They find it difficult to understand why their physicians consider their symptoms to be caused by stress. They are further disillusioned when little help is gained from seeing psychologists. By contrast, allergy therapy gives considerable relief from a restricted or modified lifestyle and food selection. Patients wish they had tried an allergy work-up before the psychological and psychiatric assessment. They no longer trust the "medical proof " scientific medicine because it failed them, and nonscientific medicine relieved their symptoms.

Do not let the experiences of these people change your mind about conventional, or scientific proof, medicine. You may need it for another illness in the future. Be aware that all who had help from virus-allergy therapy had a recent conventional medical clearance and examination before starting at the clinic. From time to time, someone's responses to clinic therapy raise the suspicion that they are harboring an underlying serious disease. These patients were referred back to their family physicians, who found they had the early stages of a serious disease or cancer (pp. 177-178).

"Scientific" or approved medical therapy places obstructions in the way of those who obtain no benefit. Scientific physicians cannot offer homoeopathy, bio-electrical medical therapy or acupuncture, because these therapies do not meet scientific medical standards. If a successful therapy is not on the approved treatment schedules, the Insurance Companies will not pay out on claims. Enquire of the college or academy promoting the unapproved therapy that successfully cleared up your illness, if they can help you to present a claim against your medical insurance cover.

### The Preemptive Syndrome

I told Mrs. C, "I would like you to go back to your family physician/ medical clinic to have your back passage and cervix checked out." "I am not going back to my family physician/medical clinic," she said, "not after all those long frustrating years of symptom suppression drugs, change-of-site symptoms and the expense. I am not going to let them tell me my symptoms are neurotic and give me the same old drugs as before." Her progress at the clinic greatly improved her health. She knows her neurotic symptoms and fatigue were caused by allergies and latent viruses. One of the meanings of preemptive is to forestall. She said to me, "Please suggest another family physician/medical clinic. If I go back to my old family physician, I will be told the improvement from the clinic is a placebo effect, and the physician will put me back on those nasty drugs."

I asked, "Why do you think this way?" She explained, "Whenever I went for an appointment I felt my physician had made up his mind what treatment to give me, before I stepped into the consulting office. It was all because of that visit to the psychiatrist/psychologist and the antidepressant drugs she gave me. It was an awful experience. What is more, I am not going to tell the physician and medical clinic what your treatment has done for me. They will not believe it is for real."

Hundreds of women and many men who attend the clinic show signs of the "preemptive syndrome." Most of them would go back to their family physician/medical clinic, if they could lay their hands on their medical folder or computer disk and throw away or delete the out-of-date and useless notes they know condemn them to a neurotic personality diagnosis. They would replace the case notes with an account of their successful therapy and a personal explanation as to why they thought it was effective. They would all like to see a change in the legislation on medical confidentiality that would allow them to supervise their clinical record notes (see The Preemptive Syndrome in Chapter 2, pp. 64-66).

**IK** The fatigue and dominance syndrome affects female patients who are worn out by food allergies, *Candida,* and latent viral illness. They give up and submit to their healthy male partners. Trouble develops when they recover their health, their figure, and take a part-time or full-time job. No longer will they submit. Domineering men lose their power over their partners. This may lead to divorce and separation. The men seem unable to accept the challenge to their authority. They are impervious to reasoning and logical explanations. The women tell me there was no dominance in the early years of their marriage, but that it gradually occurred during their long illness. Because their partners supported them and their families during the illness, and did not start another relationship, they wish to continue the marriage or partnership.

*Meet Wanda*

**IK** My Tuesday virus-allergy clinic got off to a great start when I opened the door. "I am feeling great, like I used to ten years ago. I do not believe it! What is to be tested today?" Wanda, a 35-year-old married woman, could not wait for her sixth visit to begin. I noticed the changes—more confident, more active, more alert, more body strength, more attractive skin and hair, more dress style, and other "mores." She read from her

Neurotic Notebook the mental and body changes since her last visit three weeks ago. "Look at my face—how it has improved. Will it stay improved? Will the dark circles and those small bags under my eyes return? Thank you for all you have done." What could I say? She had said it all. She is a changed person. Only months earlier she was despondent, tired, moody, and unable to function properly. I suggested the lifestyle changes and tested her responses to minimal amounts of sterile extracts (foods, molds, dusts, some microbe toxins, *Giardia* and *Candida,* plus a selection of viral extracts). All credit goes to her for the difficult changes to her way of life, but she loved it and was thriving on it. I will say no more because her case notes are in the Identikit (pp. xxiii-xxxv).

*Meet Jane on Her Third Visit*

"I'm having real difficulty and stresses doing this ecology stuff, but mother and dad are helping me at home. I feel worse when I am doing housework. It's terrible at lunchtime—oh, how I long for a slice of French bread, with my favorite honey piled on it, so that it drips off as I eat. When will I be able to eat that gorgeous food again? I know now why I feel so depressed and tired, and aching all over, and cannot remember—and, oh, my intestines are driving me mad with pains, noises, bloating, and smelly motions."

I cannot help feeling sorry for Jane, as she is experiencing a nasty burn-off of symptoms. She seems brave and determined to finish the work-up. You have to admire her, for I know of others who have given up at the third visit. Jane takes her place in the clinic and attempts to read, but the virus provocation makes her emotional and moody. She cannot remember a word of what she has just read. When the session is over and she is sitting in my office, she takes out her Neurotic Notebook and lists the symptoms and improvements for the past ten days. "There is some good news, Doctor, I had a great day—let's see—it was five days after I began the wheat and grain exclusion. Then there was another good day, the fourth or fifth, after starting the nystatin powder." A personal question finishes the session and she departs.

Three weeks later I answer the telephone. Jane, who did not attend the fourth appointment, speaks in a saddened voice, "I am worse than when I began the therapy. I was so excited after the second visit when for a few days I felt normal and strong again. I can't go on feeling so depressed, tired, and smelling so awful. I want to stop. My family physician wants me to start on antidepressants." It is a difficult situation. I have already warned her about antidepressants, and how they depress the organ cell immunity and detoxing (excretion), and often prolong the illness. I again explain that if she can stand the depression and other symptoms of excretion for another six to eight weeks, by then she should be well on the way to recovery. I remind her of the mirror medicine analogy (p. 135). I caution her, "If you stop now you will soon feel fit and well, but may relapse within one to six months." I invite her to telephone me at any time, if her depressions become worrisome, and to make a future appointment, but she does not return to the clinic. Nine months later she returns to the clinic, having given up Prozac, and is now determined to complete the full work-up. This time she is markedly improved, almost recovered, in six months.

Eight weeks later she comes to my office. "I want you to see how fit and well I am. I have a new job and am just loving it because I am full of energy and can remember details now. My motivation is great. Mother tells me I hardly ever get mad or moody these days. I'm so relaxed. If my friends talk about their problems and complaints, I just let them rave on. I sympathize, but do not get involved. I have so much energy I do not need to go to bed until 11:00 or 12:00. I love parties because I do not have to go home before they finish. I have given up all hope of eating wheat and grains, but I know a lot about cooking. The wheat and grains are no good for me. I get so tense and irritable. My friends envy my slim figure and complexion. Oh, by the way, has Liza seen you yet?"

"Yes," I reply, "Liza has attended twice, hasn't she told you? Please help her through any difficult periods of detoxing." Jane consults her Neurotic Notebook. "I won't ever forget the six weeks after finishing the course. The EBV symptoms were terrible, I knew there was no other therapy that would help me, and I did not want to try antidepressant drugs again. Mother says she never wants to have that glandular fever smell around the house again." As she stands to leave, I contrast her charming manner, confidence, figure, and complexion with the sad depressed Jane of eighteen months ago.

## DIAGNOSIS AND THERAPY METHODS

### Tell Me About the Preliminary Work-Up and MLV

"But what is the treatment, Doctor? I can learn about these viruses later." I give them a short explanatory pamphlet. "You have already had some, or most, of the preliminary work-up with the investigations and blood tests you told me about. Thank you for the old laboratory reports you brought for me to review."

The preliminary work-up includes allergy investigation and testing of dusts; house dust mites; inhalants, such as mold spores, pollens, foods, and chemicals; CRC and other molds; *Giardia;* and a number of bacterial toxins.

> "We check the methods and test results of your treatments before coming to the clinic. Some tests need repeating in a different way. Some new investigations could detect further causes. Much of your previous testing will not need repeating. We use the tests and treatments that appeared to help you to reduce the number of testing sessions. The three or four main foods in your diet are tested again, using provocation of delayed provoked symptoms."

Two or three clinic visits complete the preliminary work-up. Patients early on called it "preliminary" because it is completed before virutherapy.

Multiple Latent Virutherapy begins with polio, influenza, hepatitis, and morbilli, each tested separately by provocation. MLV can take from three to six clinic visits. During the first three years of the clinic, several groups of patients had MLV before "all that allergy testing." Nothing much happened, and all agreed to the preliminary work-up and a repeat of the MLV. This time all patients received help. Some were restored to normal health. I cannot explain why this order, the preliminary followed by the MLV, of investigation gives better results.

Active viruses are different. Immediate virus provocation and neutralization stops the symptoms of a flu infection (see Staving Off the Flu, p. 169), or the vesicles of herpes on the lips, as well as the hearing loss, tinnitus, and unsteadiness when the hearing and balancing organs are affected by a flu.

### The Interaction of Food Exclusions and MLV

Please understand that the variable intensity and type of symptoms are at first due to the food exclusion and mold treatments. The exclusion of foods, especially the Old World grass grains, wheat, barley, oats, rye, rice, and millet, may start an explosive and severe symptom withdrawal. *Candida* toxins are released when the levels of *Candida* in the bowel are lowered by exclusion of sugars, processed carbohydrates, and anti-*Candida* drugs, such as nystatin/Triazole drugs. A typical response is depression, crying bouts, and the onset of familiar symptoms. But keep telling yourself, there is no social reason for the depression and crying. As the excess allergic food molecules and *Candida* toxins come out of your body, they stimulate the changes in behavior and symptoms of your illness. When the overload of latent food and mold toxins is reduced, the viral provocation becomes significant, allowing for more accurate doses in the detoxing shots. MLV brings further aggravations and then a gradual clearing of symptoms. By now, the body's immunities and detoxing are improving, so you experience days when you feel great. It is disappointing when CMV, EBV, dengue, or another virus adds a fresh crop of symptoms and increases detoxing smells. Regular saunas and heat therapy boosts detoxing, and it is at this stage that petrochemicals are recognized by their chemical smells. Those who used recreational drugs in the past are surprised when their bodies detox the familiar smells and they experience sensations of the drugs. Cannabis detoxing has a sweet grass or fresh hay smell that pervades the testing room.

This is not the time to make a food indiscretion, as the progress of improvement and detoxing may be halted for a week or more. When the symptoms are severe, try to resist the impression that the therapy is failing. Now is the time to tell yourself that if nothing was happening, the treatment would be useless. Beware conventional medical logic that suggests the improvement should continue, as it does with symptom suppression drug therapy, unless there are "side effects." Logic is not easily applied to biology and the workings of our mind and body.

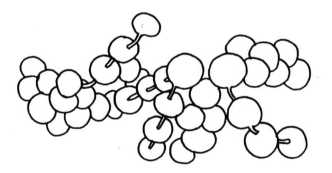

### Tell Me About MLV Methods

Latent viruses are different. They are detected by the provoked or stimulated symptoms from very dilute doses. They cannot be detected with accepted allergic testing methods, e.g., skin scratch or prick tests, RAST/ELISA/ALCAT testing, and skin endpoint titration (SET).

Virus proteins are concentrated and purified by fractionation and sterilized by heat, chemicals, and gamma radiation. The much altered viral concentrate is mixed with glycerin to preserve its potency. The concentrate is diluted in a series of vials, each one five times more diluted than the previous one (see discussion under Treatment Station Supplies, p. 6, and Serial Dilutions Chart, p. 36). To start testing the patient, a dilution is chosen that fits the examination results and questionnaire regarding the illness. The insulin syringe is filled to 0.05 to 0.1 ml, and the dose is injected into or beneath the skin for adults. For children, two to five drops of the chosen dilution, and five to ten drops of glycerin, as a sweetener, is placed on the tip of a teaspoon. The tip is then placed or slipped under the tongue. The timer is set for ten to fifteen minutes, and you should note any clearance or aggravation of symptoms, especially those you recognize from your illness, *provocation of symptoms.*

The testing is continued with more-dilute doses of the same virus, which may cause the symptoms to change, until the health professional is satisfied a suitable dose is reached and the provoked symptoms relieved, *the neutralizing dose.* The next virus is tested in a similar manner. An average three- to four-hour testing session allows four to five viruses to be tested. Instead of provoking symptoms, some patients begin to smell, as the body starts to detoxify in response to the provocation.

Latent viruses bring on delayed provoked symptoms at (a) four to twenty-four hours, *delayed;* (b) during the next three days, *extended delayed;* and (c) five to seven, even ten, days, *prolonged delayed.* Delayed responses are the important indications for the first treatment doses. *You must contact the office* on the *following day* and report any body changes and the provoked symptoms' severity and duration. Your memory can let you down after a provocation session at the clinic, so record the symptoms in the Neurotic Notebook (see Chapter 4, p. 156) when they occur.

The treatment dose is worked out from the delayed provoked symptoms and, to a lesser extent, from any immediate provoked responses. Some days later you receive a 2 ml or 5 ml vial with 2 ml sterile treatment fluid. Each vial contains thirty-plus doses, each of 0.05 ml.

At the next testing visit you are shown how to give yourself treatment shots, similar to diabetics who self-administer their insulin shots.

The number of office treatment visits are two to three for the preliminary work-up, and six to seven for the multiple latent virutherapy testing. The visits are at one- to two-week intervals, with three- to four-week resting periods after every two visits.

Testing sessions of three to four hours pass quickly. There is plenty of reading material at the clinic to help you understand and get to know your illness and the therapy. This is the time to ask the health professional any questions you may have. You can ask others attending the clinic about recipes and how they have coped with their symptoms and treatment to date.

If your illness is moderate and easy to investigate, you will notice improvements by the third to fourth visit. More severe illnesses and symptoms take longer for the return of remembered health.

If you were unlucky enough to develop your illness after one of the herpes virus illnesses, e.g., herpes, chicken pox, cytomegalovirus (CMV), glandular fever (EBV), or dengue fever, your recovery will take six to eight months, or longer.

Beta-blocker drugs can cause unpleasant reactions. If you are not sure about the drugs you are taking, ask your physician. For your own information, look up in the medical drug handbook the side effects of *all* the drugs you are taking.

MLV is a mirror image of conventional symptom suppression drug medicine, except that when recovery occurs, it persists.

### What Is Required of Me?

The very nature and variety of subjective, psychosomatic, and functional symptoms, together with the variety of suggested treatments, means there are many causes. Some causes will elude detection because medical technology and clinical expertise are not exact sciences. Be honest with yourself and with the physician. Both parties must be frank about symptoms and treatment. There can be no "pulled punches." Recovery depends 80 to 85 percent on *your* compliance, understanding, and reporting of symptoms. The physician's 15 percent is the selecting of testings and treatments until you recover.

I tell patients, without apology, "Carry the Neurotic Notebook with you wherever you go. Get into the habit of jotting down your symptoms and the provoked effects that come on after testing sessions, or if you make a food indiscretion." These symptoms could be meaningful. The early stages of treatment can upset your memory recall and motivation, so jobs around the house or at work are neglected. Do not be afraid; jot down what is happening to you, any bizarre symptoms or strange dreams that you have experienced in the past, which are frequently provoked by latent virus activity. Once treatment is under way, you and your physician will forget to use the words neurotic, hysterical, functional, and psychosomatic because you and the family physician discover your symptoms have real causes. Read all that is available on the subjects of allergy, CRC, *Giardia*, and information on latent viruses that your physician recommends. Ask if there are notes available from the clinic's office. Read them several times, with care, as local conditions are important in the treatment and are not considered in this book.

A difficult period awaits you while the allergy, mold, petrochemical, toxin, and multiple latent viruses are detoxed and return to safe levels in your body. This process cannot occur overnight. The clinic does not use symptom suppression methods or drugs because they depress, or halt, detoxing. There are no treatment magic bullets. A change of lifestyle is required and you will be asked to eat a different selection of foods for three to six months. During the work-up and treatment, a small number of people do not suffer any symptom aggravation and continue to improve until recovery. The majority suffer aggravation of some, or all, of their known symptoms and must withstand detoxing and symptom aggravation that continue for weeks. In desperation, some begin to regard the symptoms as worse than the original disease and want to quit. *But hold on!* Consider the following:

1. If testing and treatment were having no effect, you would agree that the treatment should be stopped.
2. An improvement or worsening of symptoms means the latent viruses and toxins within your organ cells are being affected and detoxed by shots of very high dilutions (i.e., very weak) of viral protein.
3. Your partner and relatives notice, at times, strong smells coming off you when symptoms are aggravated because the toxins and viruses are leaving your body. You notice that your urine and motions have strong smells.
4. Detoxing is an encouraging sign that the treatment is working, even though symptoms are aggravated.

Complying with the treatment regime and dealing with the temporary aggravation of symptoms eventually brings about recovery of your body and mind. You continue the important instructions and food exclusions, while maintaining your new lifestyle after you recover. Many patients believe the best reward for their putting up with these restrictions is no more severe or frequent relapses. I commonly hear from people after they complete the work-up, "It is just how I remembered my health and mental activity before the awful illness began."

If after reading this book, the list of "You must do this or that" is too much for you and you put the book down, I will understand. About 20 percent who request investigation and treatment discover after a month and two or three visits that they are not prepared to make the lifestyle adjustments necessary for full recovery. The successful patients are those who are determined to get started, as they are suffering ill health, moods, and depressed feelings. Many determined, compliant people know a friend or relative who recovered with virus-allergy link therapy.

Read about how you can help your body to restore its immunities:

1. Be patient and complete the work-up.
2. Nutritional supplements (Callem, 1993; Galland, 1988).
3. Lifestyle changes (Rousseau, Rea, and Enwright, 1988).
4. Exclude from your diet fast foods, soda/soft drinks, alcohol, sugar, food chemicals, and foods devoid of nutritional content.
5. Healthy home ecology (Rapp, 1996; Rousseau, Rea, and Enwright, 1988; Shepherd, 1989).
6. The environment and workplace (see Chapter 4).
7. Hidden infection (see pp. 46-47).
8. Petrochemical and heavy metal exposure and toxicity (Huggins, 1993).
9. The immunities of the bowel or food tube and microbes, food toxins, xenodrugs, and antibiotics (see p. 181).

### The Virus-Allergy Link's Mirror Image

A woman who suffered CFIDS/ME for many years visited the clinic a year after her successful treatment and return to normal health. She recalled the symptoms and suffering she had experienced for six to seven weeks after the last visit. She had heavy detoxing from OWGGs, *Giardia,* and glandular fever. She likened her old illness to a *mirror image* of her recovered health. Everything about her was the opposite to the days when she was ill and on SSD therapy. Most people who recover identify with the therapeutic mirror image. The same symptoms or syndromes are treated by conventional medicine with SSDs. At every stage of the treatment, the responses to conventional medicine's SSDs, are the mirror image of responses to virus-allergy link (VAL):

1. Conventional SSDs quickly suppress most of the symptoms. VAL: preliminary work-up and MLV cause an aggravation of known symptoms after provocation testing and during treatment.
2. At three to four months, conventional medicine's SSD therapies may require increased dosage to keep symptoms suppressed, or a change of drug or different drugs may be used to control the side effects of the antidepressant or other drugs. VAL: preliminary work-up and

MLV at three to four months has brought about a detoxing of allergic food molecules, mold toxins, excess petrochemicals, and excess latent virus from the organ cells; the patient at this stage may feel much worse or is beginning to have days of recovered health.

3. At six to nine months, the SSD therapy of conventional medicine continues, if it does not require adjustment at three to four months. Now the patient suffers sufficient side effects for adjustments of the drug therapy and is resigned to a long period on drugs and to side effects that cannot be suppressed. VAL: the preliminary work-up and MLV patient is now off all drugs, has stopped using most of the virus shots, but may need to continue glandular fever and *Candida* shots every six to eight weeks for another year to a year and a half.

4. It is significant that nearly all patients attending the clinic who suffered one or more years of illness tried SSD therapy and, in time, began to hate it. They feared future years of SSDs, or resuming drugs for a relapse or return of symptoms. They are determined to try VAL therapy to be free of drug dependence. A small number of patients are so addicted to the antidepressant drugs they were given before attending the clinic that, despite several attempts to quit the drugs, they need to continue a low drug dosage, such as one-tenth or one-fifth of the recommended daily dose, for months or years.

A male contractor, age 46, had been an asthmatic for fifteen years before responding to latency therapy. He no longer needed asthma drugs but was unable to stop the antidepressants he had been taking for the past six years. Three and a half years and several attempts later, he broke his Prozac habit.

### How Do the Treatment Shots and Drops Work?
### Specific Latency Therapy

The physician decides on the treatment dose, not so much based on what provoked symptoms occurred during the testing session, but more on the delayed provoked symptoms you experience up to five to seven days after the testing session. *Surmise:* The empirical treatment dose jump-starts the excretion or detoxing of an increasing wave of *similar* latent virus from the body organ cells holding excess virus. As the virus is detoxed, symptoms are provoked, and most people notice body smells, often foul odors. The smells and stinks are in the sweat, breath, urine, or motions. Often the person who is detoxing cannot detect the odors because the body adapts or suppresses the sense of smell for what is being detoxed. Be careful not to offend others, and if possible, ask a trusted relative or friend to tell you if you are exuding stinking smells. Many people have to postpone social occasions during detoxing periods.

The testing and treatment viral shots are many hundreds, often millions/ billions, of times more dilute than the public health vaccination shots (see influenza A and B, p. 175). By law, a vaccination shot must contain a sufficient amount of virus protein to stimulate a person's NIS to form antibodies. Latent viruses, however, have little to do with the blood immunity system. They slip by the NIS and take up residence in our organ cells (genomes). This is why people suffering severe fatigue and symptoms from latent viruses have negative blood tests for virus antibodies (see Appendix I).

An amazing area, hidden away under the tongue (sublingual), samples almost everything passing our teeth. Minute amounts of substances pass through the thin overlying epithelium and enter the bloodstream, which distributes them throughout the body. These minute amounts alert the brain and body and, in particular, the gut and digestive organs to the makeup of the incoming meal and harmful/helpful substances. Latent toxins and microbes use the sublingual entrance to the body (see p. 198).

The sublingual area was used by ancient Greek and Roman physicians. Modern allergists have taken advantage of its effectiveness in testing young people for suspected allergic foods and inhalants and in drop therapy.

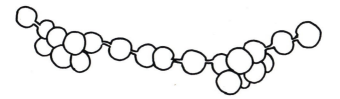

## *The Basics of Detoxing, or Ridding Your Body of Toxins and Latent Viruses*

Latent viruses forgot to ask for an antibody, but left a smelly visiting card.

A patient, 1994

Detox has many meanings in alternative health descriptions. The body chemistry reduces or neutralizes the toxic effects of a great variety of harmful substances entering our bodies. Excretion or elimination is the removal of harmful or detoxed substances from the body. Detoxing is the way the body rids itself of the numerous toxins and harmful substances it comes into contact with during life. Bacteria and single-cell organisms detox. It is a universal protective activity of all living things. (For a full account of detoxing [excreting] by VAL therapies, see pp. 184-188.)

*Nonspecific Detoxing*

*Heat detoxing.* Physicians of the ancient world knew sweating and heat treatments eliminated body toxins and vapors, hence, the old saying, "Sweat it out of your system and get rid of head colds and influenza." Before the antibiotic era, physicians could diagnose infections by the smell on the patient or in the patient's bedroom. Urine was intensely studied by ancient physicians.

*Natural detox.* We all know elimination occurs through urine, motions, vaginal discharges, the mucus and breath from the chest, and perspiration. You can tell you are eliminating something because of the different and, at times, nauseatingly strong smells. A small number of patients do not detox smells, yet they feel they are detoxing because of the provocation of known symptoms. I surmise that detoxing latentees of microbes, toxins, and other foreign materials are neutralized by antilatens (antibodies). *Surmise:* The latentee-antilaten complex has no detectable smell.

*Autosauna detoxing.* Fit people eliminate the day's noxious substances with the autosauna, in addition to the other methods of detoxing. You get into bed and fall asleep, and 2 to 3 h later your body heats up. You sweat profusely as the toxins are detoxed, sometimes so severe you wake in a bath of perspiration and have to change your night wear, even the sheets. Children detox through their scalp with the autosauna. If profuse, the damp and tainted pillowcase is changed and the pillow protected with a plastic cover. A few people have their autosauna during the day and change their clothes after a shower. Did you enjoy that hot chili meal? You may not enjoy the autosauna that follows, as the body detoxes chili toxins in the sweat and breath.

**IK**    The toxins of CRC, some molds, and latent viruses suppress the autosauna detox. *Candida* treatment and virutherapy will restore the autosauna. It is a common complaint. Women recovering from CRC resume autosaunas that make their beds smell like mushroom farms. You need a very strong desire to become tender and loving in a mushroom farm environment! If *Helicobacter* is being detoxed, the bed and urine smell like kitten urine. *Legionella* detox smells like dog or pig feces. If EBV is detoxing, the bed and bedroom take on a nauseating sick animal smell.

EBV and CMV bring about a false type of severe depression that makes you cry floods of tears. Patients collect the tears in sterile laboratory pots. The tears smell of EBV/CMV. These viruses eliminate in the increased clear nasal and chest mucus, and from the fingernail and toenail quicks. Some people notice that their mouth suddenly fills with smelly saliva, which lasts for 1 or 2 h. The back of the throat becomes painful, and medications do not relieve the pain. EBV is detoxing from the throat through the saliva and breath. No wonder EBV was originally called the "kissing disease." It is difficult to tell when natural autosauna detoxing or virutherapy detoxing is occurring during VAL therapy. Autosauna detoxing may not occur until *Candida* and virus shots are started. Even then, nothing may be detoxed until regular saunas are begun. A woman who suffered CFIDS/ME had three months of cautious VAL therapy before autosaunas began. The third MLV shot triggered the detoxing.

While elimination is occurring, your symptoms and smells fluctuate, until you suddenly realize that you have not been smelling for a week or more. In another three to four weeks, the smells may return for short periods, and then you feel very well, just as you remember before you became ill. A return of familiar smells and CFIDS/ME scary dreams, months or years later, warns you of a relapse. Be on the lookout so you can prepare a "relapse" treatment.

*Xenodetoxing.* Most xeno-SSDs are detoxed. Difficult xenodrugs are pesticides and herbicides. Xenochemicals do not occur in nature, which may account for some people being unable to excrete them, leading to accumulations with marked toxic effects. Examples are women who cannot tolerate the pill, and hyperactive children whose mothers find the pillowcases stained yellow from the yellow dye in drinks and foods they are consuming.

**IK**  A hairdresser who specialized in hair tinting for middle-aged women developed CFIDS/ME and retired, spending the next five years seeking a relief or cure, to no avail. She attended an ecology clinic and began the work-up. Two months later, on waking in the morning, she became alarmed when the sheets and pillowcases were a heliotrope color. It took six or seven weeks of detoxing the dye before she recovered her former health (refer to the green urine detoxing, p. 186).

Should you be accidentally exposed to paint or formalin fumes, head for the nearest sauna. The important effects of nutritional supplements and antioxidants in aiding and modifying detoxing are discussed elsewhere (see p. 186).

## The Bathroom Towel Test

Wash the bath towels with a nonperfumed detergent, and at the end of cycle, do two more water rinses. When doing a simple nonperfumed bar soap hand wash, use one or two water rinses. Hang out to dry. Take a long hot bath or shower using nonperfumed soap or shampoo. On getting out, shake or wipe off the excess water droplets from your skin. Dry your hair with a hand towel. Dry the rest of your body with a bath towel, taking 3 to 5 min and going over the body areas two or three times.

Sniff the towel; it may smell. Get dressed and sniff the towel again. If there is a smell, try to describe it as musty, chemical, sweaty, or animal. If no smell is present, hang out the towel to dry for use again on three or more occasions, if no smell detoxing occurs. The smell on the towel gives you the glad tidings that suddenly you are detoxing; thus, the therapy seems to be working. The smells vary from day to day. You may relate your symptoms and moods to the different smells on the towel. When you are down and depressed there may be a baneful bouquet of smells. As the toxin lessens, the smells decrease or disappear, and at the same time, you notice an improvement in your health.

## Virus Fears and Reassurances

We all know something about viruses, especially the HIV and influenza viruses. At an early age we are vaccinated to protect against active viral infections. Many of us experienced unpleasant childhood illnesses. No longer do we see the terrible complications of childhood active virus infections that past generations of parents feared. Here are comments I jotted down during interviews:

- I distrust viruses. I do not want any in my body.
- Viruses scare me, even though I know head cold and flu viruses are not dangerous.
- You do not know what is happening in your body when viruses affect you.
- The news media have stories on viruses that cause cancer. Could hidden viruses do that?
- I do not like the idea of living viruses like polio and flu being put in my body by vaccination shots or drops.
- Viruses give me the creeps. I read of a young woman recently whose heart was damaged during a viral infection, and she had to have a heart transplant.

- What about those children who died or were maimed by vaccinations?
- The AIDS virus scares me, I'm afraid other viruses will increase my chances of catching it.

I will indirectly answer some of these fears.

The good side of viruses does not get much publicity in the media. Reporters prefer to dramatize the disasters to grab the headlines. An example is a recent Ebola virus scare and the improbable implication by the media that we could be facing a pandemic. Confusion arises because latent viral infection is mistakenly thought to be similar to active viral infection. The previous eight comments are related to active viral infections. I convinced nearly all patients who expressed similar ideas about viruses to proceed with the preliminary work-up and MLV. No one suffered any permanent aggravation of symptoms from provocation testing or the detoxing shots. Latent virutherapy has a clean record. The hundreds of patients seen over the fourteen years had no persistent or permanent provoked symptoms. All who temporarily suffered marked or severe provoked symptoms recovered to their level of health before the provocation testing and went on to improved health or full recovery.

The testing dilutions contain dead, inactivated, and modified viral proteins. Common dilutions for treatment doses are $5^8$, a dilution of one part of altered viral protein to 390,625 of water, or $5^{12}$, one part to 244,140,625 of water (see Dilutions Chart at the end of Chapter 1, p. 36). These huge dilutions, by themselves, cannot bring on symptoms and cause you to excrete strange smells. The symptoms and smells are caused by the release of quantities of the same or similar latent viruses or toxins in your body cells. This is confirmed as the detoxing continues. The levels of latent virus symptoms and smells decrease. You begin to notice improvements in health and mental activity. The viruses and toxins coming out of you may have been in your organ cells for years, following a vaccination or an active viral infection in childhood. Organ cells appear to have a fantastic memory for past infections because they harbor, in a latent form, the virus or toxin. The blood immune system retains a memory of the infections through the blood cells and antibodies. In time, many of these memories disappear. It is unfortunate that conventional medicine depends on the antibodies for evidence of past infection or exposure. *Surmise:* Latency therapy gives superior memory recall. The problem, with latent memory requiring some of the original infectious agent or toxin to be held in the organ cells, is the ability of the latent organisms to increase if overall immunities are depressed. Patients may ask, "But what proof have you,

Doctor, that latent viruses exist and can cause the illnesses you talk about?" A reassuring explanation takes time.

Patients and physicians involved in virutherapy are frustrated by the lack of "scientific" proof of latency diagnosis and treatments. There is no response in the blood immune system and difficulty with arranging controlled and double-blinded studies. Over the past ten years I have been unable to get patients to agree to act as controls. They rightly refuse the delay of nine to fifteen months before their treatment starts. Patients participating in controlled studies were put off by the financial or other inducements and the personalities of the supervising physicians (Skaloot, 1993). The cost of controlled studies restricts the numbers. Can forty or fifty people's results, even the pooled results of 1,000, be applied to 100 million people? For every 100 people taking part in the controlled study, a few (i.e., three to four or more) will experience aggravation of their symptoms or drug side effects. If 100 million treatment doses are put on the world market, 3 or 4 million people will have no benefit or complain of symptom aggravation and side effects. Some of them will start litigation. In time, the amount paid out for litigation reduces the profits, and the drug is withdrawn. Controlled studies attempt to standardize the drug dose. Modern medicine is far too busy to bother about fitting the dose to the patient because of the short consultation times. By contrast, provocation neutralization sets the individual treatment dose. As treatment progresses, further neutralizing doses are found. If the original drug was matched to the patient's symptoms, there would be no need for a new expensive replacement drug. The rigidity of government drug regulating systems, the $80 million to $120 million for a single FDA approval of a drug forces pharmaceutical companies to favor the development of more expensive drugs rather than the tried-and-tested cheap drug that helps the majority of patients.

Latent viruses cannot be diagnosed without clinical testing using provocation neutralization, which was discovered by Dr. Carlton Lee in the late 1950s. Despite the lack of "scientific" proof, this technique has given relief to hundreds of thousands of allergy sufferers, with very few alarming responses. It is used by physicians in North America and Europe and has spread worldwide. As millions of patients in the future obtain benefit from the technique, the scientific proof argument will probably fade. There was no scientific proof testing when the pill was first introduced in Puerto Rico in the 1950s. In no time, it was gratefully accepted by women throughout the world. Little has been heard of the women who could not tolerate the pill, or who developed the various side effects and complications. A diagnosis of stress, psychological, or psychiatric symptoms, in most instances, is not scientific proof. Patients who experienced good results from the technique and MLV commented that they were "not interested in attitudes and arguments about scientific proof or the methods of conducting controlled clinical studies."

Latent viruses are not "xeno" or man-made, as is true of most of our symptom suppression drugs and antibiotics. Latent viruses seem to accumulate slowly in the cells that make up the organs, muscles, and fat of our bodies, often entering during infections, both serious and mild. Vaccinations using living viruses deliberately place latent viruses or genomes in our organ cells to help our various immune systems' defenses. A virus genome is the central part of the virus that has shed its outer shell or covering, called the capsid. Research work suggests that virus genomes are wrapped up and made harmless by certain proteins within our cells, possibly the heat shock proteins or stress proteins. If we neglect our level of health, or it is depressed by other means, latent viruses will increase and further interfere with the organ cells' activities, bringing on a variety of functional symptoms. The cell immunities are aided by the viral genomes. If similar wild viruses enter our body they cannot infect the cells because the inactivated genomes are present. The blood immune system eventually expels the wild viruses from the body. Sometimes the blood immune system has lost the memory for a particular virus or toxin. *Surmise:* If organ cells retain the original viruses they may be used as a template for the production of NIS antibodies.

Physicians' textbooks now recognize viral latency. The medical cumulative index listed a new heading, "VIRUSES, LATENT." The clinical results I observed during the past fourteen years lead me to predict that future editions of these references will include latency therapy, latency immunity, and latency diseases.

## THE PATTERNS OF BODY IMMUNITIES

### *Multiple Latent Virutherapy and the Body Immunities*

If you read articles and books on CFIDS/ME, you will know about the blood immunity activity, its white cell types, and antibody formation. Later books repeat this subject, adding a little more to your knowledge of the blood immune system, also called the natural immune system (NIS). When I ask patients about what they learned from the books, they reply, "It is all very interesting. There is very little useful therapy and no specific therapies." Some request expensive immunoglobulin therapy and interferon therapy, but few receive it. Others ask for antiviral drugs but are told there are dangers and considerable expense involved with their use. Most patients had courses of *Candida* and *Giardia* antibiotics, often with relief. The treatments are expensive, and the good result from the first course of therapy may not be repeated with further courses (drug resistance).

Leukocytes, the white cell warriors, with the help of complement and antibodies, kill the invading microbes or remove the foreign toxins and proteins from the NIS. Few books tell you about the fate of the gallant white cells and their broken-down or digested victims. Are they detoxed in the bile, from the urine, motions, or where? CFIDS/ME patients do not suffer from influenza or head colds while they are ill. Researchers found an increase of some immune activities in these patients, in particular, cytokines. Because cytokines are not found in all of these patients, another explanation could be the CSR (change-of-site response). *Surmise:* The immunity of the nose, chest, and muscles is so good that influenza appears as different symptoms in other susceptible organs. Instead of typical influenza symptoms during a community epidemic, CFIDS/ME patients suffer an aggravation of muscle pains and weakness, IBS, increased depression, faulty memory, and mood changes. They suffer no high fever, as would be expected, but their sweat, motions, and urine become increasingly smelly.

Provocation neutralization testing and virutherapy provoke smells in the sweat, urine, motions, breath, tears, and fingernail quicks, of all places. What is more, the smells vary: musty for molds, e.g., *Candida;* chemical for SSDs and petrochemicals; and animal-like smells from latent viruses. During an active viral infection such as influenza, at the height of the fever, the bedroom smells of influenza. Virutherapy and testing for latent hepatitis seems to jump-start the organ cells of the body to excrete some of their excess latent hepatitis, which has a fecal smell. Latent bacterial toxin from *Helicobacter* smells like cat urine. At times, there is a mixture of excretion smells.

The alimentary canal, call it what you may—food tube, bowel, guts—is a meeting place for microbes, foods, toxins, petrochemicals, and our Me and My immunities. Every effort to discipline and comply must be made by patients, if they want to regain normal bowel activity and levels of organisms (biosis). My patients are convinced that recovering normal bowel activity enhances the immunities of other parts of the body. If their bowel activity remains faulty, food allergies and toxin absorption will continue out of control. No amount of immune-boosting therapies, applied elsewhere to the body, will ensure a return to remembered health.

Active viruses are controlled by public health measures, vaccines, and, occasionally, antiviral drugs. Latent viruses do not respond to these methods. The provocation neutralization technique of Dr. Carlton Lee is a useful tool against latent viruses, some bacterial and mold toxins, and food allergy symptoms, such as the food immunization technique of Dr. Joseph Miller. The organ cell immunity probably began when bacteria and single-cell organisms (protozoa) developed protection against the environment. Multicell organisms later added tissue fluid and vegetation sap systems, and higher animals, blood systems. The immune processes became more elaborate and sensitive as evolution proceeded. Our blood immune system is a complex wonder, as are our "computer" brain activities. We are beginning to explore the wonders of our organ cell and resonance immunities.

### One or Several Immune Systems?

Blood tests are no more than a nuisance—a short, sharp prick in your vein and your dark blood is sucked into several plastic syringes. The blood goes to a laboratory machine for processing, and the results are back at your physician's office in no time. Your blood immune system, the NIS, makes antibodies to an amazing variety of substances that invade or enter your body. The media and television frequently report on new discoveries related to the NIS. The reliance on blood tests and other medical technology, X rays, scanning, and magnetic resonance imaging (MRI) gives the impression of "scientific medicine," which leads to "proof" diagnostic medicine. Scientific has a different meaning for physicists and chemists. A better medical term would be *sci* (science) + *dotal* (anecdotal) = *scidotal.*

If your symptoms and illness fit into the natural immune system, you can expect treatment. But what if they do not? What if the physician practices "proof" medicine and diagnoses your symptoms as functional or "all in your head"? The patients I see appear to have insufficient NIS activity to aid their symptoms. They complain that their symptoms were fitted to the laboratory machines instead of the machines being fitted to their symptoms. This is a tragic weakness of "proof" medicine because more and more people have symptoms that cannot be explained by laboratory machine results or medical technology, even though patients are positive their symptoms are real. "No proof" clinical medicine helps most of these people. Other immune system activities could be the reason for their successful treatments. Difficulties interpreting the reports of laboratory and medical technologies occur when the patient's illness/symptoms lie outside the affirmed scientific medicine description, for example:

1. RAST, ELISA, and ALCAT tests for food allergies are negative, or false positive, despite obvious food reactions, which are conveniently called intolerances.
2. The PCRT for DNA recognition is not always reliable. It requires body secretions or fluids, even a biopsy (a small piece of tissue from your body). Few, if any, patients are going to agree to a removal of tissue from their organs.
3. Physicians have difficulty interpreting the blood laboratory antibody results from chronic infections, such as CRC, *Chlamydia,* and the herpes virus group, in particular, CMV and EBV.
4. Because antibody tests for active viruses are negative, patients are told their symptoms are not caused by viruses. There are no blood tests for latent viruses. MLV detoxes excess latent viruses, and the patients recover their health.
5. Dr. Oettgren and his team bred mice with no Ig E. The mice developed asthma despite past "scientific" proof that Ig E must be present before asthma can develop and that the drugs used for asthma influenced patients' Ig E. This new discovery questions the accepted mode of action of asthma drugs (Mehlhop et al., 1997).
6. Problems occur in identifying the microbes of unusual or infrequent infections because the physician may misinterpret the clinical signs or the organisms are difficult to identify or culture.

*Surmise:* During evolution a primitive NIS evolved for multicellular animals and plants. The individual cells did not surrender their immune capabilities. At present, an open mind on total body immunities is prudent, until further research work comes to hand.

Five immune systems are suggested, with many small localized body cell group immunities:

1. *Natural immune system.* This system develops antibodies against an amazing variety of substances that enter the body.
2. *Organ cell immunity.* Note, not to be confused with the NIS's cellular immunity. The individual cells of the various organs, muscles, and structures of the body retain an inherent immunity. The organ cells have a limited ability to inactivate a wide range of substances that enter the cell and reside in the nucleus/cytoplasm. The cells survive by inactivating/tolerating the foreign material (latentee). The presence of the latentee in the cell affords immunity protection against a similar latentor. Detoxing is an organ cell activity.
3. *Vibratory or resonance immunities.* The techniques of medical bioelectrics are rapidly advancing, based on modern homeopathic and

Chinese acupuncture therapies. Certain people are profoundly affected by high-voltage and other forms of electrical waves. Medical bioelectric therapy has, on occasion, started detoxing of xenochemicals.

4. *Cerebral immune system.* The microglia/astrocytes cells of the brain have the important functions of protecting and regulating the environment and nutrition of nerve cells (neurons) of the brain and spinal cord.

5. *Digestive immune system.* The powerhouse of the body's immunity uses up to 70 percent of total immunity to control the "1,001" microbes and other matter that enter the gut. It includes the gut lining with surface cells, enterocytes, NIS cellular immunity, Peyer's patches, and the sublingual or absorption area of the mouth.

You can assume that during periods of health and fitness, the immunity systems work as a team, but in times of illness, one, or more, of the systems fails to perform, and its activities may not be taken over by the remaining immune systems. Other immune systems have been evolved by insects, plants, and animals (e.g., surface secretion and saliva tongue systems of fish and frogs).

For further information on the different immune systems, see texts on microbiology for numbers 1, 4, and 5, and texts on bioelectric therapy, homeopathy, and acupuncture for number 3.

### Multiple Latent Virutherapy and Change-of-Site Response

The change-of-site response is the body's way of sharing allergic reactivity among its different organs. As one organ/area is fatigued by the chronic allergic response, another organ develops the allergic inflammation and symptoms. There are age-related organ changes for allergic people from infancy to old age (see CSR pp. 194-197). Surgical operations may cause a change-of-site response. After the removal of tonsils and adenoids, children develop allergic blocked noses, and a few, to the dismay of their parents, begin to suffer asthma two to three months after surgery. Six to nine months after a hysterectomy women report the onset of asthma, skin rashes, depression, etc. The same occurs several months after a gall bladder removal. The symptoms are skin infections, liver pain, eczema, sensitive skin, headaches, and unpleasant dreams. Responsible surgeons now recommend that obviously allergic patients undergo an allergy work-up before elective surgery is performed. If you are faced with elective surgery for chronic illness/symptoms, and you know you have allergic problems, proceed with an allergy work-up. If you get a good result there may be no need for the surgery.

Asthma symptoms and its prognosis when treated with Csds have changed so much that it is almost as if there is a new type of asthma today. Lowering the surface immunity with Csd aerosols allows bacteria, molds, viruses, and other microbes to invade the linings of the nose and chest. Their presence, together with the toxins they make, reduces some of the initial improvement from the Csd therapy. The microbes exert further damaging effects over the months and years of Csd therapy. Clear mucus changes to yellow, brown, or green, and attacks of influenza-like infections become more frequent. Other problems arise too. For example, since SSDs are man-made, in time, the body immunities react against them, bringing on mild toxic symptoms or side effects.

Some physicians deny that change-of-site response symptoms have an allergic basis. I am careful to describe symptoms of patients who responded and cleared with allergic exclusions, ecology measures, and withdrawal of drugs that brought on CSR. CSR can mimic or aggravate the symptoms of CFIDS/ME, especially when the brain and muscles are involved. The CSR effect is unmasked when Csds and other drugs are withdrawn. Csds and other drugs, by suppressing symptoms in one area, speed up the procession of allergic symptoms elsewhere. As one area's symptoms are suppressed, treatment is started on the next CSR body site, which in turn induces a CSR in another organ. So many CSR areas are being suppressed that the patient spends 40 min twice a day applying Csds and other drugs to various parts of the body. If the drugs are discontinued, and causes sought for the allergic symptoms, a reversal occurs. Sadly, many who started using nasal and chest Csd treatments did not recover from some of the induced CSR symptoms, such as asthma and skin rashes.

So extensive is the use of SSDs that the CSR concept is not recognized. The CSR symptoms starting in other areas or organs of the patient are regarded as new conditions that are in no way related to the original one. The increase in symptoms is thought to be due to a decrease in the individual's immune responses. Very soon you get into a specialists' circuit. Each specialist endeavors to suppress the symptoms in his or her special area. A common result is that overall health and mental activity deteriorate. I have not seen a CSR warning put out by a manufacturer of SSDs. Numerous papers by physicians and drug advertisements in journals and popular media keep a clean image of SSDs before the public. Texts on nasal allergy are published with drug company grants, so there is no mention of CSRs. The CSR is not described, only hinted at or implied, in medical and allergy books available to the public. If you think the description of CSR fits you, inform your allergist.

**IK**    A woman was given a "depot" Csd shot in the buttock because of severe pollinosis that resisted a desensitizing course of shots. It gave her relief for the season. The next year two injections were required, and she noticed a little chest wheezing. The following year three shots were required, and the wheezing returned, together with a mild skin rash. Toward the end of the season she developed hives and was given antihistamine drugs. The pollen season finished, but she noticed increasing mood changes for no apparent reason. Her memory and recall were deteriorating so much that she became anxious about holding her job. The job went when she suffered five attacks of influenza, each of which needed an antibiotic course. She attended the clinic for the preliminary work-up and virutherapy. She had a marked allergy to OWGGs and lost a lot of fat and the water retention over the following five to six months of exclusion. She returned to the slim figure of her early twenties but was shocked to find several inch-wide craters on her buttocks where she had received the depot injections. The scarring and fat absorption of the craters had been hidden by her fluid retention problem.

**IK**    The conjunctivitis that went "roaming." A woman was prescribed Csd eyedrops and a Csd nasal aerosol for conjunctivitis and nasal obstruction of three months' duration. Within another three months she required a Csd aerosol for asthma. Over the next three years she attended several specialists, as other CSR symptoms appeared and were treated (skin rashes, IBS, urinary tract symptoms, fibromyalgia, CRC, personality changes, and unexplained fatigue). The cost of the investigations and treatments was a huge burden on the family budget. The last two winters were a constant battle against chest infections and recurring flu. After a preliminary work-up and virutherapy course, she experiences only an occasional wheeze, controlled by salbutamol. She is free of CSR symptoms.

A patient who became frustrated with SSDs independently sought a preliminary work-up and MLV courses. After four months all her symptoms were gone. She is outspoken in condemning the therapies of her physicians and specialists who failed to recognize CSR. She accuses them of practicing "lazy medicine," sometimes called "defensive medicine." This harsh criticism is echoed by hundreds of others who have been successfully treated at the virus and allergy clinic.

### Multiple Latent Virutherapy and a Cancer Link?

Cancer continues to resist our attempts to control its onset and successfully treat its victims. The clinical findings with provocation neutralization suggest a possible diagnostic test for some types of precancer conditions, and temporary relief of cancer pain and symptoms. There is no evidence, however, that these clinical findings could be a basis for a cancer therapy. Eighty years ago, a New Yorker, Dr. P. Rous, transferred sarcoma (a cancer) from sick to healthy chickens in a cell-free filtered serum. The medical and research establishments of those days ignored the discovery for fifty years. Rous was eighty-five when awarded a Nobel Prize. Dr. Carlton Lee, in the 1970s, discovered a control/relief of cancer patients' pain by serial dilution (SD) neutralizing shots of sterile extracts of surgical biopsies of the patients' cancers. Some cancers temporarily stopped enlarging, even shrank in size. His discovery has been ignored.

Could there be a connection between the relief experienced by Lee's patients and SD provocation and neutralization with human *Papillomavirus?*

**IK**   Provocation with *Papillomavirus* 4 causes urethra, prostate, or bladder symptoms in men over age 50. *Papillomavirus* 14 and 16 provoke similar or more intense symptoms. Some women over the age of 35 have noticed vaginal, bladder, and, occasionally, loin sensations. Other symptoms were small electric shock sensations in one or both breasts; similar sensations in the chest, with alteration of peak flow readings; nasal sensations, including excess watery mucus airway changes, with nasal dripping; pain and tenderness of the colon, with or without a sudden passing of feces. *Papillomavirus* 14:16 virutherapy can relieve the symptoms.

The medical literature confirms the presence of *Papillomavirus* in cancer of the cervix and bladder. Researchers have discovered *Papillomavirus* in cancer tissue from the urinary tract, breast, colon, lungs, and nose (Hansen, 1996). Most of the world's virus-induced cancers are caused by EBV, hepatitis, and *Papillomavirus.* A large number of minor viruses cause unusual infrequent cancers. Latent virus infection in the precancerous stage is difficult to detect because there is no NIS antibody stimulation, nor previous active illnesses. By the time the cancer is detected, NIS antibody formation may still be insufficient. The media describe tragic cases in which the biopsy was negative or hastened the spread of the cancer. "Scientific" papers, with their statistics, prove no connection exists between cervical and prostate cancers because there are few, if any, positive NIS antibodies to the viruses (Buchwald et al., 1996). The practical aspects of the act of coitus, together with latent viruses not stimulating NIS antibodies, raises doubts about the scientific papers' conclusions. Virus-allergy clinic patients who provoked to human *Papillomavirus* are certain there is a connection. Compare the scientific papers' conclusions with negative viral antibody findings in CFIDS/ME patients who are told nothing is wrong with them and are given SSDs for their spurious psychological diagnoses (refer to health books on CFIDS/ME).

A localized area that provoked sensations or symptoms with provocation neutralization may harbor a buildup of virus in the precancerous or cancerous growth. This is probably the best site for a biopsy. The crude cancer biopsy serum Dr. Lee used may have contained one or more cancer-causing viruses. If cancer of the cervix, prostate, or bladder is suspected, human *Papillomavirus* multiple latent provocation and neutralization is indicated. The simple and inexpensive viral provocation technique could not be patented. Provocation of human *Papillomavirus* 14:16, a noninvasive vaginal technique, could compete with Papanicolaou stain and other invasive vaginal smear procedures. Latency therapy will not interest the pharmaceutical industry because it reduces long-term SSD therapies and there is no patent. By contrast, the new patented anticancer drugs on trial are expensive, but they do cure cancer in inbred mice. Let us hope the human drug trials will be as successful. We should not forget the brave cancer patients referred to Dr. Lee twenty-five years ago. From their experiences, morphine-befuddled, dying cancer patients should be offered multiple latent neutralization because it may improve pain relief. "Scientific" and controlled statistical studies would be unethical for the group that receives no treatment and would probably not be welcomed by cancer victims (Mandell, 1979).

## *A REVIEW OF TREATMENT FAILURES*

### *Latent Virus Overload, Failures, and Their Causes*

The preliminary work-up and virutherapy ask the suffering patient to improve lifestyle, home and work ecology, and diet, and to anticipate aggravation (or improvement) of symptoms as the treatment proceeds. After the last clinic visit, with detoxing well under way, symptoms may become worse (90 percent) or better (10 percent) than when the treatment was begun. Two or three months later the promise of improved health is realized. I think it is unfair that some patients who complied and finished the course must be counted as failures because the means available at the time were inadequate to deal with their many causes of fatigue and mañana illnesses. ("There is no justice or fairness in the outcome of medical therapies"—a disappointed patient.)

Impatient people do not want to change their lifestyle. They are happy to continue with SSDs and therapies, hoping for a spontaneous recovery or the yet to be discovered "magic bullet." Their reluctance is understandable, for conventional medicine downplays any patient participation. There is no need for public health or allergy advice; instead they are told not to upset their lifestyle because "symptom suppression drugs and therapy will fix your symptoms and get you right." The advice may have worked in the 1950s and 1960s, but in the 1990s, it failed many who complied but later stopped SSDs because of severe toxic side effects. How do other therapies fare with failures and successes? Pick up any health book and look in its index for "failure," or less alarming terms. The nearest you will find is "fainting." There is no need to list "success" in the index, as that is what every health book is proclaiming, in chapter after chapter. Patients with long, expensive experiences of therapies hand me lists of failed therapies when they return the completed virus-allergy clinic questionnaire. Honesty is the best policy for these "bruised, hardened, and frustrated" people.

No punches are pulled when patients ask for explanations. The people with CFIDS/ME and mañana symptoms divide into three clinical groups:

1. Severe, prolonged, fluctuating illness of three or more years' duration; long periods of bed rest with muscle wasting; numerous symptoms and complaints
2. Recent to medium duration of one to three years; three to eighteen months of bed rest with little muscle wasting
3. Recent duration of nine to eighteen months; fluctuating short periods of bed rest

The three groups may have varying memory, mood, and depression symptoms. Those in group 1 are difficult to treat because they are on drugs, often antidepressants, and are reluctant to give them up. When detoxing occurs it is severe, and the symptoms become almost unbearable. A few have slowly recovered over months and years, with protracted therapies. Those in group 2 respond well to therapy, but progress is slowed if EBV, CMV, or dengue are important, as treatment shots will need to be continued at five- to seven-week intervals, for up to eighteen months, to reduce the risk of relapses. Those in group 3 do best; most return to remembered health.

## Failure Groupings

### Did Not Comply

1. Treatment too difficult
2. Refusal to stop symptom suppression drugs
3. Cannot afford treatment
4. Home ecology problems that cannot be fixed
5. Animals that must remain in the household
6. A present or past cannabis drug habit that is not completely stopped
7. No family support, only criticism and ridicule
8. Personal beliefs
9. Vegetarian lifestyle
10. Religious beliefs about foods and lifestyles

### Complied, but Improved Less Than 20 Percent or Failed

1. No response because chronic petrochemical toxicity cannot be controlled or is detected after the work-up: (a) the home is new, with outgassing of petrochemicals, in particular, formaldehyde; (b) new carpets are outgassing; (c) unflued gas or kerosene heaters in well-sealed homes; and (d) home hobbies or vocations involving oil and petrochemicals. The patients complied as best they could but could not get others living in the house to change their lifestyle.
2. Long-term medication suppresses skin responses, provoked symptoms, detoxing, and the body's immunities (evidence from hundreds of virus-allergy clinic patients).
3. Very good compliance, but no provoked or neutralizing symptoms occur. Most in this category visited tropical countries where hygiene was poor or absent. While there they contracted undiagnosed infections. Many of their symptoms are suggestive of arboviruses. There was little response from those who visited the Amazon River Basin, the jungles of Central Africa, the Far East jungles, and similar areas in Indonesia and the Philippines. (No malaria parasite protein concentrate is available.)
4. A favorable response to the preliminary work-up, but disappointing response to MLV. The problem is no response to herpes, EBV, hepatitis, and mumps, despite symptoms suggesting their latency.

5. Recurring infections that do not respond to therapy, such as drug-resistant *Candida* or *Giardia*, a chronic bacterial infection, a difficult to detect dental root abscess (see CMV and *Helicobacter*, p. 100), chronic chest infection, or suspicions of a chronic disabling medical condition. Some diagnoses are made after the work-up is completed because of the removal of latency symptoms.

6. The person has a long, complicated illness. Progress is slow and many give up in favor of the "comfort" of symptom suppression therapy.

7. Recovery is interrupted by repeated relapses. The immune response pattern is peculiar to the individual or could be due to unrecognized latentees (unavailable viral concentrates).

8. "Therapeutic butterflies" insist they are complying with diet and ecology but, in fact, are continuing with their faulty lifestyles and in-house animals.

9. "Psychosomatic": an abnormal interest in allergies and viruses, but no improvement or provocation during the first three visits, so therapy is stopped. A follow-up, three to six months later, reveals, for no apparent reason, that all symptoms disappeared and there is no longer any interest in allergies or viruses.

10. *Misdiagnoses:* the general medical examination requested before a patient can enter the preliminary work-up and MLV course did not detect a medical or surgical problem. If no provoked responses occur during the complete work-up, or there are unusual responses, and a review of the questionnaire raises doubts, the patient is referred back to the family physician. Over the years, fifteen people had early cancers detected. Sadly, most eventually died.

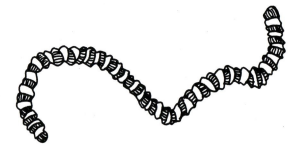

# Chapter 4

# Lifestyle Changes
# for Virus-Allergy Link Therapy

This chapter offers advice for two groups of readers:

1. *Readers who already know about allergies* will know how to change their surroundings where they move, live, and eat.
2. *Readers who are new to allergies* will be confused at first, but the practical and logical measures will in time make sense to you.

Physicians should encourage the new patient to attend an allergy support group or put them in contact with someone who was helped by allergy treatment. In time, what you, as a patient, are about to do becomes reasonable. You will need to read other books for more ideas and explanations of the treatments. Before long you will recover your remembered health and be able to help someone who is starting allergy treatments. Popular health books include descriptions of allergy illnesses and treatments. Some sections of these books contain "scientific" medical expressions that are tossed about without adequate explanations. This book contains some abbreviations or acronyms as part of important discussions. The Abbrekey© Bookmark, found in the front of the book, helps those with poor memories who need to read about allergies and ecological measures. This bookmark was suggested by those attending the clinic because they preferred abbreviations to the repeated long medical terms, which take up 5 to 15 percent of the words on the page.

You cannot be lax with home or workplace ecology if you want to get a good result from the treatment. It is an effort, but you are rewarded with meaningful provocation testing results that make the treatment so much easier for you and the physician. Complying with treatment will enable you to feel healthy sooner. The physician's office provides notes on how to improve your surroundings at minimal cost and suggests a book on allergies that suits local conditions where you live and work (Brostoff and Jamlin, 1989; Crook, 1996; Goldstein, 1993; Mandell, 1979).

## *HOW TO USE YOUR NEUROTIC NOTEBOOK*

Years ago, an unforgettable patient recovered her health, personality, and mental faculties on attending the clinic. She had suffered for years and was given a Neurosis Conversion Hysteria diagnosis:

> "Wasn't I a fool to believe that neurotic nonsense? I'm taking my revenge by calling my symptom notebook the Neurotic Notebook."

Henceforth, the clinic used her fun title for all symptom notebooks.

It makes sense to *record, record, record* changing and provoked symptoms from the day you decide to have the work-up treatments. Select a small pocket/purse notepad or a larger school notebook and make it your constant companion for the next three to five months until you have recovered or feel greatly improved.

Your unreliable memory varies during treatments, but what you jot down in your Neurotic Notebook are facts of the moment. Bring your Neurotic Notebook to treatment sessions and refer to it while answering your allergist's questions on progress. If you do not understand a section in this, or another book you are reading, record your questions in the back pages of your Neurotic Notebook so you can discuss them with your physician at the next visit. The Neurotic Notebook records sensations, thoughts, and symptoms. You know your symptoms and feelings are real, and eventually the work-up will show you that most of them are explained by food allergies, mold toxins, and multiple latent viral infections. Some physicians, believe it or not, still diagnose "hysteria." Hysterical diagnoses began in the nineteenth century with the belief that the uterus influenced "all in the head," "neurotic" symptoms suffered by so many Victorian women. This belief has since been discredited, and today, hysterical diagnoses and descriptions are also applied to males.

Some people suffer a relapse in the months or years after completing the work-up and MLV. If you should suffer such a relapse, get out your Neurotic Notebook and start the diet and ecology lifestyle again; then make contact with your allergist. Fortunately, most relapses, if treated promptly, last only a few days, or a week or two at most.

### *HOME ECOLOGY*

The house, and especially the bedroom, should be as dry as possible, with no smells or signs of mold. The best-case scenario would be a house facing the setting sun on land with good drainage. Large trees or shrubs should be 10 to 15 feet (ft) (3 to 5 meters[m]) from the walls of the house to allow good air movement around the house. Whenever possible, open up the basement for better air circulation. Keep the rain gutters clear of debris and obstructions, so the down pipes do not become blocked, causing water to leak into the walls of the house.

Do not move into a house or flat where the previous owners kept cats, dogs, or other pets inside. If such a move is necessary, the carpets should be thoroughly cleaned. If an animal smell remains after cleaning, the carpets should be lifted, the underfelt inspected, and, if stained/dirty, removed and discarded. Sticky animal saliva is the most important animal irritant. It is difficult to clean from carpets, furniture, and walls. Animal motions (feces) and urine persist in carpet fibers and underfelt. If the old carpets cannot be used and new ones are purchased, have them steam cleaned and hung in the cleaner's warehouse to dry to reduce xenochemical odors before they are laid in your house. It is better not to put carpet back in your bedroom if the flooring is of high-quality tongue-and-groove timber, heavy plywood, or chipboard. Consider sealing it and using throw mats and rugs. If the tongue-and-groove timber floors allow dust and air through gaps, put down a vinyl floor. Vinyl seals the surface, and all house dust accumulating on it can be washed away. In hot climates, a concrete or mosaic floor surface is easy to keep clean.

Your house should not have natural or artificial indoor plants or flowers, or fluffy lacy ornaments or furnishings. Get rid of plastic reflectors and light shades that outgas when heated. Keep television sets and other electrical appliances out of the bedroom because of outgassing of chemical fumes. Do not use household deodorizing/perfumed products or long-term slow-release chemical insecticides. Natural fly sprays may be used, but some sensitive people cannot tolerate them during treatment. Keep three or four fly swatters around the house while treatment is under way. Gas and kerosene heaters should be banned from the house or flat if the patient has serious symptoms from allergies and suspected latent viruses. Many patients are able to tolerate gas appliances vented outside. Avoid buying or living in a house or flat by a busy road or highway because of the vehicle fumes.

**IK**    A woman who was unable to garden at home because of the traffic fumes, finally convinced her husband to change homes. This improved her response to treatment, and she recovered from her chronic "neurotic" illness. With her improved energy, her garden is a picture of color most of the year.

Problems with mold occur in basements because of moistness. Water tracks under the house and permeates the surface, where it evaporates and encourages mold growth. This evaporation also removes heat from under the house, increasing heating bills. Covering the exposed earth under the house with agricultural black plastic sheeting will cause the mold smells to disappear from your home, and you may save 10 to 15 percent on your heating bill. Tacking or attaching reflector insulation aluminium sheeting to the under-floor beams of the house is less effective, and subject to damage over time by small animals and birds. The improvement of the home ecology makes treatment easier and reduces medical expenses.

### The Bedroom

Your bedroom should be a safe refuge with the best conditions because a third or more of the day is spent there. Allergic and chemical factors are important, and if not attended to, they will interfere or reduce the relief gained from allergy and MLV shots/drops of mixed molds and house dust. Your bedroom should be a place to retreat to when your symptoms are severe. Unsuspected allergic dusts and chemical fumes may not be detected until the bedroom has been cleaned. Bedroom suites with bathrooms have high mold levels from the steam and plumbing. Curtains should be laundered and aired frequently. An old bedroom should have the walls and ceilings scraped clean, sealed, and redecorated. Put up with a bare floor and use throw mats/rugs if the carpet is old and you suspect molds, house dust, and house dust mites are embedded in it. Wait to install a new carpet until you are fit and well for over a year.

To clean the bedroom, start at one side of the doorway and work around the room back to the doorway again. Check everything in the cupboards and remove articles in the room that could be creating dust, fumes, petrochemicals, smells, and mold. A special warning is given here about books, as they give out petrochemicals, smells, and mold spores. As you doze off to sleep, put the book you are reading into a clear plastic bag and close the bag with a tie. Keep cosmetics and medications in the bathroom. Another good idea is to store your shoes in a different room. Some people need to avoid water beds because the plastic water bag outgasses, and the covering over the plastic water bag can harbor dust mites.

It is my experience that patients are reluctant to make drastic changes to the bedroom, often for sentimental reasons. I suggest you obtain several allergy books and raise the subject at the local allergy group to see how other sufferers deal with their allergic problems in the bedroom. The main stumbling block is putting off the final decision to take up the carpet. This can wait until the main allergic problems in the bedroom are attended to

(Mandell, 1979; Rousseau, Rea, and Enwright, 1988; Winderlin and Sehnert, 1996).

> I visited a young woman's home because she was not responding to dust, mold, and CRC shots and food exculsions. I pleaded with her to take up the carpet and send out the curtains for cleaning. She complied and was surprised and impressed with the dramatic response to treatment during the next four to six weeks. By the time she finished MLV, she had returned to her remembered health and energy.

### The Other Rooms of the House

Health books on allergies give detailed instructions on kitchen cleaning and cooking methods. Gas cookers are a major cause of aggravation of your symptoms. Until you feel a lot better, turn off the outside gas meter and use electricity. You will have to do a lot of cooking for yourself, as you may not be able to eat and enjoy the same foods as the rest of your family. Packaged foods are not the answer when you are ill because of the dangers associated with processing, adulteration by chemicals and preservatives, hidden ingredients, high sugar content, and foods that cause a reaction. Check the refrigerator contents and make sure all foods are covered to stop contamination by mold. Regularly clean the defrosting unit, which has a collecting channel and tube that drains the water to a metal evaporation plate under the fridge. It is difficult to clean, but this is a common source of mold contamination of your food. Check from time to time, if the refrigerator is old, to detect, by smell, whether cooling or refrigerant gases are escaping.

Chemical cleaners for the kitchen and laundry can affect you. These should be kept in the garage or shed, and remember to tighten their stoppers and caps. Many people told me they could not clean with chemicals, and their partners or relatives took over for two to three months, until they began to feel better. When you start sweating and detoxing, the smelly clothes and sheets need frequent washing. If the washing cycle is under way, get out of the laundry room and close the door. Several people told me they could not use the laundry detergents but were able to tolerate soaps. A friend or relative willing to do the laundry at his or her home is a useful arrangement, until you begin to feel better.

Mold is a major problem in the bathroom. The room may be clean but still has a moldy smell because unsuspected molds are in the carpet surrounding, or in the toilet. After cleaning, you can take a hot bath or sun sauna to aid the excretion of the cleaning chemicals.

Those who sleep in a room over a garage may develop symptoms from the outgassing of stored petrochemicals in the garage and car. These petrochemical fumes penetrate through wood and fiberboard walls and flooring. Adults with CFIDS should change bedrooms. Before moving back to the bedroom above the garage, clean up the garage and remove all unnecessary petrochemicals, such as paints, fuels, solvents, and gardening supplies. Do not clean the garage yourself. Should suspicious symptoms recur when you move back into that bedroom, a detached garage is necessary.

The family automobile affects many people, causing them to fear a trip to town or a social visit. Keep the engine block clean and check the exhaust and muffler pipes. It is impossible to thoroughly clean a second-hand car that carried pets in the backseat, or a tobacco/cannabis smoker.

Ask someone in the family to sort the trash and food wastes for recycling. Empty kitchen scraps into an exterior waste container as soon as possible after the meal to avoid moldy food smells in the kitchen. Store the waste can in an outside shed if possible. Do not store it in the garage while waiting for trash collection day.

### IN-HOUSE PETS

Animals chew and lick unspeakable filthy things when outside and then carry infection with them into the home. Dried saliva contains spores of molds and bacteria. Panting and the licking of their coats to control body temperature result in heavy contamination by minute dried saliva particles, which can be seen clearly when sunlight pours through the windows. During the winter, heaters, and particularly fan heaters, circulate these fine particles. Elderly dogs or cats, because of lowered immunity, are greater sources of infection, especially if they have uncontrolled slobbering and sneezing. While you are receiving treatment, if you go on a business trip or holiday, ask for a nonsmoking room. Hotels do not allow animals in these rooms. Do not stay with relatives or friends who have in-house pets. The effects on memory and moods can be devastating and interfere with important business decisions.

It is distressing to interview an animal lover whom you know would respond to virutherapy but refuses to put the pets in kennels outside the house. During the first two or three years, I treated many patients who kept animals in the house. Results were disappointing, with low levels of response and frequent relapses. On checking my early records of treated animal lovers who retained their in-house pets, I found that nobody gained a useful or full recovery. Since then I have treated the occasional animal lover, but with a similar response. It came as no surprise that the following were provoked during testing: CRC, *Giardia*, hepatitis, rotavirus, *Helico-bacter, Parvovirus, Listeria*, toxoplasmosis, and Q fever. Other patients, without in-house animals, frequently provoked to some of these microbes because they had a cat in or on the bed during their childhood and teenage years. I no longer treat patients who wish to retain their in-house animals, as they are wasting time and money. The response to a total exclusion of OWGGs is disappointing or patchy. Patients may declare the animals are outside, but when the preliminary work-up results are disappointing, they confess, admit the truth, and start a cleanup of their homes. Four to six weeks later they are responding to MLV. Asthmatics attending the clinic would like to stop the inhaled corticosteroids. There is little chance of this occurring with in-house pets.

If you still suffer ecology problems in your home, your physician can supply a list of recommended allergy books. Do not nag or blame others in the house until you have done your homework from the ecology books. A reasoned request, supported by these facts, goes further than getting mad and shouting. It is difficult when you are renting or are restricted in what can be done because of financial stringency. If the problem persists in spite of your best efforts, it is better to look around for another flat or house.

## WORKPLACE ENVIRONMENT

Office working conditions affect those with chronic fatigue and lack of motivation. By the end of the week, fatigue can be marked, and those who suffer may need the weekend to recover. When others in the office are affected similarly or are complaining of headaches, irritable eyes, recurring flu symptoms, and have short tempers, you and your co-workers may be suffering from "sick building syndrome." The blame may lie with an old air conditioning system, the lack of air filter maintenance, or a copier whose fumes are circulated by the air conditioner. Do you complain? If so, ask others who are affected to make up a complaint group.

IK   A woman, age 35, was suffering from symptoms that she thought were due to office conditions or, as her physician suggested, a viral infection. She attended the clinic for fear of losing her job. She missed out on a promotion because of erratic work performance and, at times, poor memory recall. Her organization was about to be restructured. She worked hard at complying with the preliminary work-up. Four weeks after starting MLV, her incentive to work improved and her memory began to return. With the help of provocation findings and information made available to her, she and two other workers submitted a report on office conditions. It was received, and improvements were instituted. Over the past eighteen months, she suffered two relapses, but they were quickly controlled by "staving off the flu" (see p. 177). She was not dismissed from her job and survived a further restructuring of the company. She is now supervisor of her section.

The moral of this and many other stories is that if you suspect office conditions are affecting you, do not complain to the supervisor at first. Make a rough plan of the office to take to your allergist or physician, and get his or her opinions before approaching the management. Now you are in command of the facts, and your complaint will probably convince the management.

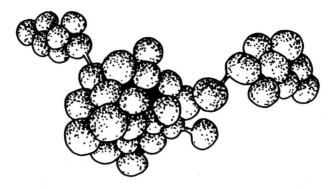

## *WHAT DO WE MEAN BY FOOD ALLERGIES AND INTOLERANCES?*

It is confusing for people to be told by one physician that they have a food intolerance, and by another, usually an allergist that it is a food allergy. The confusion began in the medical world in the 1960s, when trace amounts of a blood immunoglobulin (called E) were discovered. Ig E antibody has an important role in allergic reactions to dusts and other substances known as inhalants. Some physicians thought they had found the allergic agent and declared that allergic reactions and symptoms provoked by Ig E were "scientific" allergies. Typical allergic reactions in other people could not be called allergic because they lacked Ig E. A previous declaration of "scientific allergy" occurred early in the twentieth century following the discovery of skin testing. Unfortunately for the concept of Ig E scientific allergy, some of the highest Ig E levels occur with parasitic infections, in particular, worms in the gut, and in a few individuals who inherit high Ig E blood levels. The next discovery was that blood immunoglobulin G plays a role in food reactions and intolerances. At present, RAST and ELISA blood tests for Ig E and Ig G food antibodies are not reliable for food intolerances because they give too many false positives and negatives. RAST tests identify the foods that cause immediate reactions, but usually the patient already knows about them. About 7 to 10 percent of all food reactions are detected by the RAST test. As a rough guide, allergies provoked during the preliminary work-up are regarded by physicians as intolerances. The allergy immunoglobulins may or may not be present in your blood, as most responses appear to come from the organ cells of the body. Latent immunity does not provoke antibodies.

At first I went along with the idea of "scientific" Ig E food allergy, but my clinical results and what patients experienced soon convinced me to call all food reactions "food allergies." My patients find it easier to regard all unusual reactions from foods as food allergies. In your reading of allergy books and in discussing allergies with your family physician and specialists, keep in mind the two concepts of food allergy, one realistic, the other contrived.

Food addiction defeats many patients who at first resolve to exclude a harmful food due to an allergy, and it frustrates their allergists, who are unable to prevent their sneaking the addictive food and confusing the provocation symptoms and treatment results. Many give up the treatment because they are unable to overcome their great desire for the allergic food. Others suffer severe withdrawal symptoms and cannot last the four to five days' disruption of their lifestyle and body functions. Severe food addiction can occur with dairy, beef, and poultry products; spices; and the xenochemicals, such as preservatives, synthetic flavorings, and artificial colorings. I advise patients who cannot stop eating an addictive food to abandon MLV. Those who are able to continue the food exclusion must not reintroduce addictive foods into the diet until the gut viruses, polio, hepatitis, adenovirus, CMV, EBV, and rotavirus, are provoked and treated. Patients responding to the work-up stay off the addictive foods for a further eight to ten weeks after the last virus testing session (Collison and Hall, 1989; Feltner, 1990; Heller, 1992).

**IK**　A Dutch man, born in Java, came to the clinic with a fifteen-year history of chronic diarrhea and an invalid's pension. He bravely suppressed his great desire to eat wheat, but the chronic diarrhea continued until he reluctantly eliminated rice, his favorite food.

## Rotary Food Diets

An important food allergy interferes with treatment of the patients who come to see me. The offending food and other foods in that food family are totally excluded for three to four months. This allows time for testing and treatment and ensures a high degree of accuracy for provocation and treatment, especially MLV. The less popular members of the food groups are cautiously introduced when health and symptoms improve. If related foods cause a return of symptoms and decrease in response to MLV, a rotation diet is started. A rotation diet introduces a food every three to seven days, with less risk of developing symptoms. Consult health books on rotary diets and ask the clinic or your physician for rotary diet forms. Make a rotation list of household chores and rooms to be cleaned, and then allocate days. In time, cleaning and the maintenance of the car, together with jobs around the house, can be placed on the rotary chores program. They will not be forgotten or postponed, and you will not become exhausted trying to catch up on housework (Davies and Stewart, 1989; Gittleman, 1993; Golos and Golos, 1983; Lewis and Blakeley, 1996).

## The Old and New World Grass Grains

Food exclusions, caveman diets, and other manipulations of food intake for detecting food allergies, are very well described in allergy health books. The Old World grass grains (OWGG) breads made from wheat, barley, oat, rye, rice, and millet are "the staff of life." These grains come from the Old World, as opposed to maize, amaranth, and quinoa, which come from the New World. The OWGGs have attractive texture and taste and can easily be processed by the food industry's modern machines. One or more of the OWGGs are eaten several times during the day by people of developed countries. It is only to be expected that grain allergy is now an important and serious food allergy, affecting 4 to 6 percent of the population of developed nations. Some authorities suggest up to 10 to 12 percent of this population is affected in other ways by OWGG allergies (Schmid, 1994).

Those who react to OWGGs must forgo their old habit of rushing to work after a five-minute meal of a piece of toast and two cups of coffee. They now must prepare a more substantial meal for breakfast. Some at first say their stomach will not tolerate a cooked meal for breakfast, but once the offending food group is removed, these people find they can indeed tolerate a small to moderate cooked breakfast. Furthermore, they feel more alert and energetic during the day. You need to spend a half hour the previous night preparing breakfast, or, better still, prepare a number of breakfasts and keep them in the freezer.

Allergy health books contain recipes and methods for making flat breads from the alternative flours (see the recipe index in Chapter 6, beginning on p. 260). As soon as these breads are cooked, they should be sliced and placed in the freezer, as they rapidly become moldy at room temperatures. If you are making a stack of waffles or pancakes, separate them with waxed paper before putting them in the freezer. For years the benefits of a diet rich in whole grains and bran have been touted in the media and by the medical community. For those of us with OWGG allergies, however, this roughage may be far from healthy, possibly damaging the intestinal lining. The phytic acids of grains may aggravate osteoporosis by preventing the absorption of iron, zinc, calcium, magnesium, selenium, and chromium salts. Deficiencies of these important trace minerals can reach dangerously low levels because the processing of most supermarket foods depletes or removes them.

An OWGG-free diet requires supplementing with vitamin B complex tablets, zinc capsules or tablets, and occasionally vitamin $B_{12}$ shots. Your family physician will advise the correct dose (Callem, 1993).

### Maize, Potatoes, and History

Let us briefly review the historical influence on Europe, Asia, and Africa of these valuable foods cultivated by the Aztecs and Incas of the New World. The introduction of these crops to Europe was followed by a population explosion. People now had an easy-to-grow and prolific source of cheap food that was not susceptible to native plant diseases. Three centuries later, the potato crop failed due to viral disease, and famine returned. Millions of Europeans emigrated to the New World, where they grew an assured food supply. Population growth in Europe slowed for a while but began to increase again with the great public health advances of the nineteenth century. The peasants moved into better housing and no longer slept and lived with their animals. As the mechanisms of making water safe became known, access to fresh water supplies increased, and waterborne epidemics no longer killed off the poor. As a result, infant mortality was markedly reduced, and the peasants lived twenty to thirty years longer. The diet of corn and potatoes, with little or no OWGGs, produced a lean, wiry, active peasantry.

The accounts of two British aristocrats' journeys throughout Ireland and Europe in the 1700s and 1800s suggest that the difference in body shapes between OWGG eaters and potato and corn eaters was recognized. The wealthy, who could afford the OWGGs, developed plump figures. Rubens' magnificent paintings show the popular body images of his day. Tuberculosis made its victims thin and emaciated, as it slowly killed them. No husband seeking a healthy wife would contemplate a thin maiden. She had to be plump, obvious proof that she did not have tuberculosis. But how could peasants become plump on a diet of potato and corn, with wheat bread beyond the income of the family? Small amounts of OWGG foods and fat were given to the marriageable daughters. Wheat and fat dumplings were the answer to the maidens' prayers. (For more interesting historical facts, see Rapp, 1992; Wright, 1990.)

The plump body concept is no longer valid in developed countries. Today, industries are built on rapid excess fat removal by dieting and surgery. Few, nowadays, know that eliminating OWGGs for five to eight months will get rid of unwanted plumpness, leaving behind the modern desired trim body shape. Multinational food companies promote and keep OWGG consumption popular by constant advertising and marketing of grain foods with new shapes and flavors. With the frightening increase in allergies and intolerances to OWGGs, it cannot be long before far-sighted companies will be exploring the non-OWGG food sources. You do not have to wait for the food companies to move into the non-OWGG food market. A Mexican cookbook and Chapter 6 (pp. 260-294) will introduce a new world of attractive dishes.

Many patients told me they were allergic to buckwheat or other grains, but it was the mold in the grain or flour that caused their reacitons. A reaction to medium-grit maize, cornmeal, and buckwheat flour may not indicate that you have a maize and buckwheat allergy. Do the four-day exclusion and test meal, with the food purchased elsewhere, to confirm the apparent food allergy is false. If it is, you are reacting to the contaminating molds. In the future, buy small packs of the foods and store them in the freezer. The low mold content of most packaged foods will not affect you, and you will discover that your supposed allergy is false. Women suffering from CRC need to take particular care in choosing low-mold or mold-free foods. Fortunately, most CRC patients have a heightened sense of smell for mold, not only in homes, but also in foods. Should you suspect your sense of smell is depressed, however, ask one of your friends to check the food before you purchase or consume it. The "Victorian" atmosphere of some health food stores, with bins of grains, peas, dried and preserved produce, is a trap for the inexperienced shopper suffering from mold allergies or CRC. The foods in the bins, especially those grown organically, may be heavily infested with mold. A good test is to put your nose almost into the bulk supply barrel and take a sniff or two. Some mold-sensitive people develop marked symptoms, and that is the end of their shopping day, but they avoid a provoking meal.

Always remember that gluten-free wheaten corn flour is made from wheat grains. After chemical extraction of the gluten, between 0.4 and 0.9 percent remains. The gluten-free corn flour retains traces of chemicals used in the twelve to sixteen stages of the gluten extraction process. I know of many frightening gluten-free wheaten corn flour reactions in people with petrochemical, OWGGs, and mold allergies. Gluten-free wheaten corn flour is best avoided until you are much improved in health and your allergy responses and reactions are diminished. Even so, this processed preparation could, at times, provoke marked reactions.

### Meat, Molds, and Candida

Healthy free-range meats from different animals and birds are necessary if you are to recover your immunities and remembered health. Yet the opposite is occurring in industrial countries because of a flood of poor-quality, xenochemical-laced, and hormone-ridden meats and meat products. *Surmise:* The movement against red meat consumption in Europe and North America is due, in part, to women suffering from mold allergies, such as CRC and vaginal (thrush) discharges, of *Candida, Torulopsis, Giardia, Trichomonas,* and *Cryptosporidium* infection of the gut. After eating red meats, they are nauseated, with increasing fatigue, lassitude, and mood changes or suffer delayed symptoms the following day. When they find they are also affected by the additives in battery chicken (commercially raised poultry), they turn to fish and vegetarian meat substitutes for the family diet. Birds do not accumulate mold toxins in their tissues. Birds have fed on grains for millions of years, and their bowel lining rejects mold toxins, which are held in the bowel contents and excreted in the motions. Grass-eating animals, herbivores, are not accustomed to grain eating; they have no protective bowel activity against mold toxins. Although there may be little or no mold toxin, the battery bird meats have high levels of xenochemicals, antibiotics, and hormones (Duncan and Smith, 1993).

In 1983, I began to suspect that there were differences between New Zealand meats and those produced in North America, Japan, and Europe. At that time, I was treating several diplomatic corps wives with allergic work-ups. Three of the women returned to their homes in North America and Europe for four to six months of holiday. All had problems eating local red meats in their countries. They developed recurrences of vaginal itching and thrush discharges, skin rashes, tiredness, and mood complaints. They changed to a white meat and fish diet for the remainder of their stay. On returning to New Zealand, they ate red meats again without any problems. Their children also had problems when abroad, refusing to drink the local milk, spitting out local cottage and soft cheeses. They complained of "tummy pains" and at times had diarrhea, especially during the winter months in the Northern Hemisphere. On returning to New Zealand, their children ate these foods and enjoyed them. Since that time, patients who had received *Candida* therapy at the clinic have reported experiencing problems with meat dishes while on holiday in the United States, Europe, and Japan.

Silage, grain-fed, and feeding lot animal and bird meats and meat products affect people who suffer or have suffered from *Candida* viral infection. *Surmise:* The animal meats accumulate mold toxins and xenochemicals are present in the silage and grain meal feeds. The feed stock contains high levels of preservatives and antimold chemicals. Grains fed to animals may be those not fit for human consumption because of their high mold contamination. It is suggested that a comprehensive examination be made of feed lot and chicken battery meats to assess for mold toxin residues in muscle fibers. A comparison could then be made with free-range meats. If mold toxins that can produce symptoms and illness are found to be present, ways could be devised to remove them or to prevent the toxins from accumulating in food stock. The liver accumulates xeno- and toxic chemicals so I advise patients not to purchase chicken livers or paté made from pig liver.

Beautiful green pastures, glistening in the sun, can harbor molds that, under certain seasonal conditions of warmth and moisture, attack animals. Facial eczema in sheep causes ulceration around the mouth and nose, liver damage, and poor health, even death. Facial eczema also attacks cattle and calves. The sight of emaciated, ulcerated dying sheep confirms the frightening toxicity of some mold toxins. The treatment and prevention of facial eczema is Zinc Sulphate supplement.

The unexpected emergence of mad cow disease (bovine spongiform encephalopathy) has brought about increased demand for free-range red meats. It took a national disaster to bring about government action on poor-quality meats.

During treatment for latency illnesses, and while recovering, make a special effort to pay a bit more for a small supply of different free-range meats. Free-range red meats are beneficial and may not contain the xenochemicals present in pig and chicken meats. Two dessertspoonfuls of cooked free-range meat every, or every other day, is all you need.

### The Husband or Partner Test

**IK**  *Test A:* "Why is my wife a lump of ice in our bed? Can't you warm her up?"

I outline the treatment and the symptoms to be expected in simple terms and ask for an understanding of her illness. Often the husband cannot sleep under the load of blankets or duvets his suffering wife puts on the bed. It is better to move to another bed, but hopefully not for long, if the treatment is completed successfully. The test then becomes negative with his return to the marital bed.

**IK**  *Test B:* "You have made my wife into a bag of bones. Why can't she eat good healthy food like I do? When will she get plump again?"

I explain the fat loss when gluten is freed up and excreted. Little or no weight will go on until it is removed from her body. She will then put on a normal amount of fat. Has he noticed she is more active, less affected by moods, and a lot happier? This is often grudgingly admitted. When she recovers and puts on a little more weight, the test is negative.

I leave it to the reader's imagination to work out what happens when the sex roles are reversed.

### Staving Off the Flu

You had a good response from your preliminary work-up and serial vaccination treatments. The community and the people in your workplace are coming down with influenza. You feel you may have the flu and dread its onset, as it could reverse the improvement you are experiencing. It may bring on or aggravate the past known symptoms that you fear. When you are sure flu is beginning to affect you, draw up a dose from your flu vial and inject it. Note the time you do this. You may have a feeling of relief within 2 to 30 min; however, symptoms may return within the next 12 h. Space the next three injections at 12-h intervals, and by the third or fourth injection, there is an 85 percent chance that the influenza symptoms will clear. The 15 percent of patients who obtain little or no response from staving off the flu should be aware that their symptoms are not severe and their influenza infection is shortened compared to others suffering at home or in the workplace. Many patients have controlled their recurring winter flus. The most benefit was gained from completing the preliminary work-up and MLV. Patients used the "staving off the flu" technique whenever they suspected the flu was recurring. The following winter they were advised to use a flu shot every three weeks until head colds and the flu had disappeared from the community.

### The Provoking OWGGs Test Meal

Four days before the test, completely exclude OWGGs. Stop as many drugs as possible, especially antihistamines and nasal preparations. On the fifth day, instead of breakfast, drink three to four glasses of bottled water. Relax during the next hour and prepare the OWGG flours you have purchased (wheat, rye, rice, millet), with water and heat to make a slurry, or mix. When an hour has passed after taking the bottled water, eat two tablespoons of the flour mix. Take water as needed during the testings. Be prepared to continue the same dosage every hour until symptoms are provoked. You will recognize the symptoms; they could be a headache, a feeling of tenseness, or unexplained fatigue, an inability to read because of visual effects, or a deterioration in your handwriting. If important symptoms have cleared by the fourth day of total OWGG exclusion, they will be provoked to return during the testing. I have known patients who have persisted with this test and finally obtained provoked symptoms they recognized after eight hours and eight dosages. If you are disappointed because nothing has happened, ask your physician whether you are suitable for a five-day water fast. If not, ask around for an allergist who is prepared to advise you during the fasting and provocation. The five- to seven-day water fast is the gold standard for OWGG food allergies.

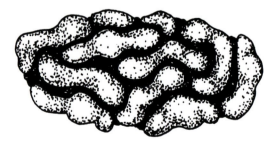

# Chapter 5

# Descriptions, Explanations, and Therapy

## *VIRUS FAMILIES*

Viruses are a disorganized bunch. The International Committee on Classification uses the shape, the weight, and the structure of the proteins' DNA (deoxyribonucleic acid) and RNA (ribonucleic acid). Viruses use either DNA or RNA. Retroviruses, discovered in 1970, change RNA to DNA with a reversing enzyme. HIV is a retrovirus. Virus classifications are not set in concrete. The committee reserves its right to change classifications as new discoveries about viruses are reported (Feltner, 1990; Garrett, 1995).

### *The Latent Virus Symptom Checklist*

Active infection or toxicity symptoms are not listed. Many latent symptoms are similar, with differences, to active symptoms. Active symptoms have no corresponding latent symptoms, and different latent symptoms are not present with the active conditions. I cannot offer an explanation for the marked or, at times, subtle differences between latent (enclosed in brackets) and active (normal text) symptoms. The listed latent symptoms are repeatedly provoked, both immediate and delayed, and have been recorded at the clinic and by patients over the past fourteen years (refer to Table 1.1). *Surmise:* The latent symptoms appearing during detoxing/excretion may be from the sudden onset of detoxing from overburdened organ cells. Frequently, other symptoms are provoked in sensitized cells that have little to contribute to the detoxing. When detoxing smells are present, the provoked symptoms are more marked or severe. The presence of poorly defined symptom and smell patterns suggests other latent viruses are being excreted. If the symptoms and smells are not those usually associated with the first provoking virus dose, suspect another virus (or viruses) has been provoked, known as shadowing symptoms (see pp. 16-18). Record these symptoms or sensations, as they may help the clinic in selecting further agents to test.

Circle your symptoms with an erasable lead pencil. If detoxing smells occurred at some time while the symptoms were present, check the box. This is not a diagnostic points scoring list (see the Virus-Allergy Score-card, p. 115). The detoxing smells are a guide to clearing or improving symptoms, even aggravation, during the treatments at the clinic. They may continue for three to six months after the last visit. If important symptoms not experienced for some years are provoked, underline the symptoms (refer to Table 1.1, pp. 9-10).

## DNA — *Herpes Viruses*

*Herpes simplex type 1.* Affects the lips, mouth, throat, eyes; skin rashes and tingling; sensitivity around the mouth and face; sexually transmitted herpes symptoms.   ☐ Detox

*Herpes simplex type 2.* The principal sexually transmitted disease; herpes vesicles, frequency, and burning; skin rashes below the waist; irritable behavior and fatigue; varying degrees of pain in the genitourinary area.   ☐ Detox

*Varicella-zoster, herpes type 3.* Children—chicken pox. Adults— *herpes zoster;* eye and corneal ulceration, deafness, vertigo, tinnitus, and facial nerve paralysis; shingles of the face; pains in the face, head, and nose; tic douloureux; chest symptoms; itchy eczema; moods and depression.   ☐ Detox

*Epstein-Barr virus, herpes type 4, glandular fever.* Headaches, fatigue, unable to get up and get going or mañana fatigue; chronic sore throat on the back of the throat; enlarged glands in the neck or elsewhere, enlarged or tender liver and spleen; deep bone pain; fibromyalgia, variable muscle weakness, tender spots, back pain, leaden limbs; moods and depression for no apparent reason. *Note:* depression can be severe, with suicidal thoughts, poor memory, excessive sleepiness and sleeping, disturbing dreams, and skin rashes.   ☐ Detox

*Cytomegalovirus, herpes type 5, glandular fever.* Urethra, bladder, and kidney functions, bed-wetting; genital area symptoms and libido; fibromyalgia, [increased muscle strength and coordination], lumbar and sacral pains; pain and reduced activity in pre-   ☐ Detox viously severely bruised or injured muscles; moods, depressions, and memory changes, for [better] or worse; symptoms of the liver, lungs, and intestines; heart symptoms, chest pains, heart racing and palpitations, irregular heartbeat.

*Herpes type 6.* A facial rash of infants; [mental stimulation]; ☐ Detox chronic fatigue symptoms.

*Herpes type 7.* Mild symptoms similar to EBV. ☐ Detox

## *DNA—Adenovirus (Originally Adenotonsilvirus)*

*Adenovirus.* Children—sinusitis, bronchitis, asthma, headaches; ☐ Detox enlarged tonsils and adenoids, enlarged neck glands, enlarged and painful abdominal lymph glands; glue ear of children, variable deafness and ear pains, pressure sensation and tinnitus. Adults—headaches, inflammation and itching of the whites of the eyes, photophobia; congested nose, sinusitis, enlarged tonsils, enlarged neck glands, and sticky mucus conditions such as bronchitis and asthma.

## *DNA—Parvovirus*

*Parvovirus.* Children—red facial rash; urinary symptoms. ☐ Detox Adults—joint aches, fibromyalgia, muscle weakness, headaches, fatigue, and chest symptoms.

## *DNA—Hepadnavirus*

*Hepatitis B.* Liver, gall bladder symptoms, loss of appetite, diar- ☐ Detox rhea or constipation; skin rash, skin sensitivity, skin itching, "creepy crawly" sensation under the skin; depression, moods: for men, aggressive and antagonistic thoughts of physical injury or sexual assault for no apparent reason, and for women, love/hate moods and fear of physical injury or sexual assault for no apparent reason; joint and muscle pain; sinusitis, chest infection; variable jaundice, with fluctuating yellowness of the whites of the eyes and the skin of the hands and feet, varying dark yellow to orange-colored urine and/or painful motions, prostate pains; for children: boys, aggressive behavior and nightmares, and girls, fearful sensations and nightmares.

**IK**    She was the last to leave the clinic. "Whew! What a night, the second one after the clinic visit and those symptoms I got from the hepatitis tests. I dreamed I'd been chased and feared I'd be raped. I was desperately calling to my partner to rescue me, but he wouldn't come. I suddenly woke up in fear, trembling. He was next to me, and I grabbed him. He said, 'That is the worst nightmare you have ever had. You were screaming my name and kicking me.' It's been years since I had a being-chased terror dream; I don't want any more. I lay awake for a long time, scared to go to sleep. Will I have any more?" I reassured her, explaining that the hepatitis nightmares can be scary, but it would probably be the last one, as she was starting to detox the excess latent hepatitis, probably from her brain cells. I did a follow-up by phone several months later and confirmed she was fit and well. "I haven't dared to sleep in a single bed yet; that nightmare was so vivid I don't think I'll ever forget it!"

## DNA—Poxvirus

*Vaccinia.* Headaches, fatigue, and skin sensitivity.                    ❑ Detox

## DNA—Papovaviruses

*Human* Papillomavirus 1 *(plantar warts).* [Disappearance or im-    ❑ Detox
provement of plantar warts].

*Human* Papillomavirus 4, 6 *(common warts).* [Disappearance of    ❑ Detox
or decrease in size or number of skin warts]; [urethra, bladder, and
prostate symptoms]; [enhanced libido].

*Human* Papillomavirus 14, 16. Genital symptoms; [enhanced    ❑ Detox
libido and male erection]; [urethra, bladder, and prostate unease/
pain]; [frequency and burning on passage].

The three types of *Papillomavirus* may provoke chest sensations or pain; abdominal sensations or pain; bowel motions, if constipated, to looser motions, or the reverse; provoked sensations in the cervix of the uterus, and breast nipples.

## RNA—Picornaviruses

*Enterovirus:* Poliomyelitis—[improved tone and strength of    ❑ Detox
muscles and joints, in particular, in the chest and depth of breath-
ing]; fibromyalgia, neck pain, middle and low back pain; [IBS,

constipation, diarrhea, and liver pain]; skin sensations, numbness, tingling, loss of sensation to touch; nasal symptoms, smell, vision, hearing, and tinnitus; headaches, bands around the head, memory, moods, and spacing-out sensations; disturbed sleeping, falling or crashing (fearful) dreams. Coxsackievirus—fatigue, depression, moods, skin rashes, headaches, sleepiness, conjunctivitis, chest pains (pleurisy), fibromyalgia, muscle weakness, abdominal pains.

*Rhinoviruses.* Head colds, watery, drippy noses, increased chest mucus, headaches. ☐ Detox

*Hepatitis A.* Jaundice, fatigue. ☐ Detox

## RNA—*Togaviruses*

*Eastern equine encephalomyelitis.* An arbovirus, or insect-borne virus; headache, muscle weakness, visual effects. ☐ Detox

*Rubella (German measles).* Skin sensitivity, redness of the skin, urticaria, hives; headaches; arthritis, joint, and muscle pains; racing heart, irregular pulse, and chest pains; halitosis; hearing, balance, tinnitus, and conjunctivitis, visual disturbances; fibromyalgia. ☐ Detox

## RNA—Flavivirus

*Dengue.* An arbovirus, insect-borne virus; chronic fatigue, fever, muscle and joint pains, liver pains; skin rashes, unexplained sweating bouts, [skin sensations of mosquitoes biting the limbs]; depression; intense fluctuating headaches, pain behind the eyes; nightmares. *Note:* no patients attending the clinic had a past history of severe hemorrhagic dengue fever. ☐ Detox

## RNA—Reovirus

*Rotavirus.* Diarrhea, abdominal upsets and pain, pelvic pains, pelvic discomfort; pain at the bottom of the spine and over the sacrum or tailbone; fatigue, depression, poor memory, irritability. ☐ Detox

## RNA—*Myxoviruses*

*Influenza A and B.* Chronic recurring or persistent nose and chest infection, coughing; weakness, fluctuating fevers, chronic ☐ Detox fatigue, depression, decreased mental activity, poor memory; fibromyalgia, muscle aching and cramping; neck, chest, and thoracic back pains, joint aches.

*Mumps.* Painful, tingling swollen saliva glands, excess saliva or ☐ Detox
a dry mouth; liver tenderness, [pain in the pancreas, ovaries, testes, and prostate gland]; aggravation of skin rashes, skin itching; depression, [mental activity]; [smell, vision, and hearing symptoms, vertigo and tinnitus]; significant [changes in blood glucose levels] during provocation; insomnia, racing of the memory, and recurring fears and worries.

*Morbilli.* Nose, chest pains and sensations, coughing; sensitive, ☐ Detox
itchy skin; fibromyalgia, muscle aches, reduced muscle strength, unexplained chronic fatigue; loss of or depressed mental activities, variable moods, impairment or loss of memory; headaches, migraines, constant pain headache; visual changes, light intolerance, and tinnitus.

*Respiratory syncytial virus.* Children—sinusitis, asthma, bron- ☐ Detox
chitis; loss of memory and ability to do school work; personality changes. Adults—sinusitis, wet drippy nose, bronchitis, asthma, difficult to treat cough; chest pains, itching or prickling deep in the chest, increased production of clear mucus; skin itching, skin color changes; eye symptoms and visual disturbances.

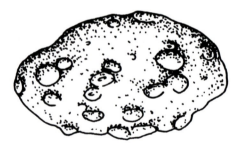

### Serial Vaccination and Cell Changes

Virus Fears and Assurances (see Chapter 3, p. 140) attempts to explain aspects of viral therapies of concern to the average person. Vaccines stimulate antibody formation in the blood. A dose of viral protein is taken by mouth, or injected, once, maybe three or four times. The dose of active viral material is weakened (attenuated) but still "alive." A common attenuated or killed vaccine is the yearly influenza shot that gives protection for the coming winter. About 20 percent of the elderly cannot tolerate the influenza shot; they develop continuing flu symptoms, severe headaches, coughing bouts, fatigue, and fibromyalgia, to mention some of the worst side effects. For these people, the single dose delivers too great a quantity of active influenza virus. Virutherapy uses treated (chemical-, heat-altered) influenza protein. The dose is a miniscule fraction of the amount of virus contained in a conventional single-shot immunization. Influenza serial virutherapy relieves vaccination side effects suffered by the elderly. Many obtain better protection during the winter from serial dilution shots of influenza, without side effects. A further advantage is that the vial can be used to "stave off the flu" (see p. 169) (McTaggart, 1996).

**IK** It should come as no surprise that twenty to forty years after a vaccination reaction or a severe virus infection, the same virus in a latent form turns out to be the principal cause of a person's functional subjective symptoms, or CFIDS/ME. Protesters from antivaccination organizations believe vaccinations may increase the risk of cancer later in life. Do they mean that the chances of a cancerous change in organ cells that hold excess toxins and latent viruses for many years are greater than in organ cells with little or no latent virus? If their surmise is correct, successful MLV should decrease the risk, if in fact it existed. Certain human viruses cause cancer. Seventy years ago, Dr. P. Rous discovered viruses in animals' cancerous cells. The medical establishment and research of those days ignored the discovery for over thirty years. Dr. Rous was eventually recognized with the award of the Nobel Prize (Feltner, 1990). Most people know that the last stages of AIDS/HIV infection bring on a cancer called Kaposi's sarcoma. Cancerous or precancerous cells have altered or depressed immunity responses, raising some interesting questions. It is possible that many of the viruses entering cancerous cells are latent and not cancer inducing. Just because viruses are found in a cancer cell does not mean they are the cause of the malignant change.

An ex-patient, who is grateful for her return to normal health following the preliminary work-up and MLV, installed a hot tub in the basement of her home. Two or three afternoons a week she invites terminal cancer patients living in the neighborhood to take heat treatment and massage. All agree it helps in coping with their cancers. All have outlived the prognosis of their life expectancy following cancer therapy.

### Latent Glandular Fever, EBV Symptoms, and Treatment

Active glandular fever is caused by the almost perfect parasite, human herpes 4, the Epstein-Barr virus, and the human herpes 5 virus, CMV. EBV is difficult to diagnose, causes bizarre symptoms, and has no specific treatment. All people can do is rest and wait for the viral symptoms to go away. But that is not all; latent EBV resides in our body cells for the rest of our lives. Latent EBV causes relapses of "functional" mood and fatigue symptoms that are often considered psychological because latent EBV avoids diagnosis. It has a sinister role in chronic hepatitis, even in cancers such as lymphoma and postnasal carcinoma.

In the third world, poor hygiene causes infants and young children to become infected with EBV. In more developed countries, teenagers often become infected. Long called "the kissing disease," the story of Epstein-Barr virus began with its discovery over twenty-fives years ago. Glandular fever symptoms were recognized over a hundred years ago. (For symptoms commonly associated with EBV/glandular fever, see p. 172.) If you have EBV symptoms, either active or latent, you cannot turn your back on them and hope they will go away. For many, the symptoms continue to fluctuate after a period of apparent recovery. Relapses occur, sometimes worse than the original illness.

You might say, "These symptoms are those of CFIDS/ME" and you would be correct. For years, EBV was regarded as the main cause of these illnesses. Throughout this book, the dominant role of EBV in the tiredness illnesses becomes obvious to the reader. Researchers working with the blood immunity patterns of CFIDS/ME people could not find sufficient evidence in the blood to support EBV as a cause of the illnesses. Physicians reasoned that the incubation period was (1) of short duration in glandular fever and (2) of long duration, if in fact present, in CFIDS. The mistake was confusing active and latent forms of EBV. Active EBV is not involved in the symptoms of CFIDS patients, although antibodies from past active EBV infections may be present. Latent EBV has long periods of fluctuating symptoms that would be described as an incubation. If researchers had used EBV provocation neutralization, they would have discovered the presence of latent EBV without accompanying blood antibodies (Buchwald et al., 1996). The expensive PCRT detected the DNA of EBV in the blood of one woman while she was suffering severe detoxing symptoms.

If CFIDS/ME medical authorities continue to restrict their requirements for proof, it will be difficult for patients and laypeople to take them seriously. Perhaps the same can be said for HIV researchers. The mistaken view that EBV is not a factor in the tiredness illnesses continued the hunt for the "true" CFIDS/ME virus. To date, there are claims of five or six "new" CFIDS viruses. Dr. W. John Martin of Los Angeles has cultivated and identified a new group of viruses with many similarities to latent viruses. He calls them *stealth viruses*. Sadly, this discovery has not led to any useful practical treatments. Perhaps many of the 1986 Lake Tahoe, Nevada, CFIDS epidemic victims would have provoked latent EBV symptoms if provocation neutralization testing had been available. CFIDS is a multicause complex illness, with considerable variation in the principal and supporting latent microbes (see Appendix I).

### The EBV Strike-Back Response

The EBV provocation ends the MLV work-up. The provoked symptoms are those of EBV, and some lesser symptoms from other latent viruses stirred up by the EBV provocation, called "shadowing" symptoms. EBV is tricky, so I ask patients to use drops under the tongue, at three- to four-week intervals, to start. You should learn not to overprovoke symptoms, and to avoid reactions that cause you to miss work. Most suffer some provoked symptoms and the EBV smell for two to three months. The smell stops, and four to six weeks later, they felt better than at any time in the past months, even years. EBV is treacherous, however, and when you have finished treatment and at last expect a return to remembered health, it can strike back with a nasty relapse. Before EBV virutherapy was available, relapses were often worse than the original illness. Most relapses are now controlled and checked within one to three weeks, provided the preliminary work-up and virutherapy are started. The terrible relapses of the past meant another loss of job and lifestyle. So bad was the associated despondency and depression, that suicide was attempted. I suggest that EBV and cannabis should be looked for in the bodies of teenage suicide victims, before a psychological explanation for their suicide is accepted by the coroner.

### The Autodetoxing Mode

Occasionally, a patient is provoked and begins detoxing with symptoms and smells typical of the provoking microbes. But instead of the detoxing symptoms fading away in a few hours or days, they continue. No serial vaccination treatment is required. After three to four weeks of autodetoxing mode, other symptoms and smells not associated with the original provoking microbe will appear. The nonspecific autodetoxing mode indicates the body's immunities are recovering (refer to the case notes on the lady who passed green urine for six weeks, p. 186). The autodetoxing mode can be a terrible experience for a few people. It cannot be stopped by neutralization, and symptom suppression drugs are needed to reduce the severity, even though their use prolongs detoxing. If the provoked symptoms are tolerated, people report a strange chemical taste and chemical smells from past xenopetrochemicals and SSD residues. Let us imagine that some, yet to be discovered, molecular dating method is available. I surmise some of the detoxed latentees' smells would be as old, or older, than the duration of the person's chronic illness.

**IK**   A woman suffering from CFIDS/ME and depression of eighteen years' duration began an autodetoxing mode from *Trichomonas,* a single-cell organism related to *Giardia.* Six months prior to the provocation test she stopped the seventeen-year continuous use of antidepressants and enjoyed reasonable health for four to five months. The *Trichomonas* detoxing mode was severe and lasted four and a half months, followed by the clearing of symptoms within a week. Since then she has felt better than at any time during the previous twenty years.

Severe autodetoxing mode continuing for longer than six weeks occurs in one out of every fifty patients.

A recovered and grateful classical music buff imagined a viral orchestra. The players are twenty-five viruses and the microbes *Candida, Giardia, Helicobacter,* and *Chlamydia.* Their instruments are our organs and muscles. The orchestra leader, influenza, provokes the nose, chest, and muscle virus sections. CRC, *Giardia,* and *Helicobacter* are the percussion or drum section because they are so good at rectal noises. The conductor, EBV, provokes all virus players. The orchestra plays the "Latency Symphony," but its duration is not for forty minutes or an hour; it continues for months, sometimes years.

## THE 1,001 "FRIENDS" IN OUR GUT

People think of their body as that part enclosed by the skin. It upsets many to discover there are two living compartments: one part is all within the skin and soft linings of our food, air, and water tubes, and the other is the 1,001 microbes and uncounted viruses that inhabit these tubes. It is estimated that 70 percent of our immune effort keeps these two parts in balance. When your asthma is making you struggle for air, do not get the idea that most of your immune effort is being directed toward your chest. Our 1,001 friends are not having a free ride in our gut. They make it difficult for one or more microbes to dominate the others and for outside invading microbes to become established in their territory. In other words, under normal conditions, the 1,001 microbes actively restore their numbers and position in our gut. Ninety trillion microbes live in or on our bodies. Most are enjoying the hospitality of our gut, without our conscious permission. Our useful friendly bugs enjoy close relationships with the cells of our gut lining, the enterocytes. When antibiotics all but wipe out our friendly microbes, the enterocyte cells keep the site free of intruding microbes, until their friends return. New and exciting research is revealing (1) how our friendly (commensal) microbes prefer sites and niches of our gut lining, (2) how they communicate with our gut cells by chemical messengers, and (3) how they turn on the gut cells' genes to consolidate the cell-microbe relationship. Our interactive gut community evolved over millions of years. Are we risking its disruption with the new supermarket processed and preserved foods? If so, the damage has been inflicted over the last forty to fifty years. Could there be a connection with the increase in IBS, obesity, and inflammatory bowel diseases?

Latency provocation and neutralization may have a role to play in detecting excessive and abnormal levels of friendly (commensal) microbes. Normal levels will not provoke symptoms. If there are cozy microbe-gut cell relationships with interchange of chemical messengers, any excess holding of the microbial messengers could provoke to latency testing. *Helicobacter pylori* may be a friendly helpful microbe until it multiplies and gets out of control (see *Helicobacter* provoked symptoms, pp. 50-51). Scientific medical therapy sets out to eradicate *Helicobacter pylori,* but this may be ineffective. If *Helicobacter pylori* is shown to inhibit or remove unfriendly invading bacteria, then practical therapy would be to reduce its excessive numbers by serial dilution therapy rather than antibiotics and chemicals (Hamilton, 1999).

The effect of antibiotics on our friendly microbe population can be as devastating as the invasion of foreign microbes. Friendly microbes help us to absorb essential elements and nutrients. Some even make vitamins that we absorb and, by altering our food, aid our digestion. Before antibiotics, most of us had a balance of microbes in our gut that has changed little during evolution. Our second *ME* gut compartment microbes invade and digest us when our personal *ME* dies. (Garrett, 1993; Hamilton, 1999).

The speciality of gastroenterology does not accept that latent viruses are present in our gut. The problem is negative laboratory printouts. Scientific medicine requires proof, not clinical anecdotal evidence. Latent viruses and microbes causing symptoms are in the gut and show their presence when provoked by latency therapy. Furthermore, MLV reduces or clears the symptoms of IBS and other gut conditions that resist conventional therapies. Satisfied patients have no doubt that latent viruses and microbes were in their gut because they experience the various symptoms and different smells during detoxing of excess individual microbes. When a minor relapse occurs, it is not difficult to identify the offending microbe. The renewed interest in latent viruses is illustrated by the increased volume of related medical research and clinical papers, and the addition of latent virus as a new classification in published and online world medical indexes.

Britain's foremost surgeon, Sir A. Lane, wrote in the *British Medical Journal,* 1919, that many body illnesses were associated with, or caused by, bacterial toxins formed in the gut. He popularized the *toxic* or *focal sepsis* concept. Enemas and bowel washouts were in widespread use at that time because they often gave relief, despite critics calling the practice "the colon fixation habit." Thirty years later, when antibiotics arrived, the enemas bulbs were removed from the medical chests. Nowadays, enemas and bowel washes are returning to favor among those who cannot obtain relief from antibiotics or gastroenterology therapies.

Those suffering from the effects of broad-spectrum antibiotics should get to know how their bowel companions were damaged, how to protect them, and how to keep the unwanted invaders, such as CRC, *Giardia, Helicobacter,* and disrupting viruses, at tolerable levels. The unwanted microbes use the nutrients for themselves, depressing our gut absorption and damaging the gut lining, leading to *leaky gut.* They will also help themselves to any nutrients and nutritional supplements you are taking. You may develop mild deficiencies or more serious ones, such as *Giardia* malabsorption.

### Are We Eating the Right Types of Roughage?

A new area of anthropology research is focusing on what our forbears ate. Anthropologists discovered fossilized motions in Middle Eastern and Iranian caves, dating from 200,000 years ago to 5,000 to 7,000 years ago. Buckwheat, a plant of the rhubarb family, is always present in the fossilized motions. Peas and beans did not appear in motions until after our ancestors began cooking with fire (the poisons in peas and beans are destroyed by cooking). The OWGGs appear 12,000 to 10,000 years ago, becoming important food items from 8,000 to 7,000 years ago. They are *very new foods* that we eat often and in large quantities. Could this explain the high rate of OWGG allergies and intolerance? Much is made of OWGG roughage in today's diet, but until 7,000 to 5,000 years ago, most roughage came from vegetables and the chitin from insects and fish (chitin is a polysaccharide similar in structure to cellulose found in the hard shell of insects and the scales of fish). We regard our forbears eating huge quantities of live insects with disgust and disbelief, but perhaps our descendants 10,000 to 100,000 years from now will regard our huge intake of OWGGs with disbelief. "Who is for a dish of cooked locusts, moths, and spiders with a spinach or lettuce salad, flavored with powdered fish scale chitin?" (Hyde, 1992).

OWGG wheat bran is promoted by the food industry and health specialists as a healthy source of diet roughage. Why then do some IBS or chronic constipation patients suffer aggravation of symptoms, even passage of blood, with their motions? Wheat bran damages and ulcerates the lining of the gut of those allergic to celiac and OWGGs. Maize bran is just as good as the highly promoted OWGG bran. If you have an OWGG allergy, or you are suspicious that OWGG bran is upsetting you, look for a supply of commercial maize bran. If you need proof, examine your motions 12 to 24 h after eating corn on the cob! If you cannot get a supply of maize bran, cut the softer roughage off the corncob. Boil the roughage, then drain and store it in the freezer. Soft boiled bran is more appetizing than the dried flakes. Begin with a tablespoon of maize bran a day and slowly increase, if required. Because of the expense of fresh vegetables, and the time required for preparation and cooking, fried chips, with their preservatives and yellow dyes, and wheat pasta have taken over the vegetables' place on our plates (Brostoff and Jamlin, 1989; Gottschall, 1994; Heller, 1992).

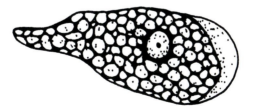

## DETOXING AND SAUNAS

Detoxing and saunas are briefly explained in Chapter 3.

Excretion or elimination involves the removal of harmful and unwanted substances from the body. A popular term is *detoxing*. Detox has many meanings, but we will liken it to a living sewerage treatment plant and its effluent. Body and liver chemistry reduces or neutralizes the toxic effect of many harmful substances that are made by, or enter, the body. The lungs, kidneys, and the large intestine remain the main detoxing outlets throughout life. Detoxing or excretion of excess allergic food particles, the toxins of organisms, latent microbes, fungi, bacteria, viruses, and toxic xenochemicals is important for maintaining normal immunities and for recovery from latency, functional, or subjective illness. As we age, our body uses different outlets; for example, older people perspire less. Try to recognize and improve the means by which your body carries out detoxing activities. Detoxing speeds up recovery, but too much detoxing brings on too many disabling symptoms. Latent detoxing treatments are adjusted to increase or stimulate normal detoxing, while giving some control over the increased symptoms. Detoxing usually has a smell or odor, but some people detox without this occurring. I postulate, from clinical observation of several hundred patients, that 80 to 85 percent of people have smelled an odor during detoxing. Those without odor may inactivate the substances being detoxed by altering them or wrapping them in a protein covering (latentee-antilaten).

### IK Preliminary Work-Up Detoxing

A distinctive pattern of weight loss confined to patients with OWGG allergies was observed at the clinic (1974). Patients with confirmed allergies to OWGGs begin total exclusion, with no dietary lapses, for four to five months. After five to fourteen days, patients usually experience an aggravation of symptoms that often becomes intolerable. Many withdraw and resume eating OWGGs and taking SSDs. The aggravation of symptoms from withdrawal may be sudden and alarming. If depression occurs or is aggravated, contact the clinic at once. Moods may be aggravated or changed and reasoning affected. The exaggerated symptoms of withdrawal clear after two to three weeks.

*Surmise:* Patients with OWGG allergies have immune systems that are slow to detox and excrete OWGG undigested proteins, which pass through the leaky gut. The gluten and other grain proteins accumulate in the body fat and provoke increasing obesity.

Clinical observation and the comments of patients indicate that there is a clearing of symptoms during OWGG exclusion. This clearing suggests that gluten is held in the fat until the brain, organs, and muscles are detoxed. Gluten held in the fat of the brain, organs, and muscles is detoxed before gluten held in the fat of overweight or obese people. Following withdrawal of OWGG foods, a weight loss of excess salt, water, glycogen (animal sugar), and some fat occurs for two to three weeks, then stalls until the body structures reduce their excess gluten. The weight loss resumes at three to four months and continues until gluten detoxing is completed. As the amount of gluten excretion rises, there is a temporary increase of symptoms, with a simultaneous decrease in fat and body fluid. By five to six months, the gluten has disappeared from the body. Body weight returns to normal and the symptoms of OWGG allergies become a memory. Do not become concerned if you "go to skin and bone" because the body weight your genes programmed will return in a month or two, but the old obesity will not return. Three to four weeks after excluding OWGGs, "burn-off" symptoms appear from the decreasing CRC population in the bowel and the release of *Candida* toxins. The symptoms are further increased by nystatin taken orally and as an enema. Symptoms decrease by the sixth to eighth week. *Giardia* activity temporarily increases as the CRC burn-off symptoms decrease. If bowel symptoms are severe, a three-day course of tinidazole, or a week's course of metronidazole, will control the worst symptoms.

The following are three main concepts/methods of weight loss and control of obesity by dieting:

1. Decreased fat, increased nonprocessed carbohydrates, and a program of physical exercise
2. Increased fat and protein (meat) and markedly reduced nonprocessed carbohydrates to control excess insulin production
3. Drug therapy using hormone and stimulating metabolic compounds

*Surmise:* Total exclusion of OWGG foods is necessary when an allergy to these foods is present.

Obese and overweight patients attending the clinic nearly all provoked to OWGG foods and CRC testing. All previously attempted many diets with small to moderate improvements. They developed the yo-yo response when they stopped the diets. A total OWGG exclusion diet is difficult, and most people need encouragement and instructions on implementing it. Despite the difficulties, hundreds of patients adopted the diet, changing their figures and improving their personalities.

We experience natural food detoxing when we eat beetroot or asparagus and notice the color or smell in our urine.

**IK**    The preliminary work-up and virutherapy program failed. His terrible breath (halitosis) persisted. He had no social life. His mother kept her distance from the foul breath. He began a water fast, and on the fifth day, "the breath" disappeared. He ended the fast on the seventh day. He introduced two foods a day, and on the fourth day, the breath returned after eating dairy and beef. He has not eaten these foods since that day. He is married and enjoying a full social and sporting lifestyle. *Comment:* About one in a hundred patients are advised to do a five- or seven-day water fast because their preliminary work-up and MLV program fail or are disappointing. A fast requires days off work and tedious reintroduction of foods. This is justified when the program's treatment fails (see the case notes on the man who had a tracheostomy, p. 47).

**IK**    A woman suffered CFIDS/ME, with fluctuation of energy, mental activity, and muscle weakness, for a period of eight years. No cause was found, and she was resigned to "tender loving care" and SSD therapy. At the clinic she provoked to OWGGs and CRC. Her hair was dull and slack and she had a dry scalp. Imagine her surprise when detoxing of CRC and other molds caused her scalp to become oily, requiring washing once or twice a day. Allergists recognize such changes are frequently related to food and mold allergies.

Xenochemicals do not occur in nature; they are man-made. Some people are unable to excrete them and suffer from their accumulations and toxic effects.

**IK**    A CFIDS/ME sufferer alarmed by green urine after the fourth clinic visit was reassured when an urgent liver function test was normal. For years she had enjoyed a green lime cordial, but she stopped drinking it after the first visit. The green dye colored her urine for the next eight weeks, then appeared for short periods over the next month. Her natural detoxing of the xenodye, brought about by the general detoxing effect of the therapy, aided her recovery.

Health books describe the important benefits of nutritional supplements and antioxidants in aiding and modifying detoxing. Excellent books on this subject are available. Ask your physician or allergy group for local preferences. The recent recognition of right-handed (dextro) and left-handed (levo) spatial arrangement (three-dimensional) of chemically identical drug molecules, both natural and man-made, explains acceptance or rejection with side effects. For example, natural vitamin Bs absorbed from our food are readily accepted by our bodies, whereas synthetic vitamin Bs, with different spatial or structural arrangement, are less effective. A potentially dangerous food industry practice is the destruction of natural vitamins and mineral combinations in foods, and the so-called "enrichment" with substitute synthetic products. Before accepting man-made nutritional substitutes for natural products, state authorities should inform the public whether long-term exposure will interfere or depress immunity and resistance to infections. Numerous studies demonstrate the superiority of natural nutritionals over their man-made substitutes. Should the public consumer who buys supermarket food suffer possible long-term immunity depression because the food industry views long shelf life and the addition of synthetic preservatives as good for business?

### MLV Detoxing

Latent viruses are eliminated by MLV in strange ways, other than those already mentioned. Elimination of EBV produces a nauseatingly sick smell in the bed and bedroom. A sudden unexplained false type of severe depression brings on floods of tears. If the tears are collected, they smell of CMV and EBV. Virus elimination occurs in the increased clear nasal mucus and watery discharge. The breath has a peculiar smell or is offensive. The fingernail and toenail quicks stink from CMV and EBV. The mouth suddenly fills with smelly saliva that persists for an hour or two (EBV, CMV, and mumps). Some patients are sure their stomach detoxes smells after their treatment shots, but most patients feel the smells come from their lungs.

During elimination, your symptoms may get worse or, occasionally, much better. Elimination continues until you suddenly realize you have not been smelling for a week or more. In another three to four weeks, the smells and symptoms return for short periods, and then they stop; you feel well, often just as you remembered before you became ill. A return of the smells which you or your partner recognizes, months or years later signals a relapse in one to three days, giving you time to prepare the relapse treatment.

### The Microbes' Response to Detoxing

We should not be surprised if the microbes that infect us have developed countermeasures to our immunities' defenses against them. The toxins of microbes and the latent viruses depress the body's temperature regulation center in the brain. They reduce body temperature or stop a high temperature or fever from developing. They slow the thyroid gland's activity and lower the daily body temperature below normal. They stop or reduce body sweating and depress absorption of essential oils, proteins, and minerals, including zinc and iron, from the gut. This further cripples the immunities' response to microbes. Bacterial and fungal toxins and the latent viruses accumulate in organ and muscle cells, reducing an individual's cell activities and immunities. Patients attending the clinic for relief of fatigue illnesses are told their body immunities are unable to mount a recovery against such heavy odds. The methods used in the clinic can only be successful against the microbes by detoxing them and their toxins and, in time, raising the patient's natural body immunities. Sadly, some chronically ill or disabled patients will not respond. The microbes have such a hold on their bodies that it not possible to stimulate the return of normal body temperature and detoxing.

Symptom suppression drugs and, in particular, antibiotic courses do not get rid of these hidden latent toxins and organ cell parasites. Any improvements from the drugs in time fail, and the body's immunities and latency responses of organ and muscle cells are further depressed. Antibiotics against the nonlatent (active) viral microbes may give patients variable improvement or fail because of resistance. Many antiviral drugs cannot penetrate organ cells to affect their latent viruses. Other antiviral drugs enter but fail to eradicate intracellular latent viruses and bacteria. Detoxing methods developed over many centuries were dismissed and forgotten when antibiotics appeared in the late 1940s. From the evidence of an increasing incidence of fatigue illnesses, it is possible that enema bulbs or disposable enema units will become household items by the year 2010.

### Body Temperature, Microbes, and Toxins

"Frozen" patients are investigated by other physicians before coming to the clinic. The thyroid gland activity tests, thyroxine dosage, and vitamin B complex did not affect the sensations of coldness. From clinical observations and responses of many patients, I believe this type of body coldness is caused by food and mold allergies, petrochemical toxins, CRC, *Giardia* toxins, and latent viruses. Could it be that latent viral genomes and toxins are depressing the nerve cells of the temperature-regulating centers of the brain? Most CFIDS/ME patients with lower body temperatures do not develop a fever when infected by influenza. Their temperature-regulating centers are unresponsive.

> Jane, on recovering from CFIDS/ME, put it this way: "You slowly climb the treatment mountain. At the pass, the temperature control center begins to function, you warm up and begin to sweat, then start the descent to the recovery plain below."

**IK** Although the clinic room was a little too warm from the late summer sun, during provocation and neutralization with a virus, a woman suffering from chronic migraine, put on her coat, walked over to the heater, and turned it on. Her hands were white and blue. Her face was drawn and pale. The forehead thermometer registered normal. She experienced the coldness during earlier testing sessions with *Candida* and *Giardia*. Influenza was worse, but *Morbillivirus* froze her like a lump of ice. Twenty minutes later her coat was off, the heater turned off, and she felt warm. She neutralized with morbilli $5^8$. Ever since the sudden onset of her illness years ago, she often woke at 2:00 to 3:00 a.m., feeling she was freezing to death Moribilli virutherapy helped her to recover remembered health and took away her chronic migraine.

**IK** "I feel like an animated ice maiden from Peru. Why can't I warm up?" She sat in the warm spring sun, her hands and the tip of her nose were white and bluish in tinge. Her feet were like lumps of ice, and she was wearing enough clothes to be out in a blizzard. A skin thermometer on her forehead gave a normal temperature reading. Six months later, she completed the treatment course and her husband joined her again in the double bed.

Heat therapies are as old as medicine. Hot springs and pools became centers for treatment of the ills of those who lived in the past. Saunas, a Scandinavian word for heat treatment, became popular worldwide after World War II. With the arrival of SSDs in the 1950s, heat treatments again fell into disrepute because they were not a "quick fix." They remained popular in Scandinavia and Japan. Saunas are staging a comeback because they promote detoxing and improve athletic performance. The old advice to those with fever or influenza is a hot bath and good night's sleep to "sweat it out." But do not take the aspirin and brandy nip. Increased body temperature (1) slows down the invading microbes, (2) increases the flow of blood in the small blood vessels and capillaries, (3) stimulates the activity of the blood immune system's activities, especially the white cells, and (4) increases organ cell activity and detoxing. Most microbes that attack us cannot tolerate feverish temperatures. Aspirin and a nip of brandy lower the temperature. So why give the microbes a second chance to get at you?

As you sit in a sauna or hot bath, ask yourself two questions: Why does this aggravate my symptoms and then improve them? Why does heat make my breath and sweat have such a strong smell? Scientists believe it is the activity of mitochondria, called the powerhouses of the cell, and heat shock proteins present in every cell of our bodies. Heat shock proteins are able to remove excess toxins, and probably latent viruses, into the tissue fluids. The blood immune system carries them to the excreting areas of our bodies. Cells lining the gut and lungs detox from their free surfaces. When millions of our cells are stimulated to rid themselves of excess toxins or latent viruses, the amount excreted is sufficient to stimulate known symptoms and to make the person smell, even stink. Because the treatment dose is extremely dilute, it does not have any smell. It seems reasonable to assume, then, that the large amount of mobilized and excreted latent virus is causing the provoked symptoms, not the minute amount of processed viral protein in the treatment dose. All this occurs without any antibody stimulation by the blood immune system.

I ask all patients to record the type of smells coming out of them and the symptoms occurring at the same time. Detoxing is a continuing activity, even when we are fit and well. Each person has his or her individual pattern of detoxing. Before you get out of the sauna, ask yourself the following questions: Where does all the sweat come from? Why are many of my symptoms coming on? Why am I beginning to get irritable, moody, and depressed? Why do symptoms from the sauna clear away two to three hours later? Why do I feel more energetic and active when the symptoms clear? This book attempts to answer these questions.

**IK**   Several women recovering from severe CRC detoxed such musty smelling sweat that their partners refused to sleep with them. Hepatitis, EBV, *Legionella,* and *Trichomonas* have very unpleasant smells that "reserve" the double bed for the patient. The smells vary from day to day; for example, one smell may persist for a few hours, then disappear, only to be replaced by another smell. The first smell may detox from the skin through sweat, and the next smell may detox through the urine or breath. Complex smells suggest several toxins and microbes are detoxing.

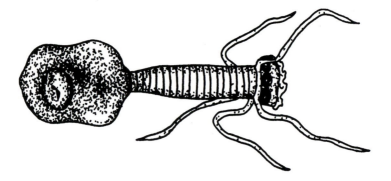

## Heat Treatments

### Saunas and Sun Saunas

Saunas and sun saunas stimulate detoxing. Autosaunas can distress your partner if you sleep in a double bed. Keep to a regular sauna routine while you are receiving treatment from the clinic. Keep away from sauna houses using pine or eucalyptus oil, as the tree oils (terpenes) are irritants and will aggravate any chemical sensitivities you may have. If you cannot sweat during your first two or three sauna visits, take a lukewarm or tepid shower to chill the skin and then reenter the sauna. The temperature differential of the skin will jump-start sweating. Do not persist after three tepid showers. Keep a watch on your salt losses during sweating. The loss of salt makes you tired. A crude test is to lick some of the sweat off your arm. If it is salty, you are in salt balance. After the sauna take a warm or hot shower to remove the sweat. *Do not take a cold shower or plunge* after a heat or sun sauna. *Surmise:* The cold turns off the heat shock protein effect and detoxing symptoms stop. Your sauna-induced symptoms are cleared, and you feel great for the next 2 to 3, even 5 to 6, h after. If you take the traditional cold plunge, your heat sauna is not cost-effective.

Sun saunas are taken during the hot months of the year because of convenience and no expense. Start a regular program to reduce viruses and toxin levels as soon as the sun is hot enough for sun saunas. Lie on a mat behind a glass sliding door or outside. Cover yourself, except for your face, with one or two blankets and an absorbent sheet to collect sweat. Place a sheet of black cotton material or aired degassed black agricultural plastic on top to absorb the sun's heat. Plastic sweat suits are also available. For the first two or three saunas, your body may refuse to sweat, despite getting very hot and developing headaches and symptoms you recognize. Try the tepid shower technique described previously. Tolerate awful feelings and sweating until you cannot take them anymore, then crawl inside the house. Lie on the bed, well covered, to avoid becoming chilled. Sweating may continue for another 30 min to 1 h, during which most people fall asleep, waking in 1 to 2 h feeling motivated and energetic. Do not expose your skin to the sun, as it releases histamine, a cause of headaches and muscle aches. The hot season of the year is when you truly battle with your toxins and multiple latent viruses. By the time fall is in the air, you should be feeling a lot stronger and mentally adjusted. Do not fritter away the hot summer days and forgo regular sun saunas because they will help you to feel so much better. You will regret stopping the sauna program when the cold weather comes back and you are no better, compared to how you felt last winter.

## The Autosauna

Have you ever woken up 2 to 4 h after falling asleep, feeling hot and sweaty and suffering from a headache? Women attending the clinic for chronic fatigue treatments tell me they lie awake in bed, cold as a lump of ice, and are envious of their partners who, 2 to 4 h after going to sleep, get very hot and sweat. The women begin to sleep better and autosaunas appear after about the fourth or fifth clinic visit, or after the herpes group of viruses is provoked. The autosaunas produce moldy and viral animal smells.

After 2 to 3 h of sleep, our temperature control centers start up the autosauna. It continues for 1 to 2 h most nights, until the toxins or viruses are excreted. Night sweating is normal for infants and young people. Mothers should identify the smells, especially if there is heavy night sweating. Sick children begin musty night sweating shortly after treatment is started. Infants and children also detox and sweat from the scalp. Observant mothers report yellowing of pillowcases, until cola and orange drinks with yellow food dye are stopped. Women suffering from CRC and CFIDS/ME are very sensitive to perfumes and chemical smells. They are affected by chemicals that are detoxed by their partners' autosaunas. They are unable to get up in the morning and help with the breakfast. Women who "test smell" the bedding after both have arisen in the morning report that the chemical smells come from their partners' side of the bed. These reports are too frequent to dismiss. The men are very considerate and take the clinic's advice to go to a sauna or have a hot bath before they come home from work. Are we preventing toxin excretion from many of these areas by taking SSDs such as antidepressants and using underarm antiperspirants? Blood tests are negative for viral antibodies before and after autosaunas.

## Cold Water Therapy

Reports suggest that cold water therapy helps those who cannot tolerate the high temperatures of saunas. Cold water chilling may jump-start detoxing. It was popular in the past. On awaking you take a quick cold plunge or shower, followed by a brisk rubdown with a towel, bringing about a warming stimulation of the skin and clearing of the mind. CFIDS/ME patients are not advised to have cold water therapy. If you use cold water therapy from time to time, try to graduate from a sun sauna or hot bath to a heat sauna because of the superior detoxing effects.

### Social Group Immunity

*Surmise:* A closely related group of people may aid one another in provoking the excretion of excess toxins and microbes in one or others of the group through body secretions and the breath. At detoxing, an individual contacts a second person who is not in a detoxing mode. The first person's latentees/latentors are absorbed by the second person, provoking excretion of any excess latentees the second person may be carrying. There is an aggravation during the detoxing and then an improvement of the second person's symptoms.

**IK**  A woman, age 40, was partly disabled with deformed rheumatoid arthritis joint changes of the hands, wrists, knees, and feet. During the ten years since the onset, she showed no response to conventional therapy of methotrexate and gold therapy, etc. She and her partner were animal lovers since childhood. She provoked to *Parvovirus, Mycoplasma pneumoniae,* influenza, rubella, and *Chlamydia.* MLV provoked marked joint and muscle symptoms and then a great improvement, which declined after ten days. At the next visit, *Clostridium difficile* $5^{15}$ provoked remarkable improvement in muscle and joint movements, but two days later, she experienced the worst provoked aggravation of the work-up. She went to bed for four days but, after that, had an even greater improvement in joint and muscle movements. After the fourth weekly *Clostridium* treatment shot, she noticed some symptoms the following morning, when she had a discussion with her partner, who slept in a separate room. Later that morning, he fell ill at work with muscle and joint aches and diarrhea. He returned home and slept for the next 12 h. He could not straighten his knees for 48 h. He has not taken a day off work for the past fifteen years. Prior to this, he worked with horses and probably harbored *Clostridium* in his motions. By the third day, he was back at work.

*Surmise:* Social group detoxing of latent microbials and toxins would help to maintain the group's immunity. Severe active infections would continue to kill and disrupt the survivors' NIS and latency immunity. Social group detoxing could prevent intercurrent infections becoming chronic in the group. Over the years, many women patients attending the clinic became aware that when they were detoxing, following a treatment shot, their children, partners, or close friends, developed temporary or transient behavioral changes and/or symptoms suggestive of being unwell that disappeared the next day. It could be that infected and healthy individuals are constantly surrounded by low-concentration latentee particles from self-detoxing.

### CHANGE-OF-SITE RESPONSE (CSR)

Imagine your persistently blocked nose is treated with a cortisone or Csd nasal spray. After seven to fourteen days you breathe freely. You are told not to stop the daily spray or aerosol for the next two to three months. If you do, the nasal blocking returns. During this time, you may suffer a severe head cold, perhaps a chest infection, or be exposed to a dusty and moldy home, workplace, or sick public building. You become aware of wheezing and a little chest tightness. The chest symptoms persist even though your nose is clear. You consult the family physician, who gives you another Csd spray or aerosol to clear the symptoms from the chest. Another two to three months go by, and you find you cannot stop either medication without the symptoms returning. Then you notice a red itchy rash; or a headache, such as a migraine; or irritable, blurry eyes; or repeated influenza infections and head colds; or memory recall problems, behavioral symptoms, unexplained tiredness, loss of motivation (mañana); *or* the onset of CFIDS/ME symptoms. For each of these new CSR symptoms you are given the appropriate SSDs. Read about the Csd drugs (see pp. 203-207) before continuing further. Always inspect the labels on the medications you are using to see if Csds, antihistamines, NSAIDs, or antidepressants are included in the preparations. It is important to know what you are giving your child. CSR may be severe in young children.

CSR is confined to allergic people. Nose and chest Csd aerosols and sprays do not bring on CSR in nonallergic people. Patients comment that CSRs occur in organs or areas of their bodies that suffered a viral infection, a bruising accident, past trauma, or a previous symptom suppression operation, e.g., tonsillectomy or hysterectomy. CSR varies markedly from person to person during treatment with SSD therapy. As health improves, the risk of CSR is reduced.

**IK**    Three children in a family were given Csd sprays for their blocked noses. Each experienced a different CSR, as well as asthma, headaches and mood changes, and irritable bowel syndrome. By 1978, the Csd and cromolyn sprays were widely prescribed for nasal obstruction. During that year I was consulted by over a hundred mothers because they thought the excessive overactivity or hyperactivity was due to a food allergy or food chemicals. When the nasal sprays were stopped, the nose blocked again, and in most cases, the overactivity ceased. The obstructed noses cleared with food exclusion and dust mold therapy. The parents were shocked when CSR was explained to them.

Allergic people experience CSRs throughout their lives. As an infant, food allergies cause vomiting and diarrhea, then the appearance of skin rashes as the digestion settles down. The skin rashes improve for a year or more, but the nose becomes blocked, or wheezing develops in the chest. Within another two or three years, the chest is still worrisome but the child has periods of hyperactivity. About age ten or twelve, the chest is improved, but there is a complaint of headaches, often the beginning of migraines. Some, or all, of these symptoms may persist until age fourteen to sixteen, when the teenager is said to "grow out of the allergies." But then the acne appears with a personality change. By the early twenties, there is little or no allergic activity, until ages thirty-five to forty, when migraines reappear, together with chest wheezing, and often asthma. Before this age a virus infection, body trauma, physical injury, or mental shock can bring on symptoms. From the age of forty until death there is a varying pattern of allergic symptoms. Could sharing the response among its different organs and structures be the body's response to the allergic challenge? (See the conjunctivitis that went "roaming," p. 149.)

Csd preparations, by suppressing symptoms in one area of the body, speed up the "allergic procession." As one area's symptoms are suppressed, treatment is started on the next CSR body site, which in turn induces another organ to a CSR. In time, so many CSRs are being suppressed, the patient spends forty minutes twice a day applying Csd and other preparations to various parts of the body. If the Csd and other preparations are discontinued and causes of the allergic symptoms identified, the patient is released from carrying "the corticosteroids cross." Sadly, many attending the clinic did not recover from all of their CSR-induced symptoms. Csds and cromolyn (sodium chromoglycate) reduce the inflammatory reaction and possibly increase the intake of the allergic substance or antigen by the surface cells of the linings. The drugs increase the presence of bacteria, molds, and viruses. As a result, the chest and nasal mucus often becomes yellow, brown, and even green.

Surgical procedures induce CSR. The removal of tonsils and adenoids is followed by the onset of asthma and bronchitis, weeks to months later. The onset of asthma and/or depression comes on six to nine months after a hysterectomy. After a gall bladder removal, patients experience skin itch, pain in the womb, eczema, and headaches, and in many, a recurrence of the pain in the operation scar or wound. As preliminary work-up and MLV relieve the CSR following tonsillectomy, hysterectomy, or gall bladder removal, two questions should be considered: Were the symptoms in these organs due to an allergic response? Should the allergic work-up have been performed before the surgery, as the organ symptoms were not acute? Dr. Jonathan V. Wright offers convincing evidence that CSR symptoms are not new (Wright, 1990).

> A woman described her last three years of SSD therapy using Csd skin preparations, Csd asthma aerosols, intermittent prednisone 5 to 20 milligrams (mg), by mouth, and a series of antidepressant drugs as "clobber therapy." Four months after attending the clinic, she was able to stop the last of the drugs, the antidepressants. "Why was I made to suffer those awful drugs for three years?"

I have heard the same complaint many times (see "buttock craters," p. 149).

Some physicians deny CSR symptoms have an allergic cause or basis. Numerous papers by physicians and drug advertising in journals promote a clean image of Csds. Professional articles on the treatment of nasal allergies, often supported by company grants, do not mention CSR. Patients are told the increasing numbers of new symptoms, while on Csds and other SSDs, are due to a decrease in their immune response. Many become frightened and seek alternative treatments. Other physicians use Csds extensively, as they believe the drugs aid the person's immune response against allergy and inflammation. One such Csd is called an "asthma preventer," but the catch is that it is only a preventer as long as you keep taking the Csd. So extensive is the use of Csds to suppress symptoms that the CSR concept is not regarded as a side effect of Csd drugs. Warning notices do not appear on the CSR-inducing pharmaceutical products. Instead, symptoms occurring in other areas or organs of the patient are regarded as new conditions in no way related to the original symptom.

Chronic CSR symptoms in time mimic CFIDS/ME because they involve the brain and are difficult to treat. The similarity to CFIDS/ME is further increased when the muscles are involved in the CSR effect. The CSR is unmasked when Csds are withdrawn.

A woman who independently sought preliminary work-up and MLV with disappearance of all CSR symptoms was outspoken in condemning failure to recognize CSR. She called it "lazy medicine." She wished that an attempt had been made to identify the causes of her symptoms instead of suppressing them. She complained that her family physician was more interested in manipulating the various drugs that were available for symptom relief than in making an attempt to find causes. I consider her criticism to be rather harsh because often the causes cannot be identified (see The Eczema of a Hundred Causes, p. 79).

The CSR is not adequately described in medical texts, nor in the popular allergy books available to the public. If you think these descriptions fit your symptoms, inform your allergist or family physician. A 1992 study of 328 patients attending the clinic reported 687 CSR symptoms from using Csds and cromolyn. The frequency of nasal symptoms, e.g., bleeding and crusting, sticky colored mucus, wheezing on effort or asthma, suggests warnings should be placed on all treatment aerosols and sprays. The use of Csds is a wonderful advance in the treatment of asthma, but as with all therapies, the susceptible patient must be given adequate warning of CSR, probably when the third refill is requested. Csd inhalers and aerosols are *not* preventative asthma therapy for all types of asthma. Csd preparations suppress immunity responses and local symptoms.

For many years after the Csd beclomethasone came on the market, it was believed that minute amounts of the drug were absorbed from the treated surface linings. Some people absorb considerably more and develop mild to obvious toxic symptoms. Only a fifth of the total inhaled dose gets into the air tubes of the lung; the rest is swallowed. The Csds are carried away from the nose, chest, and eyes in mucus, which is also swallowed. As the Csds are not digested, they are absorbed from the gut. It is suggested that the constant presence of spent or used nasal and chest Csds encourages some gut organisms. The drugs probably depress the activity of the gut lining mucosa, in particular, the epithelial Ig A antibodies. My patients are sure their *Giardia* was worse when they were using Csds. So marked are the effects of Csds on the mucus and function of the nose and lungs, the resulting symptoms suggest a new type of asthma exists (McTaggart, 1996; Mansfield, 1997).

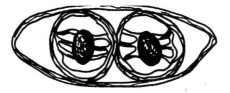

## THE SUBLINGUAL (UNDER THE TONGUE)
## DOOR TO LATENCY IMMUNITY

The sublingual organ, or area under the tongue, is a mysterious gateway to your immunities, in particular, the OCIS. This area and treatment drops are often mentioned in popular health books on allergy, but there is no mention of what happens, or how the testing and treatment drops work. It is assumed they work the same way as shots, but this may not be so. Mothers are always asking, "How do the drops under the tongue cause the upsets and improvements in my child's behavior during the testing and later treatments?" Or, "What is going on under the tongue? I can't see anything when I look there." Under the tongue/sublingual testing and treatment is a practical way of treating allergies and latency symptoms for those ages fourteen through sixteen, and for adults with seasonal pollen allergies or perennial house dust and inhalant allergies. The herpes family of viruses is treated equally well by drops or shots. Furthermore, it does away with children's dread and fear of injections. It is easy for mothers to treat younger children, and older children soon learn how to treat them-selves. Not a lot is known about absorption into the body from under the tongue; in fact, most physicians dismiss it as having a placebo effect.

Have you observed elderly folk halted in their walk by angina heart pain? They put a nitrate pill under their tongue to ease the pain. If you attend a wine-tasting exhibition, notice how the experts roll or swill the wine around their mouths, before spitting it out, and then announce their description of the wine. Some of the wine passes through the sublingual area into the bloodstream and is rapidly circulated throughout the body and brain. I suggest that it adds an, as yet, unexplored dimension to the complexity of the senses of smell and taste. You could say the sublingual organ is an opening or gate for the OCIS and the blood immune system. Everything passing the teeth is monitored and sampled. A minuscule sample of everything passing the teeth is delivered into the bloodstream, if the sublingual organ (SLO) allows it to pass. Where else in the body is there such a comprehensive warning organ? It is to the gut what the eye is to vision of the surrounding world.

The small compact area of the SLO lies under the protection of the tongue. It is in the most dependent area of the floor of the mouth. After a sample is accepted and passed into the bloodstream, it is quickly flushed away by saliva from the nearby ducts of the two saliva glands under the lower jaw. Should a food or substance persist in the mouth, the absorption is turned off. The SLO shows discrimination by allowing certain sub-stances to pass and blocking others from entering the bloodstream. From the ages of twelve to sixteen, there is increasing restriction on entry to the bloodstream, possibly because the individuals' immunities systems are approaching optimum levels. Take care of your SLO with good oral hygiene, and do not smoke, and when you reach old age, you will still benefit from an active SLO. The SLO is not surrounded by phalanxes of the NIS's protective white blood cells or lymph glands, suggesting it is an entry or gateway for the OCIS. There may be similar areas or organs throughout the gut, as some drugs are administered by enema.

Chewing a mouthful of food breaks up the food, releasing its tissue fluids, and some of the carbohydrate is converted to sugar by the saliva enzymes. A food can be recognized as having carbohydrate in it if, on chewing, it develops a safe, sweet taste. It is a far cry from our predecessors' chewing of sweet roots to the present mass addiction to sugary processed foods. Food particles pass through the SLO and into the bloodstream to circulate throughout the body, alerting the gut and its digestive organs to the nature of the food that will soon arrive. The food particles (antigens) could influence the brain to stimulate the appetite so the person continues eating. On occasion, the sublingual treatment drops are too strong, and shortly after dosing, the child will vomit. The SLO may play a role in the rejection of a mouthful of food, improving discrimination by the taste and smell senses. *Surmise:* When new or unfamiliar substances pass the SLO, minute amounts are taken up by the OCIS for latent memory or immunity templates. Larger recurring amounts may stimulate the NIS and its antibodies.

The SLO is not a recent development of our body. It evolved hundreds of millions of years ago with certain fish and amphibious animals, e.g., frogs, newts, and salamanders.

### *SLO Provocation and Therapy*

The test solution of 0.1 to 0.2 ml, with three to four drops of glycerin sweetener for the children, is placed under the child's uplifted tongue, and the timer is started. The chin is held low for 30 seconds (sec) for contact of the solution with the SLO. During this time, little of the dose passes to the back of the mouth and throat. After 30 sec the child can swallow and speak. From then on, behavior, provoked symptoms, and signs are recorded for the next 10 min. Provoked symptoms are neutralized by a weaker testing dose. Mothers are told to continue watching their children for the familiar delayed provoked symptoms, so important in determining the treatment dose. Most children can tolerate testing for 3 to 4 h, unless a particularly marked provocation occurs.

**IK**    Justin, age 6, was aggressive and disrupting at play centers and schools. He was turned away from three kindergartens and two schools. He was given one last chance to behave at a third school. Aggression toward his sister and hyperactivity occurred at home. Justin, accompanied by his distraught mother, arrived at the morning clinic. He complied with the sublingual drops and within an hour an OWGGs allergy was provoked and neutralized. There were marked bursts of hyperactivity with CRC, and at neutralization his red rash paled. Hepatitis provoked aggressive hitting of his mother and kicking of the shins of other adults in the clinic. He had to be held until hepatitis $5^8$ neutralized, when a completely different boy got off his mother's lap and started to play on the floor. Suddenly he experienced an urge to pass a motion. Other molds, house dusts, *Giardia,* and viruses were provoked and neutralized during a further testing session. Justin remained at the school, is progressing normally, and now has friends. He became hyperactive during the worst of the grass pollen season. His parents improved the home ecology with the limited funds available. Justin is unable to eat OWGGs, apples, and pears.

Older children and teenagers recognize immediate provoked symptoms. Delayed provoked symptoms are more marked and persistent. Sublingual testing of adults is patchy, variable, or completely negative, except for the herpes family of viruses. The SLO appears to select the amount of the treatment dose that passes into the body. A treatment shot of 0.05 ml CMV $5^{12}$ provoked marked symptoms, whereas a sublingual dose of 0.1 to 0.5 ml of same-strength CMV provoked a less marked, more tolerated response. Both treatment doses brought on delayed sweating. If the first shot from your new treatment vial provokes excessive, even severe, symptoms that stop you from going to work, try a sublingual dose four to five days after the provoked symptoms have subsided. The sublingual drops are given once or twice a day, or every second day, depending on the severity of the provoked symptoms. When there is no further response from the drops, start the shots again. If symptoms are too severe, return the vial with an explanatory note.

Sublingual drops can be expected to suppress symptoms and start detoxing within three to four weeks. Pollinosis sufferers should start drops four to six weeks before the pollen season begins. House dust drops, once or twice a day, are started just before the fall chills begin. CFIDS/ME people who recovered with latency therapy are advised to continue EBV drops at four-, six-, even eight-week intervals for the next two years. Frequency of drops varies greatly among patients. When symptoms and detoxing are controlled, vary the daily dose and interval between drops until a minimum dosage produces adequate control. Patients, usually women, with intensely supersensitive skin, suffer severe pain from injection shots. Fortunately, all responded to sublingual testing and therapy. After six to eight weeks, the skin sensitivity improves and shots can be tolerated.

The benefit of sublingual therapy is lost when the lining of the floor of the mouth becomes irritated and inflamed, blocking the SLO. A rest period of two to three months, during which shots or SSD therapy is given, may restore the mouth lining.

"Can you tell me how the sublingual drops improved my child's symptoms?" "My family physician says it's a load of nonsense, a placebo effect." Sublingual drops have been used for the past fifty years or more. In practice, sublingual drops activate both immune systems to varying degrees and in different manners. The strong dilutions $5^1$ to $5^5$ stimulate the NIS antibodies to the materials in the drops, and depending on the level of antibodies, there will be varying neutralizing of similar materials entering, or already present in, the body. To avoid provoking symptoms, the dose is gradually increased, slowly stimulating antibody levels. The strong dilutions depress detoxing. Weaker dilutions of $5^5$ to $5^{15}$ may not influence antibody formation but instead stimulate the OCIS to promote detoxing.

Because latency symptoms fluctuate, or have a habit of recurring from time to time, unused treatment drops and vials are stored at the back of the refrigerator to maintain their potency. Sudden life-threatening reactions to foods, drugs, and insect stings are said to occur in supersensitive people. A trace of peanuts, peanut oil, crayfish, or shrimp in a mouthful of food is enough for a life-threatening situation to occur. The response can be rapid, and the resulting swelling of tissues, effects on the heart, and, often, loss of consciousness are responses of the NIS. If the mouthful is not swallowed, how is the provoking food or drug entering the body? *Surmise:* The dangerous material passes through the SLO and is rapidly circulated throughout the body, accounting for the many organs and structures involved in the anaphylactic reaction.

**IK**  John, age 11, suddenly felt faint and his lips began to swell within 2 min of starting the sublingual test dose for soy. The provoking dose was soy $5^8$. A more severe reaction would have occurred with soy $5^2$. A large dose of antihistamine syrup and a small dose of sublingual adrenalin drops controlled the reaction. John was a difficult feeder after his mother's breast milk supply dried up when he was six weeks old. Soy milk formula affected him during the last month of bottle feeding. His mother was surprised at the severity of his reaction to soy products. Once soy products were eliminated he did not return to the clinic. His mother kept antihistamine syrup and an ampoule of adrenaline in the home medicine cabinet. The clinic does not test for soy allergy using provocation shots.

All detoxing therapies are nonspecific. They provoke microbes and toxins (latentees) that are easily excreted. Many microbes, however, especially viruses, virus-size bacteria, and some toxins, are little affected by nonspecific detoxing. Specific latency therapy doses (latentors) stimulate the detoxing of similar microbes and toxins. For example, *Candida* toxin shots stimulate the detoxing of excess *Candida* toxin and may, to a lesser extent, detox other related mold toxins, in particular, *Torulopsis*. CMV shots stimulate the detoxing of CMV and, to a lesser extent, other viruses of the herpes family, such as v. zoster and EBV.

### The Anaphylaxis Emergency

Anaphylaxis is a medical term for a life-threatening allergic reaction to foreign substances, usually foods or xenodrugs, e.g., peanuts, prawns, insect bites, injections of anesthetic or antibiotic drugs. Treatment to prevent recurrences is unpredictable. Susceptible people, even little children, need to have drugs on hand and adrenalin injections.

Patients who experienced past anaphylactic-like reactions suggest there are similarities with latency therapy. In other words, SD-provoked symptoms may be a miniature harmless copy of an anaphylactic reaction. Could there be a connection between a detoxing response and a life-threatening reaction?

### Latency Anaphylaxis

*Surmise:* All body cells hold minute amounts of a variety of latentors from the outside world, e.g., foods, chemicals, microbiological organisms and their toxins. During natural or provoked detoxing, some of the latentee overload is discharged to the tissue fluids, leaving enough for an immunity memory template. The highly sensitive allergic person may have unstable retention and detoxing of organ cell latentees. Either a large dose of peanuts, or a minute amount, such as the smell of peanut oil, can start a massive detoxing. The large meal of peanuts tends to start an immediate reaction, whereas the smell of peanut oil will cause a delayed reaction. The severity of a collapse and the symptoms depends on the number of cell deaths, the type and amount of the antigen or latentee, and the presence of latentee xenotoxins, microbes, and their toxins, held in the cell. Those prone to marked reactions and anaphylaxis may accumulate greater amounts of latentees. The detoxing process gets out of control, resulting in cell death (apoptosis). When considerable numbers of cells holding the latentees rupture, the sudden release of large amounts of latentee and the products of cell death, e.g., histamine, together with the incoming antigens, overstimulate or overwhelm the NIS.

> A patient who had suffered three mild to moderate anaphylactic responses said, "This injection is giving me the sensation of mild anaphylactic symptoms, Doctor. Will it get worse?" The virus provocation continued, with neutralizing of the symptoms and sensations.

Clinical evidence suggests an anaphylactic reaction is a combination of the NIS coping with the immediate alarming reactions and the OCIS joining it with the delayed responses.

## SYMPTOM SUPPRESSION DRUGS AND THE VIRUS-ALLERGY LINK

At present, antidepressants are the preferred drug therapy for CFIDS/ME and other fatigue and lack of motivation/mañana conditions. The new antidepressants help many patients, but few regain their remembered past health and energy while taking them. The first six months are the best, then symptoms start returning or are aggravated by a relapse, often caused by influenza. The dosage of drug is changed, but for many, the first wonderful three to six months of relief does not return. All who attended the clinic wished to get off the drugs, especially lithium, and did so as the work-up proceeded. A few were unable to completely withdraw and required very low antidepressant doses until their immunities and health recovered.

> After completing the clinic's work-up, one man reduced the recommended dose of antidepressant to one-eighth. After numerous attempts to discontinue the minimal dose, he eventually succeeded, two and a half years later. Patients wishing to discontinue lithium

should slowly reduce their dosage over a period of twelve to eighteen months. The good news: if you comply with lifestyle and treatment advice, you will slowly but surely build up your immunities and health to near-normal or normal levels. You will then be able to disengage from the drug addiction.

How do antidepressants improve the symptoms of CFIDS/ME and the tiredness illnesses? One popular explanation has the drug working through the brain's limbic system (Goldstein, 1993). The transmitter chemicals from the nerve endings at the junctions (or synapses) are boosted by look-alike, man-made copies of the natural transmitter chemicals. The antidepressants aid or supplement the natural chemicals, allowing them to work better at the junctions. They also improve the activity of the receiving end plates of the connecting nerve fibers (axons). Since antidepressants do not help, or often aggravate, CFIDS/ME and fatigue patients, does this mean the limbic system is absent or not functioning in these patients? Intracellular toxins and an overload of latent viral genomes are believed to depress cellular activities. I surmise from clinical responses of patients that latent viral activity interferes with the production of neurotransmitter compounds, with the neurons, and with the sensitivity of their receiving junction axon end plates, where the endings of the nerve processes meet each other and transfer their impulses. Boosting the levels of xenoneurotransmitters does not correct the abnormal activity. In time, the xenoneurotransmitters develop intolerance or toxicity in the affected nerve cells and their junction end plates. The individual three-dimensional spatial arrangement of antidepressant drugs may not be identical to the natural neurotransmitters. Antibodies to the xenodrugs may be present in people with very sensitive NISes. An increasing load of toxins, viral genomes, and xenodrugs increases symptoms, in spite of changes to the drug therapy. Could this be why so many, for the first few months, have a marked improvement that gradually declines, with increasing side effects?

Antidepressants dramatically improved the symptoms of a small number of patients who completed the work-up, with little improvement from MLV. It was similar to an antiviral drug therapy. The majority had their viral symptoms aggravated by antidepressants. Those attending the clinic who had unsatisfactory antidepressant therapy improved on MLV and by discontinuing the drugs.

**IK**    One woman who took antidepressant drugs for months before MLV cleared away her depressions said, "Antidepressant drugs are not logical." She had previously suffered from three types of depression and had asked her family physician to prescribe four different anti-depressants in an attempt to match the drugs to the different depressions. It was not possible.

Antidepressants depress or modify the detoxing of toxins and MLV. EBV detoxes with false depression and floods of tears and is present in tears and nasal secretions. Antidepressants suppress the false depression but block detoxing, thus delaying recovery. Before attending the clinic, patients noticed antidepressants decreased or stopped their strong body smells. As they reduced the antidepressants during the preliminary work-up the smells returned because detoxing resumed. At the same time, they began to notice an upsurge in symptoms that were no longer suppressed. The patients benefited with better provocation of symptoms and more accurate treatment doses. Patients sweated considerably more during saunas after they stopped the antidepressants. They commented that they could not tolerate the degree of sauna heat while on antidepressants. Antidepressants may interfere and depress the cells' heat shock protein activity. I suggest long-term antidepressant therapy be closely monitored because of its cumulative effect on the body's ability to cope with the accumulation of xenodrugs, latent toxins, and viruses.

## *Corticosteroids*

People with asthma can be thankful for insoluble Csd beclomethasone, for it has revolutionized the treatment of asthma. Asthma symptoms and prognoses have changed considerably since its introduction. There is a new type of asthma abroad today. After many years of use, it was discovered that minute amounts of the drug are absorbed from the nose and lungs. Here are some useful tips. Respect the powerful effects of Csds applied to any part of your body. When handed a prescription by your family physician, always ask if any Csds are present and what symptoms they will be treating. Physicians who are concerned about side effects of drugs will hand you an information leaflet.

Read the section on change-of-site response and learn of the problems some allergic patients had with Csds (see pp. 194-197). It is not surprising that a woman who suffered severely from a prolonged Csd treatment called her side effects "the corticosteroid cross" (see p. 195) and another frustrated woman angrily named it "clobber therapy."

The following are undesirable effects of "the corticosteroid cross"/ "clobber therapy":

1. There is an increase in the stickiness of all body mucus. The sex hormones have a similar chemical structure to the Csds so a similar stickiness occurs, e.g., the sticky cervical mucous plug caused by the pill.
2. The amount of watery (serous) fluid coming away from the treated surface membranes decreases. The immune responses of the treated membranes are suppressed by Csds. Infection and reduced inflammation occur.
3. Some of the following organisms are present in nearly all people who are using inhaled Csds (nose, chest) or Csd eyedrops for periods of six months or longer: *Aspergillus, Mucor,* CRC, *Giardia, Helicobacter, Chlamydia,* and multiple latent viruses.
4. The surface linings' allergic response to allergens is suppressed by Csds. The allergic response reappears in another part of the body, i.e., a change-of-site response.
5. The allergic and immune responses of the treated linings, including the gut, are suppressed. Clinical symptoms suggest there is an increased absorption of pollen and inhaled substances (antigens) through the lining membranes of the nose and chest.
6. Unduly sensitive people get body reactions to minute amounts of the Csds in asthma and nasal inhalers. They suffer increased absorption of Csds when the treated surfaces are infected by molds, bacteria, and viruses.
7. The constant presence of spent nasal and chest Csds could affect the gut organisms. Csds could depress the immunity of the gut lining, further aggravating food allergies. Csds could enhance the risk of Crohn's disease of the lower small bowel and colon.
8. An active viral infection, such as influenza, or a flare-up of glandular fever should not be treated with Csd's for fear of lowering the body's immunities. Patients believe the Csd courses they received aggravated their CFIDS/ME.

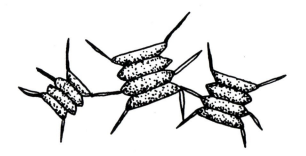

## Antibiotics

Antibiotics cope with bacteria, but not viruses. The antiviral drugs are limited in their activity against viruses. Chances are, you will be given an antibiotic if you come down with the flu. The same may happen when you have a flare-up of symptoms from multiple latent viruses. Before taking the course, consider what the antibiotics may do to your 1,001 friends in the gut.

Chronic sinusitis and asthmatic people who come to the clinic complain of persistent or recurring yellow *(Staphylococcus aureus)* or green, *(Pseudomonas aeruginosa)* sticky, "hard to cough up" mucous phlegm. Numerous antibiotic courses failed to get rid of the colored mucus. Some patients received six months of continuous antibiotic courses, and the infected mucus returned. They believed the antibiotics lowered their immunities. Ongoing inhaled Csds are responsible for chronic nose and lung infections and appear to perpetuate asthma. During the preliminary work-up, the Csds are stopped, if possible. *S. aureus* and *P. auruginosa* are added to the treatment vials. Within one to four months, the asthma has largely disappeared or cleared, leaving a whitish, moist, "easy to cough up" phlegm. These asthma patients dismiss the drug company "preventative asthma image" of inhalant Csds as misinformation. There will be times, however, when an acute asthma attack is provoked, and oral or inhaled Csds for two to four weeks will control it (Feltner, 1990; Garrett, 1995; McTaggart, 1996).

## PSYCHOLOGY AND THE VIRUS-ALLERGY LINK

Most people attending the clinic received psychological therapy, including counseling. A lesser number visited psychiatrists. One-third of patients are on or have used antidepressant drugs and are keen to get off drugs after months, even years, of taking them. They can no longer tolerate the drugs' side effects. Here are their comments:

- It is a pity the psychological therapy I received was not combined with the allergy and virus treatment I am now receiving.
- I was getting help from psychological treatment and then it fell away. It might have continued helping me, if I had started allergy and virutherapy.
- I did not stop all of the psychology advice and therapy when I began the allergy and virutherapy. A month or two later I was getting better

results from my psychological therapy. Now I am so much better I
have stopped it.

Antidepressant and antipsychotic drugs allow better control of symptoms but do not identify the causes of behavioral changes. The problem
facing the community is the lack of another treatment option. Medical
authorities refuse to accept allergy or heavy and toxic metals chelation
therapies. Patients attending the clinic receive a variable mix of psychological, allergy, CRC, and multiple latent virus factors, and a referral to
assess xenochemicals and toxic metals. They are rehabilitated by a combined approach that includes ecology. One patient called it "realistic
psychology."

Realistic psychology is a partnership of the two approaches. Psychological therapy is very useful, often essential, during the difficult detoxing of
CRC, *Giardia,* and multiple latent viruses, in particular, the effects of
detoxing glandular fever. Allergy and viral therapies are most effective for
the difficult areas of psychological stress therapy when other results are
disappointing.

Radiologists are using new technologies, e.g., MRI and positron emis-
sion tomography [PET], to explore brain activity and to identify thought
and other body function centers in the brain. An example is the amygdala
nuclei of the brain, a center for heart rate, certain organ functions, and the
emotion of fear. The amygdala nuclei are part of the limbic system, which
includes other brain centers. The limbic system has a linkup with the
hypothalamus. The limbic system controls most of our bodily activities.
Physicians suggest it is influenced by symptom suppression antidepressant
drugs, modifying the neurotransmitters to normal activity, with improvement or recovery of symptoms (Goldstein, 1993).

**IK**    Bill was in his late teens. His mother believed he experienced a
personality and physical change following hepatitis B vaccination
many years ago. He attended the clinic and recovered his memory,
physical activity, and general health. He was provoked with hepatitis
at the clinic, and that evening he had an awful aggressive dream that
woke him and remained vividly in his memory. The following day
he telephoned me and related the dream. I asked him if he had
experienced it in the past. He admitted this terrible experience had
occurred five times before. He was so ashamed of the dream that he
had not mentioned it to anybody. He became aggressive, rude, and
distant, and remained unpleasant for the next 24 to 36 h, then
changed back to being a pleasant happy young man again. "It is the
hepatitis" I told him. "You won't get that dream again, or if you do,

hepatitis virutherapy will stop it." Over the following months, Bill experienced further aggressive moods, and it was clear to his family that he did not realize they were coming on him. The family was able to warn him of their onset and he neutralized with hepatitis shot 5[6]. The episodes disappeared, followed by a marked improvement in his health and increased enthusiasm for physical fitness and body development. I am confident the dreams will not worry him in the future. Before attending the clinic he was given SSD therapy and psychological management, with unsatisfactory results. If hepatitis virutherapy helped Bill with that nasty streak and changed him from Mr. Hyde to Dr. Jekyll, it should be able to help many others with similar behavioral and psychological problems.

Provoked dreams, moods, and behavior follow viral provocation, in particular, with CMV, EBV, hepatitis, polio, dengue, and RSV. An example is the provoked dreams, moods, and behavior from CMV provocation testing or during detoxing of CMV. The dreams involve threatening animals, space creatures, and fearful or sexy episodes. I suggest that CMV is affecting the activity of nerve cells in the brain, including the limbic system. During provocation I have observed all-embracing fear and terror an immediate or delayed symptom following CMV testing. CMV provokes sexual urges, dreamy states, and fluctuations of kidney function. The fear sensations provoked by hepatitis and polio are different. *Surmise:* The sensations may be from adjacent areas of the brain (see Latency Dreams, p. 60). Psychologists and scientists researching dreaming behavior describe similar types of dreams and accompanying behavioral patterns. They have other explanations but are unable to provoke dreams, although their psychological and drug treatment is often successful. Patients who tried psychological therapy commented on the frequent relapses of fearful dreams.

A prominent New Zealand psychiatrist dismissed my views and explanations because he firmly believed he was dealing with a chemical problem of neurotransmitters in the brain. He considered the numerous scientific controlled studies of the responses to antidepressant drugs were scientific proof. He regarded allergy, CRC, MLV, and especially, food allergy exclusion and ecology medicine as nonsense. He challenged me to produce similar scientific proof. There is considerable opposition among health professionals to accept that food allergy and ecological causes play any role in psychological mental illness (Huggins, 1993). CRC and MLV could be regarded by many psychologists and psychiatrists as a threat to their area of practice. The food allergy pioneer, New Zealander Dr. Hare (1902), could not get his papers published by a medical journal. He self-published two books on his findings from controlling foods and recording the beneficial results of food exclusions for patients with mental illness at a mental asylum in Queensland, Australia. Dr. Feingold had similar problems in the 1960s, as did Dr. A. Schauss in 1981, when he described his clinical observations of the effect of food allergies on prisoners' behavior. Despite the lack of scientific proof, the methods of Feingold and Schauss are used with considerable success. I know of psychologists who test with sublingual food drops and give dietary advice to enhance psychological therapy.

If you are receiving treatment, psychological or SSD, for similar symptoms, enquire of your parents/relatives if you suffered in the past from an active viral infection, a vaccination reaction, or an unexplained infection that would suggest latent viral activity. Realistic psychology, allergy, and MLV could give better assessment of poor school performance, memory, and recall; bad behavior and mindless aggression; depression and suicidal thoughts; and home and domestic violence; and possibly provide the reasons for repeated crime by adults.

### Psychology and the New Causal Medicine

The term causal medicine includes clinical methods and therapies that suggest or confirm causes for functional, subjective, all-in-your-head symptoms and illnesses. At present, these causeless conditions are explained away by hypothetical or assumed diagnoses. Pasteur discovered that some illnesses were caused by germs and revolutionized medicine (the germ theory of disease). Causes of important illnesses and symptoms were discovered following the development of laboratory and medical technology. Improvement of laboratory techniques led to Dr. Koch's (1843-1910) postulates (assumptions). Koch's disciplines are still accepted as scientific proof of infection. Latency microbial infection, however, does not fit his requirements. Be assured that latency infection should, in time, meet these requirements. Over the past fifteen years the presence of latent viral material has, from time to time, been detected in muscle fibers and organ cells of those suffering from CFIDS/ME and fatigue illnesses. In the meantime, it is best to press on with latency therapy, for you stand a good chance of gaining some improvement, even a clearance of symptoms.

Causal medicine embraces 20 to 30 percent of symptoms and illnesses with functional, subjective, all-in-your-head symptoms as well as certain fibromyalgia symptoms and diagnoses. Psychological, psychiatric, and some alternative health therapies moved into the causeless void. Symptom suppression drugs and techniques are at present prescribed because the real causes and their appropriate therapies are not known. Conventional medicine accepts psychological management of the causeless void because it has not found any scientific techniques for detecting hidden causes.

The psychological grip on causeless illnesses is slowly but surely being challenged by new unscientific diagnoses and therapies (new causal medicine [NCM]). The last one hundred years since Dr. Freud's move into causeless illness has seen psychology retreat from those areas where real causes were found. The advent of scientific medicine and its controlled clinical studies entrenched psychology's control of causeless illness. The protection allowed psychology to move into new areas of society, such as justice, crime, and education, consolidating the acceptance of psychological therapies for emotional and behavioral conditions.

It is difficult for nonscientific, but clinically effective, therapies to challenge any part of the great psychological medicine industry, although there is growing dissatisfaction with psychology's pseudoscientific concepts, and the disappointing long-term results of therapy, including SSDs. Challenging therapies are refused publication in journals because their work is branded anecdotal, i.e., not scientific. NCM's access to research funds and community projects is refused funding. Controlling and funding authorities are satisfied with the present arrangements. The public's dissatisfaction with psychology, psychiatric therapy, and symptom suppression mind-influencing drugs is confirmed by universal complaints of those attending the clinic. Could it be that psychological methods failed because there are unrecognized causes, such as latent food, chemical and microbial toxins, and latent microbes and viruses? NCM is in the "think different" category. As such, it should not be restricted by scientific medical proof and statistic requirements, which appear to satisfy conventional medicine. NCM is capable of giving considerable clinical relief to patients and should be encouraged, even though it may threaten certain areas of psychological medicine. Such a threat to accepted medicine occurred fifty years ago, when antibiotics caused a revolution in medical therapies. Active bacterial causes were discovered, e.g., the psychological and psychiatric symptoms from syphilitic infection of the brain. When NCM is better accepted and understood, the appropriate diagnostic investigations will be discovered and made available, although they may conform to a different "scidotal" and statistical requirement. NCM requires a complete revision and evaluation of some present therapies and a change of approach toward patients suffering functional, subjective, and all-in-the-head illnesses (Webster, 1996).

"Allergy and virutherapy enabled me to finally end the antidepressant drugs I took for two and a half years. Before that, every time I tried to stop, I relapsed!"

"The 'scientific' concept of medicine has no morals. It is best for inbred mice."

A physicist and recovered patient

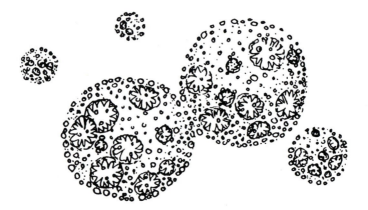

# Chapter 6

# The Virus-Allergy Link
# Eating Plan and Recipes

## *INTRODUCTION*

Mrs. Jean Rothwell, a professional teacher of food and cooking subjects, has devoted her time over the past three years to the menu groupings and the recipe index. She contributed much of the material in this chapter. She reviewed, modified, developed, and cooked to her satisfaction all the recipes. Jean suffered latency illness and got to know and experience food allergies and "functional," "psychological," latent viral and toxin symptoms and illness. The recipe index began as a few cyclostyled sheets of OWGGs, poultry, dairy, and beef exclusion recipes (1970s). A simple OWGG exclusion diet, e.g., no celiac, is no longer suitable for the range of functional illness symptoms. We acknowledge the hundreds of patients who gave us favorite recipes that helped them during their OWGGs or other food exclusions. Jean looked through the recipes, modified many, and selected approximately ninety for the recipe index. A majority of the tasty and easy to prepare recipes were used by patients during the past eight years. Before issuing the recipe index, the clinic compiled a basic non-OWGG group of recipes over twenty years. Many of the index items are similar to recipes in numerous food allergy books published during the past twenty-five years. The recipe index is different because no OWGG flours are included. We wish to acknowledge the skill and devotion of so many food allergy exclusion and food rotation pioneers. They, with some enlightened physicians, explored alternative foods, modified and developed recipes, suffered the disappointment of failed cooking results, and gave to food allergy victims their successful, tasty, nutritious substitutes. You, too, should acknowledge their achievements when you open the oven door or lift the lid of the breadmaker only to find a flat, tough baking failure. Do not give up. Try again until you get a baked delight with every attempt.

## OUTLINE OF THE VIRUS-ALLERGY LINK
## EATING PLAN

What to eat? That is the question after you get home from the first testing, or 24 to 48 h later, when the provoked symptoms you know so well convince you a food must be excluded from all meals. After an evening meal on the testing day, you are probably tired and suffering provoked symptoms, so go to bed. Waking the next day, the real difficulties begin because you had immediate and delayed reactions to provocation with the OWGGs. What to eat for breakfast? What to eat for lunch? OWGG allergy is the most frequent and demanding of food exclusions. The book's eating plan and recipe index does not include advice for other food exclusions. It is an extra effort, at first, to organize and prepare foods when you are suffering or recovering from the withdrawal symptoms of food exclusion and, later, provoked symptoms from microbial testings. Confine your meals at first to simple recipes with plenty of vegetables and greens.

Because of memory problems and lethargy, from provocation symptoms or withdrawal from foods, it is difficult to learn about foods and where to obtain them, let alone prepare them for meals. Try not to eliminate all the OWGG foods the day after testing, unless they upset you. You need real determination and commitment to change your old lifestyle and to comply with the OWGG exclusion. So difficult are the first three to six months, many are unable to continue the work-up; return to the comfort of the SSDs for the rest of their lives, and an uncertain future for their health, moods, and behavior. Most people, however, can organize their cooking and meals around their lifestyle routine because they soon notice an improvement in energy and memory. The VAL eating plan guides you in the choice of foods and any new cookware you may purchase. Make the most of the limited selection of alternative grains and the need to rotate them to avoid becoming allergic to an alternative grain, thereby reducing your selection. You will find new cooking methods and food preparations. The selection of non-OWGG takeout and snack foods in retail shops is limited and often expensive. Should you need to stay off OWGGs for months or years, you will need determination, patience, and an inquisitive mind to find and explore the tastes and flavors of the many alternative foods. Make no mistake, there is a large selection of alternative foods no matter where you live.

You may be dismayed because you have an additional poultry or dairy and beef, perhaps a maize/corn, allergy. At first, exclude them along with the OWGGs. Once your intestines recover from the irritation and toxic effects of the OWGGs, it is surprising how many other food allergies improve, even disappear. In the developed world, 6 to 8 percent of the population have severe to moderate problems with OWGG allergies. And 4 to 5 percent are unable to reintroduce OWGGs in their diets. Popular food allergy books have good recipes, planned meals, and important directions on how to substitute if eggs, chicken, milk, cheese, butter, and beef are excluded. For many celiac patients, the uncertain results of a wheat and barley exclusion diet (limited OWGGs) lead them to have doubts about whether they suffer from a more serious disease of their intestines. The only way to be sure about wheat or OWGG allergy is to do a complete exclusion for three to four months or, if you are over sixty-five, for six months. OWGG allergy exclusions deny you a large range of convenience and prepared foods. You no longer enjoy the wonderful taste of freshly cooked wheaten bread, or the satisfying texture of hot steamed rice. But you cannot go on being ill and unable to hold down a job or look after the family. The resulting improvement in energy, memory, and behavior becomes important, not only for you, but for your partner and family. After you have recovered "previously remembered health" and made sure of the improvement for three to four months, then you may cautiously reintroduce some of the OWGG grains, one by one, on a rotary plan.

### Fundamentals of OWGGs and Sugar Exclusion Diets

Throughout this book, complete OWGGs, apple, pear, and quince exclusions are recommended. This is the only way to discover if you are allergic to wheat and other OWGGs. By eliminating the OWGGs, the *Candida* yeasts in your bowel lose much of their food supply and return to normal levels. The OWGGs are excluded from all advice about dieting, the suggested three- and nine-week diet routines, and all recipes.

### What About Adding Rice and Millet to the Diet?

If you want rapid and complete recovery, forget about them for the next three to four months. Introduce rice (celiac diet) one to two months after you recover remembered health. If symptoms return within two to three weeks, exclude all OWGGs for the next year and try again. If you tolerate rice, do not use it more than every other day. Should the old symptoms start returning after a few months, even up to fifteen months to two years, the celiac diet is not for you. The addition of rice increases the variety and quality of baking products. You will find excellent recipes in the numerous allergy and health books. We suggest you contact your local celiac association for recipe books using locally available foods.

*What About Breakfast?*

Get into the habit of eating a cooked breakfast, as the slow release of energy from the fats and complex carbohydrates reduces the need to snack during the morning. Some people told me they vomited after their first cooked breakfast, but they persisted with small portions and gradually increased them over the next three or four weeks. They took the remainder of the cooked breakfast to work and, after heating it for lunch, noticed they had little urge to snack during the afternoon. Other patients told me they eat a breakfast larger than their evening meal. Most likely, as kids, they were given large cooked breakfasts before going to school. It is a pity these old food customs have fallen victim to the modern food industry. Remember, human intestines evolved on a large root and leafy plant intake over thousands of years. On a mixed diet with a high vegetable content you will assist your gut and the useful microbes living there to restore normal activities.

*What About Eliminating Sugar and Honey?*

Sweeteners will placate your sweet tooth when you stop all sugars, honey, sugar-containing foods, and confectionery. You cannot escape sugar, as it is present in all supermarket prepared foods. You can avoid sugar cheating during the first two months of exclusion. Cheating has had frightening results, often a relapse of the illness. Purchase the smallest bottle of liquid saccharin, not the sugarlike granules. A saccharin-cyclamate combination, when available, is preferred by many who notice a chemical aftertaste with liquid saccharin. Be aware that a person's acceptance of a sweetener may change to dislike after months of use. If other sweeteners are not acceptable, this is an opportunity to break the sweetener habit. Many attending the clinic suffered toxic effects from aspartame (Equal), such as aggravation of their preliminary work-up symptoms, in particular, headaches, memory problems, visual disturbances, depression, and confusion associated with latent viral infections. All other sweeteners are changed to some extent by heating and cooking, so sprinkle a few drops onto the food as it is being served. Chemical sweeteners give you time to explore the range of natural sweeteners, their cost, and whether they are accepted by the child or you. A serving of stewed fruit without added sugar may be all that is necessary for sweetening. The exclusion of added sugars and honey later enhances the sweetness of fruit sugars. Check out your health food shop's range of natural sweeteners. Some popular ones are a liquid glycerine derived from coconuts; Jerusalem artichoke flour, which contains FOS (fructooligosaccharides), an indigestible complex of sugars;

pure FOS; and an herb, stevia. At present FOS and stevia are expensive. Our experience at the clinic is that young children lose their sweet tooth long before adults do.

## PREPARING FOR THE EXCLUSION DIET

### A Word of Caution About Sugar and Honey

The twentieth century could be called the "sugar era." Cheap sugar from cane, beet, corn, and fruit is available for all in the developed world. Processed sugar mixes well with most foods and, being cheap, is a food extender. Sugar is in most prepared foods. It is not practical to try to avoid it. All you can do is avoid adding it to foods. Candy, confectionery, honey, and jam are avoided. Numerous patients tell me honey provokes their *Candida* symptoms more than processed sugars. Milk is avoided because lactose is not absorbed and *Candida* thrives on lactose.

Numerous medical papers and several health books describe the health problems resulting from too much sugar, yet the consumption per person is not falling. Please do not take excess sugar, as you will not get the full benefit from OWGGs and other food exclusions. If you are allergic to maize, sugars derived from maize/corn will tend to remain in the food tube. Besides their damaging bodily effects, high blood sugar levels stimulate and feed the 1,001 microbe "friends in our gut" (see p. 180). During digestion, fluid passes from our tissue and blood into the small intestine. When the blood and tissue glucose levels are high, glucose passing into the bowel will be lost to bowel microbes. It is simple to identify patients who should not eat excess sugar; they are provoked with cane or maize/corn sugar. The mothers of "sugarholic children" are impressed and convinced by under-the-tongue provoked symptoms. Birthday party foods should offer sugary "delights" and savory, spicy treats (see pp. 107-108).

### Rotation of Acceptable Foods

Rotation means eating a single food one day and again in four days when you begin the OWGGs exclusion. Rotation intervals for allergic foods are also found through trial-and-error testing. It takes time to learn to like and eat alternative foods. We suggest you eat one of the following carbohydrate foods for breakfast: maize polenta, buckwheat, amaranth, quinoa, sago, and tapioca. Tapioca and cassava appear to depress *Candida* activity. Amaranth depresses and reduces bowel parasites. We suggest you eat two to three servings of tapioca and two servings of amaranth a week. A more appetizing breakfast is a mix of equal amounts of cooked tapioca and amaranth. If cassava is available, tapioca can be excluded. At first eat pancakes, waffles, cakes, and biscuits with non-OWGG flours on the rotation day. After two to four weeks of excluding OWGGs, the gut begins to tolerate more foods more frequently. Some foods require a longer rotation interval. Use buckwheat and maize pastas sparingly, as they are no substitute for vegetables. Avoid the convenience of eating, or the desire to eat, a single food, too much, too frequently, e.g., maize/corn products, two or three times a day. This retards the recovery of your gut and, in time, may induce an allergy to maize.

If you are friendly with people from a different ethnic group, inquire about their foods and meals. Have an ethnic meal every three to four days. During the first two to three months, avoid ethnic dishes with multiple food items. Ethnic foods have different names for OWGG products. If in doubt, consult a dictionary. Single ethnic foods, e.g., okra, root vegetables, bean and chickpea dishes, give you variety and new flavors. If you eat ethnic foods or you enjoy the cooking, acquire a cookbook and try substituting acceptable flours and herbs.

### Cooking and Eating at Home, Flatting, and Rooming

Pans, utensils, and a stove are all you need in your home kitchen for the VAL recipes. You can add a blender, waffle iron, and microwave to vary the meals, especially for quick snacks. On average, two nights a week are devoted to cooking. Make one to two weeks' supply of the recipe at a time and freeze it. To reduce time spent preparing meals, the weekly diet routines incorporate three similar meals every two to three days, e.g., breakfast servings of tapioca, sago, and buckwheat. Cook two or more servings of fresh fish or meat and freeze the remaining portions after the first meal. Refrigerate unused portions in a sealed container for a day and a half to two days. Any longer invites food poisoning. Frozen vegetables ease the cooking burden when you are exhausted or going through the withdrawal and burn-off periods. Be cautious when buying the "cook and chill" foods (prepared foods heated from a frozen/chilled state). Do not leave them in your refrigerator.

IK    "I am positive it was that 'cook and chill' chicken dinner that made me ill. But how can you prove it? The poisoning has set me back ten days. I suppose that was because my immunities are below par at present. I am going to avoid all 'cook and chill' meals until I am fit again."

You cannot avoid "cook and chill" foods at restaurants and takeout places. Always remember to eat them promptly after purchase. Poor handling of "cook and chill" foods before sale allows bacteria to grow, and it is their toxins that poison us.

Older children (ages eight to fifteen) will enjoy making waffles. Show them where you keep the ingredients and teach them how to make the waffles. Make a large supply and put the leftovers in the freezer. These can later be taken out in the morning and packed in a lunch box or defrosted in the microwave and eaten as an afternoon snack.

It is difficult to do your own cooking if you live in a community flat. You will not be able to eat most of the community meal, unless it is a meat or fish and vegetable dinner. Ask if you can do your cooking at midday or after the evening meal. If not, consider eating takeout food and in restaurants, or change your accommodations. You could return to your parents' home, perhaps another relative's, for six months or until you recover. Second-hand microwave ovens and waffle irons are reasonably priced and are quite suitable for a bed-sitting room. They allow you to make a variety of snacks and simple meals. Avoid frying meats because of the smell. If you are too weak at times to go out to eat or buy supplies, ask a friend to do this for you and to cook your meal, if he or she is willing.

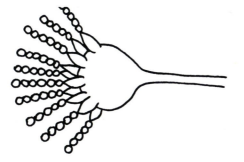

### The First Week of OWGGs Exclusion

Instead of trying to work out what to buy at the food market, what recipes to cook, or what prepared meals to buy, we suggest you eat simple, filling meals as set out in the following pages. The withdrawal from OWGGs provokes plenty of symptoms. Your activities and memory could be affected. Just as you are beginning to feel some improvement from excluding the grains, you start the *Candida* treatment with nystatin and increasing symptoms result. They are often worse than those from the OWGG withdrawal and can last three to five days or longer. For better treatment results, start the OWGG exclusion, and after two to three days, begin the nystatin powder.

*Warning:* If you suffered in the past from depressions requiring a psychiatrist's advice and therapy *do not* start excluding OWGGs and within a day or two take the nystatin therapy. A sudden severe depression can result. Discuss the problem of depression with your family physician, who will prescribe the nystatin or amphotericin B and instruct when to start taking it and at what dose.

Your physician may give you low-dosage SSDs for two to three, possibly six, weeks to get you through severe food withdrawal depression and symptoms. Sometimes the combined effects of the CRC, *Torulopsis glabrata,* and food exclusion require a short course of a mild antidepressant. Most people do not need these drugs. If you decide to start the OWGGs or other principal food exclusions, but you are put off by the possibility of severe withdrawal symptoms, contact your family physician or someone you know who has completed the work-up. Be prepared to eat a larger meal when you feel like eating. Switch the evening meal to the morning meal, or the midday meal, for there are strange swings in appetite and nausea during OWGG withdrawal.

To begin with, some of the new foods will taste strange and be unattractive foods to eat. But for the next two months, it is necessary to eat to live. Purchase plenty of root vegetables and potatoes, lots of greens, especially salad greens, have sufficient fruit to stew without sugar, and eat two pieces of fruit a day. Keep away from apples and pears. If you are on a limited budget, do not buy expensive alternative foods in supermarkets and health food shops. Some patients eat at fast food outlets or restaurants. It will be difficult to get enough to eat unless you patronize Mexican fast food outlets or restaurants. Ask for extra servings of fried potatoes and corn chips. If you are not satisfied, purchase salads and continue the meal when you get home, or start it before you go out to the restaurant. If you regularly patronize a restaurant, ask them to cook two or three extra baked potatoes, sweet potatoes, or yams. You can eat them for snacks. Plenty of green salads help to reduce *Candida* to normal levels. Many younger patients told me they survived the first month or more by eating at Mexican fast food outlets and restaurants. Many fine Mexican cookbooks can provide you with recipes. We suggest you eat two or three Mexican meals per week. As these recipes are readily available, they are not included in our recipe section. Bouts of hunger afflict many during the first one to two weeks of withdrawal. A suggestion is to take salads in a plastic bag, together with one or two cold baked potatoes for lunch.

By the fourth day of exclusion, a terrific urge to eat an OWGG product, especially wheat, will afflict you. It even upsets what you are doing, and, in fact, you can imagine the smells of the fresh bread. It is a trying time, especially for ex-OWGG-allergic smokers. We suggest you buy chewing gum, drink plenty of water, and space out the four to five cups of tea or coffee allowed each day, as a cup may reduce the hunger within two to three minutes. These difficult, testing hunger urges can recur over the next three to five weeks. Always keep some food in your bag or car to overcome an OWGG urge. If you succumb and eat the OWGGs, it will put you back several days and prolong the exclusion.

After four to five days of OWGG exclusion, little or none of these foods is left in your bowel. As the OWGGs disappear the large population of *Candida* begins to die and reduce. Most of the liberated *Candida* toxins are eliminated in the motions, but a little more than usual is absorbed into your body and will provoke symptoms. You could mistake the increase of *Candida* symptoms as a failure of OWGG exclusion, even believing that you are not allergic to them. Your partner may notice you are starting to have a strong musty smell, and you may smell mustiness after passing a motion. The motions become a lighter brown from excluding sugars and honey and they are better formed. At the time you notice *Candida* symptoms, you will get cold hands, feet, even limbs, for no apparent reason. I have seen it occur in the middle of a hot summer day. There is an annoying return of excessive tiredness, irritability, a tendency to argue, depression, and moods of varying degrees. Do not reach for the nearest antidepressant pill; the symptoms should pass in four to seven days. If not, consult your family physician (see Ngaire's experience, p. 239). The *Candida* in your bowel reduces to a more normal level. During the next four to seven days, the *Giardia* multiply and cause increased gassiness, with strong-smelling flatulence, and aching, even pain over the appendix area. There is an increase in muscle and joint aches (see p. 88).

## The First Week of Exclusion for Children

Children under five years continue their meals while gradually eliminating the OWGGs. Add the alternative foods in very small portions, gradually increasing as they are accepted by the child. Grind meat and fish into pastes that can be added to some of the alternative foods to give known flavors. A refusal to eat, or just picking at food, often occurs for two to three days as a withdrawal effect is experienced by the child. Following this there is an improvement in appetite. Keep up the fluid intake, but do not offer cow milk because the lactose sugar will encourage *Candida* infection to persist. During the three to four days of poor appetite, the child may be increasingly moody, aggressive, or whining and crying because of the withdrawal effects. Teething may aggravate these symptoms, so wait until those symptoms lessen to start OWGG exclusion. It is a great surprise to the mother when a chronically blocked allergic nose and mucus clears within four to ten days of OWGG exclusion. The child's appetite improves because he or she can taste the food. Children with blocked noses choose salty, sweet, or hot and spicy foods because they are tasting with their tongue. A child whose nose opened up so that he could blow his nose told me, in confidence, "Mum's dinners are beaut [excellent]. They do not taste like chewed up lavvy [toilet] paper anymore." During the periods of crying and irritability, do not give in and allow sugar or some OWGG food, as you will only prolong the exclusion symptoms. You have to "be cruel to be kind."

Schoolchildren between five and eight years suffering from the effects of withdrawal seek out or steal the addictive foods from other children's lunch boxes, the neighbors, and the refrigerator. I was told of young children who climbed up to the top shelf where there were hidden supplies! You will need to keep the bread, biscuits, and other OWGG grain products under lock and key. A mysterious or unexplained return of the old symptoms after exclusions are under way is suspicious. Probably, the child has found a cache of sugar, bread, or biscuits. Two to three weeks after the exclusion of OWGGs, introduce older children to the waffle iron and teach them how to use it.

### The Next Eight Weeks of Exclusions

So you survived the first seven to ten days of exclusion and nystatin therapy. Withdrawal symptoms are improving; some have disappeared. You are sleeping better, feeling more relaxed, and experiencing less bloating and little or no pain in your abdomen. Most at this stage of the exclusion are determined to continue and recover. You may not have the energy or drive to start cooking new recipes, so continue with a repeat of the first week's food and meal cycle. Begin the nine-week meal and food schedule when your energy and interest is improved. Select recipes from the index (beginning on p. 260). Two or three of them may become favorites, but avoid eating them every day. The recipes offered in this book are both simple and complicated. Choose the simple recipes to begin with, and you will not run the risk of wasting any of the food ingredients. Halfway through the nine-week schedule you may be able to start making pancakes, waffles, muffins, and scones. Keep the remaining batch of baked goods in the freezer to stop mold growth. If you are not feeling up to it, perhaps a friend or relative could cook a supply of baked cookies and bread for you.

## LIVING WITH FOOD EXCLUSIONS
## AND SUPPLEMENTS

### Eating Out and on Holidays

Excellent advice is offered by the many health books on allergies. For the first three months, do not attempt to eat any OWGGs, and question the waiter at the restaurant to be sure monosodium glutamate (MSG) is not present in the food. On holiday or overseas, insist that the travel agent books only nonsmoking accommodations for you. Hoteliers refuse to let animals into nonsmoking accommodations. When you arrive in the city ask around for the nearest Mexican restaurant or takeout place. Choose hotels that provide a cooked breakfast selection. Eat a large breakfast to satisfy you until the evening meal.

### Nutritional Supplements for OWGG Exclusion

Before, or when, you start the OWGG exclusion, purchase the following supplements (if unsure about their actions, consult a nutritionist):

- A zinc tablet that will give you 50 milligrams of elemental zinc
- Vitamin B complex tablets or powder
- Calcium tablets
- A magnesium salt
- Vitamin C powder
- Selenium tablets
- Vitamin E 200 milligram capsules
- Three cold pressed oils—green extra virgin olive oil, flaxseed/ linseed oil or sunflower oil, cod liver oil or a fish oil such as salmon or tuna

If you are taking supplements, add the larger zinc dosage and any of the three oils, if they are not included. If you are not improving on your nutritional program, here is why. Your gut lining and friendly microbes are damaged or disrupted by the OWGG gluten, xeno-SSD therapies, and antibiotics. In other words, you swallow the nutritional supplements, but you do not know if they get into your body. Your 1,001 microbe friends may get to them first, or the sick, stunted, and ulcerated gut lining cannot take them into the body despite the deficiency that exists. It takes about three to four months on the OWGG exclusion diet for your gut lining to recover, and then the supplements are absorbed in the normal way, i.e., when they are needed. Should you become allergic to one or other of the cold pressed oils, check with your chemist or nutritionist for a similar substitute. There are over ten cold pressed oils from which to choose. Take the cod liver/fish oil from the bottle, but if the taste at first is too unpleasant, change to capsules. As soon as the animal unsaturated oil balance returns to your body, the taste of cod liver oil markedly improves. If children will not take the cod liver oil, rub the dose into their skin. As they improve, the cod liver oil taste will improve and they will probably accept it. If all else fails, cook a whole fish and get three or four meals out of it. This way, the very important animal unsaturated fats and mineral complexes are absorbed. Those with a fish allergy should consult their family physician or a nutritionist as to what animal oils to take.

You may be taking excess alpha-linolenic acid (ALA), an essential fatty acid, and experience little or no improvement, unexplained fatigue, continuing insomnia, and constipation while taking flaxseed oil (Eades and Eades, 1998). Linseed allergy causes skin rashes and IBS. Consult your nutritionist for alternative oils such as safflower, sunflower, peanut, or maybe a local oil that does not contain any ALA. Flaxseed oil has many virtues, but its high level of ALA is not one of them. Patients have stumbled onto their flaxseed oil allergy after noticing they were getting irritable bowel symptoms from flaxseed porridge.

Vitamin K helped many who felt cold as a result of their allergy to OWGGs. Vitamin K is available at the pharmacy or drugstore as chilblain tablets. Vitamin K has a warming effect, which improves as the level of gluten decreases in the body. Because of the effect of gluten in the bowel, the organisms that make Vitamin K are reduced, or you are not eating enough food that contains Vitamin K. The result is bruising from the slightest injury. Vitamin K clears up this problem. It also has the effect of improving well-being and memory. (**Note:** This effect is not reported in the literature.) However, you cannot continue taking Vitamin K every day because it affects blood clotting. The dose that suits most people is one tablet every day for fifteen days, then a pause for two weeks, then one tablet a day for another ten to fifteen days, or until the tendency to bruise stops. You need to watch how much you are spending on nutritional supplements. There is no point in purchasing expensive preparations if your gut lining is damaged and your 1,001 microbe friends are under stress (see p. 180).

The following supplements will help you return to remembered health using OWGG exclusion:

1. Zinc: one tablet three times a week
2. Calcium: two tablets twice a day
3. Vitamin B complex: one tablet or equivalent powder three times a week
4. Oils: cod liver oil, one teaspoon a day; flaxseed/linseed oil, one teaspoon a day; or sunflower oil, two teaspoons a day; olive oil, one tablespoon a day
5. Vitamin C: one-eighth teaspoon of powder a day
6. Magnesium: one tablet, or magnesium sulphate (Epsom salts), one-sixteenth to one-eighth teaspoon a day

These doses may seem insufficient, but larger recommended doses could not be tolerated by many patients, and as the OWGG exclusion will last for three to four months, possibly for years, it is better to take the small doses on a regular basis. Selenium tablets and Vitamin E 200 or 400 milligram (mg) capsules are given when memory and recall are affected. They are taken together three times a week.

### Continuing OWGGs Exclusion and Reintroduction

You are feeling fit and well; your weight is down and your energy up, just as you remember before your illness overtook you. You still want to return to "normal social" OWGG foods. But can you? You do not want to slip back into poor health again. You could be one of three groups. The lucky ones return to an everyday diet after three, six, or twelve months of exclusion. They are careful about excess sugar, junk foods, and alcohol. Those in the middle group are able to return millet, rice, and perhaps rye or oats to their diet by rotating them at three-, four-, or five-day intervals. Many return to total OWGG exclusion during the grass pollen season (see p. 26). It is bad luck if you are in the fixed OWGG allergy group, or those who appear to have a genetic tendency for food and inhalant allergies, and petrochemical toxicity. You will always react, either immediately or as a delayed response, if you stray from OWGG exclusion. Console yourself by thinking of what you could have suffered from if you had not excluded the OWGGs. I have asked hundreds of continuing OWGG exclusion people about their lifestyles. One commented, "Sure, it has its problems, but you feel so *relaxed,* your body works better, feels lighter, and you have got all that extra energy."

After excluding OWGGs for months or years, certain bakery foods and recipes become your favorites. You must keep up variety in your diet. Otherwise, you could develop new allergies to the alternative foods you are eating too frequently. Such foods are onions, eggs, coffee, and tea. In time, many have to give up caffeine and alcohol. These tendencies are more likely to affect those over the age of seventy-five but can affect younger people who have suffered years of disability before recovering. If you are disabled or retired and have a plot of land, grow your own green vegetables rather than a flower garden.

Some of the lucky people come unstuck when they return to their former lifestyles and begin to suffer one or more relapses. I hear back that some did not return to the clinic because the treatment was nonsense. No doubt they opted for symptom suppression therapy. Those who return to the clinic find, on retesting, that their food allergies are more severe or that they have developed other food allergies, or *Candida, Giardia,* and *Helicobacter* problems. My honest advice to you is to avoid these food relapse situations. Should you develop mild or moderate fatigue, do the food exclusion and work-up again, just as you did when you were severely ill. You may need to contact your doctor or the clinic for further advice. Continue the exclusions for six months before you start reintroducing the OWGG foods again.

### What About Cheating?

That is up to you, for you know what the trade-off is. Keep an eye out for the slow creeping return of gradually increasing symptoms in the weeks and months ahead. If you get an immediate or next-day reaction from cheating, do not repeat it too often. If relapse symptoms are occurring too frequently, or are difficult to control, consider a preliminary work-up and MLV to control the latent microbes and toxins you may have accumulated over the years. Other therapies may help you out in this situation, provided you continue the OWGG exclusion.

### Directions for the Challenge Meal

Eat enough of the food, e.g., millet or rice, to fill you up within 15 to 20 min. Do not eat any other food at the meal, and drink only spring water. It is best to eat the meal at midday so that you can detect delayed symp-

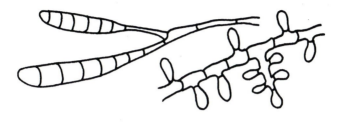

toms. A few people begin to feel ill or have symptoms they recognize before they finish the meal, but the symptoms generally start up 1 or 2 h after the meal. Most symptoms disappear after 4 to 5 h. One group of delayed symptoms you may have experienced in the past includes hives, abdominal pain and diarrhea or a single motion, muscle/joint (fibromyalgia) pains, and headaches. If you are over sixty or were very ill before the exclusion of OWGGs, you may get delayed symptoms over the next two or three days, even longer. Do not forget to watch out for unexplained tension and poor motivation. If you used to have flushing of the face or trouble writing, have at hand a mirror or a pencil and pad to check every quarter hour. One of the best ways to judge what is going on is whether you can continue reading when you may lose concentration and/or your vision becomes affected.

After exclusion of OWGGs for three to six months, it is unlikely you will experience a marked provoked symptom from the test meal. It is best to be on the safe side and to have on hand tablets of Alka-Seltzer Gold® or to purchase beforehand from the pharmacy or drugstore a small quantity of baking soda, potassium bicarbonate, or Triple Salt Powder, and five quick-acting antihistamine tablets. Refer to allergy health books as to how to use these preparations. Some of you may have suffered from asthma, diabetes, depression, severe headaches, or minor fits before you did the exclusion. Seek out a family physician who knows something about allergies and test meals before you do the test. The test meal may indicate you can eat millet, rice, and rye, but the other OWGGs have brought on symptoms within 4 to 12 h. Several weeks or months later, even though you are using the safe tested foods and enjoying them, symptoms start appearing, especially if you become ill with influenza, have an accident, or the grass pollen season begins. Stop the OWGGs, wait two to three weeks, and do the test meal again. Often, rice is the culprit. For confirmation contact the nearest allergy clinic. Would food immunization help? This is a simple therapy requiring daily injections or two or three shots a week for months, even years. It carries a risk of change-of-site responses (see p. 194).

### Reintroduction

You are excluding the OWGGs so you can test the foods you want to reintroduce with a test meal. Do not introduce two or more OWGG foods in the test meal. Keep an interval of two to three weeks between each food because some OWGG foods may give you prolonged delayed symptoms. Avoid eating safely introduced OWGG foods two to three days before you are testing the next food to be introduced. You may be able to eat two or more reintroduced OWGG foods a day, but to start with, it is better to eat one of the foods each day, to avoid confusing reactions. For instance, some people may introduce two foods, e.g., millet and rye, with no problems, but with the third food, e.g., rice, symptoms start up. If they now introduce rice and millet, with no symptoms, and later add rye, the symptoms return. If you suspect this is happening to you, select one or two of the foods you tolerate and forget about the others. People with such reactions should not eat the two foods at the same meal or on the same day.

Home testing of suspect foods through challenge meals yields useful information. Make time to test the big three foods; OWGGs, poultry, dairy, and beef. Begin with the OWGGs, and if convincing provocation of symptoms occurs, start a total exclusion using the recipe index included in this chapter. The full benefit of OWGG exclusions should be experienced in two to four months' time. Poultry, dairy, and beef, corn, potato, tomato, avocado, etc., may continue provoking immediate or delayed symptoms. Take time off to test each food group, doing one group per week. Now is the time to confirm or dismiss your suspicions and any past laboratory testing that gave positive food results. If you defer for months or years, sooner or later you will need to go through the whole exclusion process again. If suspected food allergy symptoms continue, seek further advice from an allergy professional. Exclusions carried out will aid the allergic investigations and probably reduce the number of clinic attendances.

The following are two home provocation tests:

1. On the hour test: Do not eat breakfast and drink three to four glasses of spring water. At 9:00 or 10:00 a.m. start with the first meal of two tablespoons of the cooked or heated pure food. An hour later repeat the meal and then continue every hour until recognized provoked symptoms occur. If no symptoms occur after the fifth meal stop the provocations but continue to avoid any other foods for the next 4 to 5 h as delayed provoked symptoms may appear.
2. Dr. Coca's Pulse Test (1956) has an accuracy of over 50 percent (Hyde, 1992).

A third test, applied kinesiology for food allergy, is much favored by chiropractors. The test is described in health books on food allergies.

**IK**  She took digestive enzymes for eleven years following severe mumps that damaged her pancreas at age 6. She became fatigued, with loss of memory, weak limbs, and symptoms of CFIDS/ME following glandular fever fifteen months ago. Exclusion of OWGGs and MLV, morbilli, mumps, and CMV improved her to a plateau that was not sufficient to return to school. Home testing with two teaspoons of cooked pork every hour provoked marked recognized symptoms. All these years she had hated the taste of pork, but it had sneaked into her as a medicine three times a day for eleven years. She improved with beef (cow) digestive enzymes.

### Advice to Spouses, Partners, Parents, and Family

Your attitude toward your relative or teenage child attempting a food and lifestyle change is almost as important as the therapy that person is receiving. Be as helpful as you can during the first three to four months, and you will be rewarded by seeing your loved one recover his or her old personality.

Here are useful comments made by those who won back their health and vigor:

- Please be patient.
- Spend a little time trying to understand what I am doing.
- After food withdrawals, food indiscretions, or clinic testing, I can get irritable, argumentative, fatigued, and sleepy. Please understand it is the allergies, toxins, and multiple latent viruses that are causing my behavior.
- Take no notice of my behavior while I am detoxing.
- Don't think the treatment is just like the others I have tried. I know this will help me because it brought on the symptoms I know so well during testing.
- The fatigue gets me, and my limbs won't work. I am not putting it on to get sympathy. I feel like a puppet, being manipulated.
- When I get depressed and cry, I know I am detoxing. I don't need sympathy, but because I am so exhausted, I do need help to eat and clean up after the detoxing is over.
- Don't complain about my bad breath or the smells in my sweat, urine, and motions. I've smelt them at times, but I know they will clear away when my detoxing ends and I am a lot better.

- Don't ask me to go back on symptom suppression medicines. I don't want to spend the rest of my life on antidepressants. Who knows, after ten or more years on them, my brain could be damaged.
- My detoxing symptoms were more severe when I had my PMT [premenstrual tension] symptoms. As I recovered, both sets of symptoms improved, and now I am no longer troubled by PMT.
- I can't forget how my family supported me, tried to understand the treatment, and, when I was so exhausted, baked and cooked the exclusion meals for me. When my memory was so poor, they reminded me to take my medication and kept me informed of family matters.
- Our ADD child's behavior returned to normal. My partner was wonderful and helped me so much. I don't think I could have done it by myself and would probably have agreed to take the SSD Ritilan®.
- Don't assume my irritability, moodiness, depression periods brought on by the treatment have a psychological cause, because they don't. If I take symptom suppression drugs to relieve these symptoms, they stop my detoxing. That's what cortisone does.

Following the last testing session it is difficult to understand how there could be a further increase, for three to four weeks, of symptoms and detoxing smells. The worst offenders are glandular fever and *Legionella* toxins. The next one to two months of heavy detoxing provokes aggravated symptoms, then recovery occurs.

Painful decisions must be made if you want your family member to have the best conditions for recovery. None of my patients made a full recovery from moderate to severe viral/allergy illness when pets and smoking were present in the home. Sometimes recovery occurs, but because of the pets/smoking, patients have relapses two to three months later, despite continuing treatment. In a few cases, the ecology of the home was improved, and after further treatment, recovery took place.

Please encourage your loved one during his or her treatment. If you have doubts, I suggest you discuss it with your relative and then telephone the physician who is giving the allergy and viral therapies. I have seen people improve for a while and then fail because of the persistent, hostile, and uncooperative attitude of their family members. I have treated brave people who knew their marriage or relationship was in trouble because of their illness. Spouses and partners need to be patient when waiting for their loved ones to recover. The reward for patience could be a restored relationship. Allergies and multiple latent viral illnesses, CFIDS/ME, and other neurotic symptoms have increased markedly during the past five to ten years. It is not a contagion in the accepted view, for it picks out those who, consciously or not, let their overall immunities become depressed. Such illnesses could strike you sometime in the future.

## EXCLUSION MENUS

### *The Three-Week and Nine-Week Diet Programs*

The three-week program is a weekly repetition of the same meals. The OWGGs exclusion could be bringing on symptoms, making you tired, depressed, and unable to get up and get going. Nystatin or other drugs for CRC will probably aggravate these symptoms. Cooking is minimal for the first week, but if you begin to feel more energetic, try the simple recipes that are listed for the first week of the nine-week plan. If you are doing well by the third week, select recipes you feel you can prepare and place them in your planned menu.

The nine-week plan follows, with every two weeks repeated. If you are becoming more energetic, continue selecting a new recipe number from the menu food list. The pages of the recipe index can be photocopied. Place a copy in the kitchen. Put a ring around the recipe numbers you like. Record your comments on the meal in the space below. Many people starting OWGG exclusion experience problems with recall and short-term memory. Should you need to exclude another main food, avoid excluding both foods at the same time. Instead, start on the main food and exclude the other in one to two weeks' time to avoid further aggravation of your symptoms. Once you begin to feel more energetic, and the cooking does not tire you, try recipes that are in other allergy health books or those recommended by present or past OWGG-allergic people whom you meet.

If you are housebound or not working, put aside two periods a week to do your baking and other dishes to be frozen. Those working part-time or full-time will need to cook two nights a week or wait until the weekends. As the exclusion symptoms begin to improve, about the third or fourth week, you regain more energy and are able to stay up till 10:00 to 10:30 p.m. Do not waste this opportunity. Turn off the television. Now you will have some time to get the cooking done. A word of warning for those with a gas stove. When cooking, keep the exhaust fan going, or some air circulating to carry away the fumes from the gas elements.

Hankering or longing for the foods you are excluding can lead to failure. If you can, approach the new ingredients, recipes, and types of food, anticipating their new flavors and textures and the new and interesting dishes you will encounter. It is said that "variety is the spice of life," but it could also be said that "variety of foods makes for a great life." We have done our best with the recipes included in this chapter to remove those frustrating baking failures. Remember, these recipes were tried and tested by many who suffered in the same way that you are now suffering.

A businessman with CFIDS/ME and OWGGs allergy continued working. His wife worked full-time. He contacted the local allergy group and arranged for one of the members with OWGG allergy to do their shopping, cooking, and house duties. "She's been a great help to us both, and I reckon it was one of the best deals I ever made. She knew what was best for me."

Menus are arranged for different lifestyles, various ages, and severe CFIDS/ME. As you recover, select recipes you can manage to cook and digest. If you suffer a temporary relapse, return to simpler recipes that require little preparatory effort. For lunch, packed or purchased, take hot/cold drink or soup in a thermos when away from home.

- Home menus—all cooking facilities available
- Flatting or group house menus—many or all facilities available
- Bed-sitting-room menus—few facilities and dining out
- Children's menus—ages seven or eight to fourteen years, most or all facilities available
- CFIDS/ME menus—disabilities requiring attention and help from relatives or social workers

Until OWGGs exclusion cooking courses become available at the technical colleges, you will have to rely on the local food allergy group or recipes from food allergy health books. In the United Kingdom, the Women's Nutritional Advisory Service helps patients with IBS and supplies them with useful recipes. Best to exclude OWGGs and substitute with other flours.

*Shopping List*

*Flours.* Potato, pea, and soy (buy 2 to 3 cups (c) at a time, but more of the potato flour); cornflakes or corn puffs; buckwheat groats; acidophilus yogurt; plain yogurt; cheddar, colby, or plain cheeses; olive oil and/or soybean oil; canned peaches and apricots (bottled, fresh, or frozen fruit is suitable); sago; tapioca balls; canned soups, if thickened with maize/corn flour; baked beans; canned asparagus or creamed corn (reduced sugar); eggs; unfermented white vinegar (4 percent acetic acid); corn/buckwheat crispbreads; canned pineapple pieces, or crushed, with no added syrup; gelatin powder; choice of sweetener, a cyclamate sweetener liquid, for baking, tea, and beverages; canned bean mix; butter; wheat-free and gluten-free baking powder; arrowroot or maize/corn flour; nuts, choice of cashews, almonds, local walnuts.

*Meat.* Selection of beef/buffalo and goat cuts, mince; lamb and hog, rabbit, kangaroo, venison; chicken and turkey legs and pieces.

*Fish.* Fresh whole or fillet and/or shellfish, prawns/canned tuna, salmon, sardines.

*Vegetables and salad greens.* Potatoes and sweet potatoes, onions, carrots, rutabagas and other root vegetables, pumpkin, celery, lettuce greens, bean sprouts, frozen peas, corn, tomatoes, and cucumber.

*Fruit.* Two to three pieces of fresh fruit a day if tolerated. Include local produce in the diet.

### *The Recipe Index*

The Recipe Index for no Old World grass grains (OWGGs) is arranged to help those beginning their OWGG food exclusion. The prefix **B** = breakfast; **L** = lunch; **D** = dinner; **S** = snacks. Thickenings, roux, and stocks are lettered **CB**. As the exclusion proceeds and you gain more confidence, please choose any menu that takes your fancy for a particular meal. You may be hungry in the morning instead of at dinner time. Periods of hunger and nausea may come and go without any pattern. When you are well on the way to recovery, the normal daily eating pattern will return.

### *A Menu for the First Three Weeks*

#### *Monday*

*Breakfast.* Cornflakes; unsweetened crushed pineapple; plain yogurt • Fry the leftover cooked or boiled frozen vegetables in a selection of cooking oils (corn, safflower, sunflower, or peanut) using herbs, spices, and mild curry, if tolerated; dice cold meat or canned fish; add thin soy or fish sauce and grated plain cheese when served **(B24)** • **Alternative:** Cooked or reheated baked potato; add meat/fish, yogurt, and herb stuffing. Also suitable for a packed lunch.

*Morning and afternoon breaks throughout the week.* Orange or seasonal fruit, a baked good, and 1 to 2 teaspoons (tsp) diced nuts or nut flour • Drink: thermos of hot water for soup, or cold for a drink at the workplace.

*Lunch or supper.* Salad • Cube of cheese • A slice or two of non-OWGG bread **(B10-B15)** • A cold baked potato and one piece of fruit.

*Evening or midday meal.* Meat and steamed vegetables, as many vegetables as you can eat • A commercial pasta sauce (low calorie) for the vegetables • Sago and crushed pineapple, yogurt • Cube of cheese and one or more slices of non-OWGG bread.

*Evening preparations.* Maize porridge **(B7)** • Hard-boiled egg • Half a can of soup in a thermos, hot water for soup or cold for a drink • Stew fresh fruit; put excess in the freezer • Any baking in excess of requirements, pack, date, and store in the freezer. Commercial non-OWGG pastas are a substitute for vegetables and can be added to the morning bubble and squeak **(B24)**.

## Tuesday

*Breakfast.* Maize porridge (or polenta) mixed with diced fresh fruit and yogurt, served warm or cold • Fried leftover cooked vegetables, in a selection of oils, herbs, and spices; diced cold meat, 1 heaping tablespoon (tbsp) of canned spiced beans • One slice or more of non-OWGG bread, diabetic jam or mild cheese.

*Lunch or supper.* Salad with bean sprouts and dressing containing olive oil (take daily dose of olive oil with the salad) • Cooked beans or spiced beans • Cold hard-boiled egg • Soup, if available, use a thermos.

*Evening meal or midday meal.* Potato chips and pickles (in 4 percent acetic acid vinegar) • Meat or fish • A large serving of steamed vegetables and pasta sauce, if desired • Sago **(B3)** and crushed pineapple • Cube of cheese.

*Evening preparations.* Soup, sago.

## Wednesday

*Breakfast.* Sago and stewed fruit yogurt • Large serving of vegetables and spiced beans, fried in a selection of oils, using herbs, spices, and 1 tsp fish or non-OWGG soy sauce • Fry an egg, if desired, before cooking the vegetables • One or two slices of non-OWGG bread, diabetic jam.

*Lunch or supper.* Salad, grated cheese, and dressing • Diced cold meat or fish • One or two slices of non-OWGG bread, peanut butter • Soup in a thermos, prepared the previous evening.

*Evening meal or midday meal.* Corn chips and pickles or corn maize dip **(S70)** • Chicken pieces and large vegetable serving • Corn porridge polenta and stewed fruit or diced dried fruit (dehydrated).

*Evening preparations.* Buckwheat porridge, tapioca. (The second-week menu substitutes amaranth porridge for buckwheat, and the third-week menu substitutes quinoa for buckwheat.)

*Thursday*

*Breakfast.* Buckwheat porridge, stewed fruit or unsweetened crushed pineapple, yogurt • A selection of leftover vegetables, chickpeas, frozen vegetables, fried in herbs and spices; 2 tsp of spiced beans • One or two pieces of non-OWGG bread, peanut butter or diabetic jam.

*Lunch or supper.* Salad and cold meat or chicken leftovers • 2 to 4 tsp of bean salad, canned or homemade • Soup and muffin (**B17-B19**).

*Evening meal or midday meal.* Microwaved/baked whole fish • Large serving of steamed vegetables and pasta sauce • A waffle or pancake filled with diabetic jam, stewed fruit, sprinkled with nut flour • **Alternative:** Corn porridge and stewed fruit.

*Friday*

*Breakfast.* Tapioca, stewed fruit, and 1 tbsp canned coconut cream or milk • Leftover cooked vegetables and portion of fish fried in a selection of oils, herbs and spices, and fish or soy sauce • One or two slices of non-OWGG bread, peanut or other nut butters, diabetic jam.

*Lunch or supper.* Salad with leftover chicken or fish and bean salad, prepared (**L43**) or canned • One or two pieces of non-OWGG bread and cube of cheese.

*Evening meal or midday meal.* Corn chips and corn/maize dip (**S70**) and pickles • Lamb or hog, grilled, baked, or microwave stewed • A large helping of steamed vegetables and pasta sauce or fresh mint and non-OWGGs vinegar (4 percent acetic acid) • Buckwheat porridge, stewed fruit, and yogurt • Cube of cheese.

*Saturday*

*Breakfast.* Tapioca, stewed fruit, yogurt or coconut cream • Leftover vegetables fried in a selection of oils, herbs, and spices; add 1 tbsp of cooked lamb/beef liver or cold fish • Fish/soy sauce • Muffin and diabetic jam.

*Lunch or supper.* Salad with canned fish • Sweet corn chowder (**D51**) • Muffin or non-OWGG bread and cheese.

*Evening meal or midday meal.* Roasted, fried, or microwave stewed beef and large serving of steamed vegetables with pasta sauce • Buckwheat porridge, stewed fruit, and yogurt/coconut cream • Cube of cheese.

*Sunday*

*Breakfast.* Buckwheat porridge, stewed fruit, yogurt/coconut cream • Fry an omelette (**B23**) • Leftover vegetables, sauces, herbs, spices, and a selection of oils • One or more slices of non-OWGG bread, jam or peanut butter.

*Lunch or supper.* Salad and diced leftover beef or hog • Remainder of sweet corn chowder • Two or more pieces of corn crispbread, or (**L41**).

*Evening meal or midday meal.* Corn chips and corn maize dip • Spanish soup (**L31**) • Cold beef and steamed vegetables; a commercial corn or buckwheat pasta • Tapioca, stewed fruit, and yogurt • Cube of cheese.

### Menu Management

Repeat the first week's menu for the next two or three weeks, or alternate the two home menus, substituting or adding recipes from the index, if your digestion is improving. As your immunities return to normal, the number of allergic foods will decrease.

"Do I have to eat the vegetable and oil dish for breakfast? It is so boring, and my stomach will not take all these foods in the morning." I reply, "Didn't you spread margarine or butter on your toast? They are fats. Please persist because the vegetables and oil dish is slowly digested, reducing the urge to snack. Your coordination, alertness and mental activities will improve, with no more wild blood sugar fluctuations (hypoglycemia) or stimulation of CRC symptoms." Rotate the breakfast cooking oils, i.e., corn, safflower, sunflower, or peanut, or any good local oil that contains some unsaturated fats. Retain the olive oil for the daily lunchtime salad dressing. Coconut milk or cream has a pleasant flavor and contains important short-chain saturated fatty acids. Open a can and pour half into two sealed containers, and place one in the freezer. Coconut milk and cream go sour after three to four days of refrigeration.

### Home Menus

#### Monday

*Breakfast.* Cornflakes with sliced bananas and yogurt • Leftover vegetables, choice of cooking oils, herbs, and spices (**B24**) • A selection of frozen vegetables, cooked and canned/frozen chickpeas, substitute for leftover vegetables • Choice of non-OWGG breads (**B10-B15**).

*Lunch or supper.* Salad and olive oil • Baked stuffed potato served with stewed tomato • Ground mixed nuts, 2 tbsp • One or two slices of non-OWGG bread.

*Evening meal or midday meal.* Grilled midloin chops • Vegetables • Peach sago (**B3**) with yogurt.

*Packed lunch.* Baked stuffed potato with tomato • yogurt and fresh fruit • Crispbread, or one to two slices of non-OWGG bread or baking (**L41**)

*Evening preparations.* Cook amaranth; bake muffins and cornbread.

## Tuesday

*Breakfast.* Half grapefruit or stewed kiwifruit • Amaranth porridge • Baked beans • Choice of breads.

*Lunch or supper.* Salad, olive oil • Scrambled eggs (**B22**) • Corn crispbread or waffle (**L34**) or (**L41**).

*Evening meal or midday meal.* Savory mince or cottage pie (**D54-D55**), vegetables • Peach sago with yogurt.

*Packed lunch.* Salad and olive oil dressing • Ground or diced mixed nuts, 2 tbsp • One or two pieces of non-OWGG bread or baking (**L41**) or corn crispbread • A cube of cheese • Fruit • Thermos of hot/cold drink.

*Evening preparation.* Cook tapioca.

## Wednesday

*Breakfast.* Cooked tapioca (**B1**) and stewed fruit, yogurt • Cooked vegetables, choice of oils, herbs, and spices, and baked beans to flavor • Two pieces of non-OWGG bread or baking.

*Lunch or supper.* Coleslaw salad (**L46**) with olive oil and lemon dressing • Serving of leftover cottage pie • Cube of cheese.

*Evening meal or midday meal.* Fish fillet (**D56**) • Creamed potato and vegetables • Gelatin dessert (**D63**) with pineapple, topped with diced nuts.

*Packed lunch.* Salad with olive oil dressing • Choice of non-OWGG bread • Cube of cheese • Fresh fruit.

*Evening preparation.* Salmon cakes (**B21**).

## Thursday

*Breakfast.* Amaranth with stewed fruit and yogurt • Salmon cakes (**B21**) and small serving of cooked vegetables, choice of oils • One to two pieces of non-OWGG bread (**B10-B15**).

*Lunch or supper.* Salad and olive oil dressing, topped with canned or cooked asparagus or creamed corn • Poached egg • Corn crispbreads or choice of non-OWGG bread • Fruit.

*Evening meal or midday meal.* Blade steak casserole, with tomatoes and onions, vegetables, baked potato • Gelatin dessert (**D63**).

*Packed lunch.* Salad with asparagus, carrot, celery slivers; lemon, vinegar, and oil dressing • Bread • Cube of cheese.

*Evening preparation.* Soak buckwheat and corn grits.

*Friday*

*Breakfast.* Cooked tapioca with stewed fruit and yogurt • Leftover casserole, poached egg, and serving of vegetables, choice of oils.

*Lunch or supper.* Bean salad **(L43)** with lemon, vinegar, and olive oil dressing • Canned fish • One to two muffins **(B17)**, peanut butter or diabetic jam • Cube of cheese • A piece of fruit.

*Evening meal or midday meal.* Braised pork chop and vegetables • Buckwheat groats **(B5)** with stewed or fresh fruit and yogurt.

*Packed lunch.* Bean salad **(L43)** with lemon and oil dressing • Choice of bread and cheese cube • Yogurt and piece of fresh fruit.

*Evening preparation.* Cook buckwheat and corn grits.

*Saturday*

*Breakfast.* Buckwheat with stewed or bottled/canned unsweetened apricots and yogurt • Corn or carrot fritters **(B25)** • One to two pieces of non-OWGG bread **(B10-B15)** • Cube of cheese or diabetic jam.

*Lunch or supper.* Sweet potato or pumpkin soup **(D50)** • Yogurt • Muffin **(B17)** • Piece of fruit.

*Evening meal or midday meal.* Leg of lamb or chicken roasted in bag with vegetables • Corn porridge (or polenta) with black currants or raspberries and yogurt.

*Evening preparation.* Soak and cook quinoa and dried beans or chickpeas • Make stock • Bake loaves, muffins, biscuits, or cakes for week ahead and a pizza.

*Sunday*

*Breakfast.* Buckwheat **(B5)**, fruit and yogurt • Leftover vegetables, choice of cooking oils, herbs, and scrambled egg • One or two non-OWGG bread slices.

*Lunch or supper.* Coleslaw salad **(L46)** with salmon or canned fish • Choice of baking • Ground mixed nuts, 2 tbsp • Fresh fruit.

*Evening meal or midday meal.* Cold lamb or chicken with peas and vegetables • Corn porridge (or polenta) with fruit and yogurt • Or pancakes **(B9)**/waffles **(L33)**.

*Evening preparation.* As for Saturday, if deferred.

### Flatting or Group House Menus

The following example menu is for bed-sitters and flatters who supplement at restaurants, cafés, and takeout stores. It is suitable for those with increased food withdrawal symptoms.

*Comment:* If an oven is available, bake a selection of breads when the kitchen is free in the evening. Otherwise, arrange to visit a relative's or friend's kitchen to cook a supply of breads. Your parent or an older relative may be able to do the baking, if you supply the ingredients and recipes. The night you prepare food for other residents in the house is an opportunity to continue into the evening preparing your food for the next two to three days. As you recover, you will gain energy to return home, eat a meal, and cook into the evening. If the kitchen is not used during the weekend, cook during the day. Those with a bed-sitting room select items from the menu that they can prepare with the limited means available. A waffle machine is suitable for a bed-sitting room, but before you purchase one, check your rental agreement. The waffle mix makes a reasonable crust with cheese, peanut butter, and diabetic jam filling.

"I did it. I'm off smokes and grains and it's been worth it. Look at my new figure, and I feel so relaxed."

**IK**  Ngaire (P), age 24, had an on-again, off-again food exclusion and smoking saga. The first week she constantly and irrationally ate any foods without grain. She could not get herself to feel full or satisfied after eating huge quantities of potatoes, vegetables, eggs, mince, and cheese. On the second day her resolve broke. The depression was marked. She could not stop thinking of bread and noodles. She had a meal of them and promptly vomited them back. She wished for a microwave oven. After work she would eat a pot full of boiled vegetables. She used a lot of herbs, chili sauce, curry, and onions. She would wake at 3:00 a.m. and feel so hungry that she would get out of bed, warm up some of the cooked vegetables, and fill up. For snacks she ate nuts, diced or ground, seeds, and dried fruit. When she went into the cafeteria with her lunch box, she had an overwhelming desire to throw it away and order some bread or cakes. Instead, she ate piles of salads and chips for lunch. Muscle and mental tension were so marked during withdrawal she had to continue smoking and drinking cups of coffee. During the second week of withdrawal and starting nystatin, the hunger was worse and she often overate and was sick. Improvement started suddenly on the tenth day, as the combination of nutritional supplements, nystatin, and a better selection of foods came together. By the third week, her appetite was reducing, and by the fourth, there were long periods when she had no desire to eat and yet felt active. She could go without food for up to 6 h. By then she had conquered both the smoking and the OWGG withdrawal. From then on she became relaxed and active. She moved from a single room to a flat with a kitchen. She spends time planning and cooking a varied menu. She has tried several times to reintroduce OWGGs but now realizes she has a permanent, or fixed, OWGG food allergy.

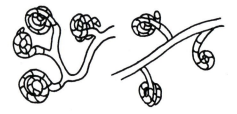

The following menu supplements meals at restaurants and cafés. Try the diet if you are ill or the OWGG withdrawal aggravates your symptoms. Avoid hot sauces and herbs until your appetite returns. Interchange meals (for example, lunch/supper) with an office worker. If he or she takes the packed lunch suggestions, plan for daily food preparation periods.

### Monday

*Breakfast.* Corn grits porridge (or polenta) and unsweetened canned peaches, a banana, and yogurt • Leftover vegetables, choice of oils, herbs, and spices • Thin clear sauce, choice of meat, fish, or savory beans • One or two pieces of non-OWGG bread, diabetic jam or marmalade.

*Lunch or packed lunch.* Baked stuffed potato with tomato • Fresh fruit and small container of yogurt • One or two slices of non-OWGG bread (**B10-B19**), muffin, or cake • Ground or diced mixed nuts, 1 to 2 tbsp.

*Evening meal or midday meal.* Grilled chops or meat with bone and fat removed, microwaved in a mild sauce • Peach sago with yogurt.

*Tuesday*

*Breakfast.* Half grapefruit or diced orange, added to serving of corn porridge • Leftover vegetables or cooked frozen vegetables, choice of oil, herbs, and spices (**B24**) • One to two slices of non-OWGG bread, diabetic marmalade or stewed orange and lemon jam substitute.

*Lunch or packed lunch.* Salad, olive oil dressing • A waffle, reheated in the microwave • Bread or crispbread and cheese cube. • One piece of fruit.

*Evening meal or midday meal.* Savory mince, vegetables, and buckwheat/corn pasta and suitable pasta sauce • Fruit sago and yogurt • A muffin or a piece of fruit.

*Wednesday*

*Breakfast.* Tapioca, stewed fruit, and yogurt • Leftover vegetables, choice of oil, herbs, and spices • Portion of cooked mince • One or two slices of bread and jam.

*Lunch or packed lunch.* Salad and olive oil dressing • Piece of fresh fruit and yogurt • One to two slices of non-OWGG bread and peanut butter, or ground diced mixed nuts, 2 tbsp • **Alternative:** A waffle to be heated.

*Evening meal or midday meal.* Baked or steamed fish, creamed potato, and vegetables • Amaranth porridge/gelatin dessert (**D63**), fresh fruit • A piece of non-OWGG bread or scone and cube of cheese.

*Thursday*

*Breakfast.* Amaranth porridge, fruit, and yogurt • Salmon cakes (**B21**) and serving of vegetables, choice of oil, herbs, and spices • Bread or a muffin and jam.

*Lunch or packed lunch.* Poached or hard-boiled egg and canned creamed corn • A small salad and olive oil • Nut flour, 2 tbsp • One or two pieces of non-OWGG bread and cheese cube.

*Evening meal or midday meal.* Blade steak stew/fried schnitzel with cheese, tomato, baked potato, and vegetables • Gelatin dessert and fruit • A muffin.

*Friday*

*Breakfast.* Buckwheat groats, stewed fruit, yogurt • Leftover vegetables, choice of oil, herbs, and spices • A little of last night's stew, and cooked chickpeas • One to two pieces of non-OWGG bread and jam.

*Lunch or packed lunch.* Bean salad with lemon, vinegar, and oil dressing (**L43**) • Fresh fruit and yogurt • Bread or muffin and cheese cube.

*Evening meal or midday meal.* Chicken pieces, braised or cooked in microwave, and vegetables • Tapioca, stewed fruit, and yogurt • A muffin or scone and peanut butter, if tolerated.

### Saturday

*Breakfast.* Buckwheat groats, mashed banana, and yogurt • Fried vegetables with a little canned fish or diced meat, choice of oil, herbs, and spices • One to two pieces of bread and marmalade.

*Lunch or packed lunch.* Sweet potato or pumpkin soup (**D50**) • Fresh fruit and yogurt • A piece of non-OWGG baking • Ground or diced mixed nuts, 2 tbsp.

*Evening meal or midday meal.* Cold chicken pieces, baked potato, and coleslaw salad • Quinoa porridge with fruit flavoring • Piece of non-OWGG bread and cube of cheese.

### Sunday

*Breakfast.* Quinoa porridge, stewed fruit, yogurt • Fried vegetables and scrambled eggs (**B22**) • Choice of oil, herbs, and spices.

*Lunch.* Coleslaw salad and canned fish or diced meat • A toasted slice or two of celery and cheese loaf (**B10**), if available • Waffle with meat and cheese filling.

*Evening meal or midday meal.* Lamb, frozen peas, and other vegetables • Tapioca with fruit and yogurt • One piece of non-OWGG bread or half a muffin with peanut butter, if tolerated, or jam.

**Important Note:** The meals appear to be very substantial, but they are planned for people with an appetite. Those with small appetites can pick and choose smaller quantities. Fried vegetables ("bubble and squeak") for breakfast and a salad at lunch helps to control CRC.

### Children's Menus

Read about the different ways to manage and arrange interesting exclusion diets for children. Adopt a method that closely fits your child's requirements (Hyde, 1992; Mandell, 1979). After two to three months of OWGGs exclusion, the majority of children experience recovery of health and improved behavior. Now is the time to try introduction and food rotation of millet, rice, rye, and possibly oats. Unfortunately, many children are unable to eat wheat and barley. Too much rice and too frequent meals of rice will bring a return of allergic symptoms. As the OWGG exclusion brings about improvement in health and appetite, larger meals are consumed. The opening up of a food allergy-blocked nose brings awareness of individual food tastes and flavors other than salty, sweet, acidic, and bitter. Now is the time to interest the child in tasty foods and to reduce consumption of the sugary ones. The following week's menu is suitable for sick children. Add recipes or items from the books you read to the recipe index (beginning on p. 260). As CRC nearly always accompanies OWGG food allergies, use a milk that is free of lactose, e.g., soy milk, coconut milk, or processed cow milk and milk formulas with or without corn. Check that the milks have adequate calcium content; if not, give calcium powders or pills. Encourage the child to drink plenty of safe, filtered water. From time to time, add a twist of lemon or orange or a little vitamin C powder. Imitation ice cream is permitted two or three times a week, once recovery from CRC is under way. Make fresh fruit jam every four to five days. Try the diabetic jams, but remember that sorbitol can cause diarrhea in some people. Refer to p. 240 for interchanging of meals and planning food preparation times.

## Monday

*Breakfast.* Cornflakes or soft corn porridge, sliced banana, and yogurt • Toast a slice of non-OWGG bread and cut into toast fingers, with a thin layer of jam or peanut butter.

*Light meal.* Baked stuffed potato or potato chips dipped in a sauce • A small amount of stewed tomatoes and/or baked beans.

*Main meal.* Diced lamb or hog meat from a grilled chop (the meat may need grinding or mincing for acceptance) • Vegetables and potatoes • Peach sago and some yogurt.

## Tuesday

*Breakfast.* Corn porridge or quinoa, stewed peaches or fruit and yogurt • Toast fingers with fruit topping or diabetic jam. • Lactose-free milk drink.

*Light meal.* OWGG-free sausage pieces • Baked beans • Corn crispbreads with cheese, cucumber, and a piece of fresh fruit.

*Main meal.* Beef/lamb/venison burgers or mince balls with peas and carrots • A few fried chips • Citrus sago and yogurt.

*Wednesday*

*Breakfast.* Tapioca, stewed peaches, and yogurt • Toast fingers with fruit topping • Lactose-free milk drink, hot or cold.

*Light meal.* Salmon cakes • Some hot chips • A piece of fruit and yogurt.

*Main meal.* Beef/lamb burger • Stir-fried vegetables with a corn spaghetti or pasta and cheese • Fruit jelly with stewed fruit.

*Thursday*

*Breakfast.* Tapioca with sliced banana and pineapple and yogurt • Toast fingers and topping • Lactose-free milk drink.

*Light meal.* A salad or coleslaw • Remaining salmon cakes • Sultana scones • A piece of fresh fruit.

*Main meal.* Beef schnitzel with corn grits batter • Potato, mashed or chips, cauliflower, and carrots • Fruit jelly.

*Friday*

*Breakfast.* Buckwheat porridge with stewed fruit and yogurt • Lactose-free milk or fresh orange juice drink.

*Light meal.* A waffle with vegetable and cheese filling • Some hot chips.

*Main meal.* Braised or roasted chicken pieces • Sweet potatoes, taros, leeks, and buckwheat pasta • Fresh, bottled, or canned berry fruit and cream.

*Saturday*

*Breakfast.* Buckwheat porridge with stewed fruit and yogurt • Toasted celery and cheese fingers with topping • Lactose-free milk drink.

*Light meal.* OWGG-free sausage pieces • Lentil and potato soup • Toasted bread fingers with cheese • A fresh fruit juice drink and piece of fruit.

*Main meal.* Baked fish with corn grits batter, chips, baked tomatoes, and silver beets • Fruit soy crumble and yogurt.

*Sunday*

*Breakfast.* Cornflakes or puffs/quinoa porridge • Corn or carrot fritters with tomato sauce and remainder of flaked fish • Toasted loaf fingers with cheese • Lactose-free milk drink.

*Light meal.* OWGG-free sausage pieces with tomato • Muffins and topping • A piece of fruit.

*Main meal.* Steak and kidney • Mashed potatoes or chips, rutabagas, and peas • Fruit soy crumble.

Select tasty rather than sweet, sugary, salty snacks from the recipe index or from other health books. Reward your child with ice cream and special snacks. As the food allergy withdrawal and *Candida* reduction in the bowel proceeds, the child's appetite will increase, leading to less fussy eating. The basic menu may need drastic altering from time to time, as children may insist on eating a similar meal every day for a week or more, and then suddenly switch. Bizarre eating is often a feature of the first three to four weeks of allergic food exclusion. Make a variety of small waffles for infants and younger children. Older children like waffles, so encourage them to get out the waffle iron when they come home from school. They soon learn how to mix and make their favorite waffles. An easy way to make nonfat potato chips is in the microwave. Purchase a special chip rack and be sure you get the potato variety that produces crisp chips. Commercial chips depend on poor-quality fat and oil for their crispness. If you can home microwave nonfat chips, your child will avoid poor-quality fat.

## CFIDS/ME and OWGG Withdrawal Symptoms Menus

Those suffering from CFIDS/ME with sleep reversal should follow this pattern: take breakfast at midday, the main meal at 6:00 to 7:00 p.m., and the light meal at 11:00 p.m. to midnight. Remember, no snacks. For nausea or small appetite, try eating half to one-third of the suggested meals six times a day at 2 to 3 h intervals. The exclusion of an important allergic food and the treatment of CRC will in time reduce and clear most hypoglycemia episodes. Light and main meals are interchangeable. Plan ahead for food preparation and cooking periods. Drink plenty of safe, filtered water.

### Monday

*Breakfast.* Corn porridge, with no sugar; cornflakes or corn puffs, 3 to 8 percent sugar • Sliced banana and yogurt • Herbal or very weak tea.

*Light meal.* Lettuce, tomato, cucumber, a little canned fish, olive oil and lemon or vinegar dressing • A piece of fruit.

*Main meal.* Grilled hog midloin chop and vegetables • Stewed fruit and yogurt.

*Tuesday*

*Breakfast.* Polenta, cornflakes or puffs • Canned or stewed fruit and yogurt • A piece or two of non-OWGG bread or muffin • Herbal or weak tea.

*Light meal.* Baked beans • Corn crispbreads, piece of cheese • Piece of fruit.

*Main meal.* Savory mince and vegetables or chips • Tapioca and stewed fruit with yogurt.

*Wednesday*

*Breakfast.* Sago and stewed fruit • One or two pieces of toasted non-OWGG bread.

*Light meal.* Baked potato with cheese and spring onion filling • Piece of fruit or cucumber.

*Main meal.* Microwaved fish and vegetables • Tapioca, stewed fruit, and yogurt.

*Thursday*

*Breakfast.* Buckwheat porridge, stewed fruit, and yogurt • One or two pieces of toasted non-OWGG bread, diabetic jam, if tolerated.

*Light meal.* Canned creamed corn with some salad greens or canned asparagus • A poached egg.

*Main meal.* Blade steak casserole and vegetables • Peach sago and yogurt.

*Friday*

*Breakfast.* Amaranth or quinoa porridge • Sliced banana or stewed fruit and yogurt.

*Light meal.* Some leftover casserole and remaining canned creamed corn • Asparagus • A piece of fruit.

*Main meal.* Beef schnitzel with corn grits batter, garlic, and onion • Vegetables • Gelatin dessert and stewed fruit.

*Saturday*

*Breakfast.* Buckwheat porridge and stewed fruit • One or two pieces of toasted non-OWGG bread and diabetic jam.

*Light meal.* Coleslaw salad and canned fish or diced schnitzel • Celery and cheese loaf—best eaten fresh **(B12)** • A piece of fruit.

*Main meal.* Chicken, vegetables, and potato chips • Gelatin dessert and fruit.

*Sunday*

*Breakfast.* Amaranth or quinoa porridge and stewed fruit or a small helping of leftover vegetables, olive oil, herbs, and cooked chickpeas • Herbal or weak tea.

*Light meal.* Coleslaw salad and canned fish, or use remaining salmon as salmon cakes • Corn crispbread and cube of cheese • A piece of fruit.

*Main meal.* Remainder of chicken, vegetables, and chips • A muffin or sultana cake.

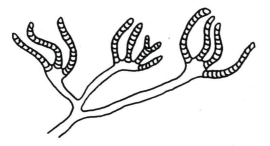

### Useful Advice for Exclusion Menus

- Eat two main meals a day: breakfast and an evening meal.
- Prepare a substantial breakfast, with a cooked dish such as "bubble and squeak," which includes fried vegetables and meat leftovers from the previous day's meals **(B24)**.
- Gradually increase the amount of breakfast you eat.
- Avoid processed foods and food colorings, if possible.
- Open canned foods and immediately empty into a glass container. Cover with a snap-on plastic lid or plastic film. Dispose of any unused portions after four days in the refrigerator.
- Eat a plain evening meal, meat or fish and vegetables, followed by fruit.
- Steam all vegetables. Be sure that quick-fry/stir-fry vegetables are *adequately cooked and heat sterilized.* You cannot risk food poisoning or infections.

- Cut meats into bite-sized pieces and cook until well-done.
- Eat a tapioca dish for breakfast or an evening dessert, three times a week.
- Soups you prepare, canned or packet, are suitable. Prepare soups and keep hot in a thermos.
- Cook enough porridges, tapioca, and sago for two to three daily helpings.
- A whole cooked fish is sufficient for three daily helpings.
- Eat salads, lettuce, spinach, coleslaw, etc., for the midday meal.
- Use chemical vinegar or preserving vinegar, with 4 percent acetic acid (not fermented).
- Use herbs and spices or OWGG-free prepared sauces on vegetables. Tomato, pasta, Asiatic clear fish, soy, and Worcestershire sauces can be used for vegetable servings.
- Eat Mexican meals two or three times a week.
- Mince your own meat in the kitchen food processor. Avoid preserved meats while you are ill and recovering.
- Avoid preserved meats because of toxic nitrate preservatives.
- Do not eat sugar or honey, but a sweetener such as stevia cyclamate is helpful until your sweet tooth is controlled.
- Purchase real fruit jams or diabetic jams. Sorbitol sugar causes diarrhea in some people. The pectin jelly or filler in commercial jams may be derived from apples and is not suitable for those with OWGG food allergies who like to eat jams every day. Small quantities are acceptable.
- Do not expect wheat (OWGG)-free breads to be soft, moist, and white. You can make a wide variety of breads with interesting flours and flavors. Nutritionally, they are excellent. The breads are best served fresh and hot, but they freeze well. Slice before freezing, separating the slices with lunch or wax paper. Put the frozen slices straight into the toaster and toast for a minute or two.
- Mashed banana improves the texture and moistness of breads. A very small amount of sugar improves the texture and aids the rising action of the baking yeast.
- Purchase wheat- and gluten-free bread mixes, but be sure there are no OWGG flours in the mix. Be adventurous and try baking fruit loaves, flat breads, pancakes, scones, muffins and waffles at home. Avoid all rice flour until you have recovered your health.
- For those excluding poultry, dairy, and beef, substitutes that do not change the textures are available, e.g., vegetable milks and cheeses and egg substitutes.
- Seeds and nuts can be ground to flour in the food processor. They are easily digested in this form. Make small quantities sufficient for three to

four days. Store in a container in the refrigerator. Local organic nuts are safe. Imported nuts are fumigated. Nuts with no information on their origin probably contain xenochemicals. Open the suspect nuts, cut into small pieces, and place on an electric or microwave tray/plate; heat the nuts but avoid browning them and damaging the nut oils. Try different temperatures and settings. Leave in the oven to cool. Test eat some pieces before grinding. If you have a reaction, repeat heating. During this heating process, sufficient xenochemicals may evaporate and you will be able to eat the nuts without reactions.

- Use corn/maize foods, such as cornflakes and corn puffs and medium/coarse maize/cornmeal porridge (polenta). Buckwheat, amaranth, and quinoa grains make tasty porridges.
- The flours to use are maize/corn flour, corn grits, cornmeal; buckwheat flour; potato flour; soy flour, soy flakes; pea flour, lentil or pea and chickpea flours. Other flours are available at Asiatic and specialty food shops. Some alternative flours have strong flavors, so combine them in baking with bland flours, thus improving the flavor of the final product. Pea, cornmeal, and potato flours go well in savory breads, muffins, and pizza bases. Soy flour goes well with potato flour for cakes and puddings. Buckwheat flour is a brownish dark color, but do not let that put you off. Corn grits make crunchy crisp batters, popular with children.
- An increasing number of commercial food products use grains without any OWGG flours. Some such products are pastas, such as spaghetti and vermicelli, and mixes for pancakes and waffles, corn and buckwheat crispbreads. Check the ingredients of corn breads, and when you take them home, slice and freeze or use the breads within two days, as they tend to go moldy.

*Cooking Suggestions*

*Wheat-free bread mixes.* These should be wet enough to make a sticky batter. Purchase wheat-free baking powder. Do not overmix, as the quickly forming gas will escape. As soon as the mix is completed, immediately put it into a hot oven. If baking powder with baking yeast is used in the recipe, a little sugar is needed for the yeast to work. If the bread tastes sweet after cooking, reduce the sugar when you repeat the recipe (**CB4**).

Modified starch usually means wheaten flour is present, but maize modified starch usage is increasing. Wheaten modified starch in supermarket food is not easily avoided. Many of you on the road to recovery will tolerate small quantities. Those with very sensitive irritable bowel symptoms will react. Selecting products in the supermarket is difficult for those with a marked OWGG allergy because so many products contain modified starch from wheat or rice flour. If in doubt, contact the manufacturer and hope you will get an honest reply.

*Potato and other flours.* Use white and sweet potatoes as often as possible. Try the numerous potato recipes. Potato flour makes light baking, e.g., sponges. Potato chips are best made at home, as commercial chips contain yellow dye or the whitener metabisulphate. Corn chips for menus should not be too savory. Use taros and yams as you would potatoes. Use a pea and potato flour mix to dust meat for braising, roasting, and in casseroles. Pea flour makes a very tasty gravy. Use soybean products no more than once daily. Dried beans are soaked for 12 h or more. Instead of an hour's cooking, use a pressure cooker. For the first four to six weeks, when progress is slow, avoid cooked red beans. Canned beans are expensive but useful for emergency meals. A small amount of spiced beans adds flavor to breakfast "bubble and squeak" or cooked vegetables. Many patients are unable to eat peanuts, but for those who can, grind them to a flour or paste for better absorption. Ground peanuts and mixed nuts, together with popcorn, are useful snacks.

*Vegetables and fruits.* As wide a range as possible should be eaten because vegetables in the bowel help to reduce *Candida* and other microbes to normal levels. Allergic vegetables and those you do not digest cause indigestion and flatulence. Eat two pieces of fruit a day. Do not eat ripe, very sweet fruit. Some fruits may upset your bowel if eaten fresh, so, if in doubt, stew the fruit, but do not add sugar. When you are considerably better or have recovered, but find you have to continue the food exclusion, preserve fruit in season, but do not add sugar. If you cannot manage bottling or canning, use a dehydrator unit. Have on hand unsweetened canned crushed pineapple. Use only canned unsweetened tropical fruit salad, as it does not contain apples or pears. OWGG-sensitive people react to apples and pears. If you mix fresh fruit with a breakfast cereal and store it in the refrigerator, it will ferment.

If organic fruits and vegetables are available, try these suggestions, which helped many who did not suspect petrochemical toxicities. If you have limited means, put aside enough money to live on organic vegetables or fruit without any chemically treated produce for six weeks. You will notice less, or no, improvement if you mix organic and treated produce. Eat organic produce for four to six weeks or until you experience seven to ten days of freedom or improvement of symptoms and health. Now is the time to provoke with treated produce, which is eaten without any organic produce for seven to ten days. By the end of the week, you will notice old symptoms returning, if you are sensitive to the petrochemicals. If you still suspect petrochemicals in the produce, return to organic foods for at least three to four months and then provoke again. I believe that some of the improvement from the five- to seven-day water fast is from the reduction of petrochemicals. After three or four months, you should be feeling a lot better, perhaps experiencing a return to remembered normal health, from the work-up, lifestyle change, and organic produce. I suggest you continue with organic produce, but if your income is limited, try rotating the organic and treated produce, avoiding mixing, for periods of two weeks. Now that your detoxing ability is near or back to normal you should be able to cope with the petrochemicals in the produce.

*Chicken.* During recovery, eat free-range chicken if possible. Otherwise, cook battery chicken until the flesh is well-done. Hold the cooked chicken in the microwave oven for 10 to 20 min after cooking stops to ensure the heat penetrates the whole carcass. During cooking some of the additives in the flesh will be broken down to less harmful compounds, and some will evaporate and leave the flesh.

*Fish.* During your illness and recovery, it is best to cook whole fish if possible. Filleted fish with the skin removed is exposed to oxygen in the air, which quickly converts the unsaturated fats to saturated fats, and the complex mineral proteins, together with tissue fluid leakage, are dried by the air. It is said that fillets could lose over 50 percent of their useful oil and mineral content. Choose a variety of fresh fish, even though some species may not be as attractive in taste and texture. Learn how to cut off the head or ask the fishmonger to remove it before wrapping it up. Large fish are cut into fillets. Choose one with the skin still attached. Prepare the whole fish by removing any remaining scales from the skin and opening up the belly flap and the large vein that runs along the backbone. Wash out the old blood. Puncture the skin on both sides before microwave steaming or oven baking to keep the fish from exploding. Do not overcook, and if the fish is fresh, try cooking it without herbs and oils. Place the cooked fish on a cutting board and remove the skin. Run a knife down the midline where the side bones are and lift off the cooked flesh, inspecting and feeling for bones. When one side is removed, turn the fish over, leaving the backbone in place for support. Repeat the removal of the cooked flesh into a containing dish or onto warm plates. Fish cooked in this manner retains unsaturated fats and complex mineral proteins. While you are ill, do not buy smoked fish, as no useful oils or trace mineral complexes are present. Avoid skinned frozen fillets if fresh fish is available. Place the frozen fillets in the oven/microwave and cook.

*Preserved meats.* Avoid meats with nitrate preservatives, such as corned meats, preserved mince, hams, tripe, tongues, sausages, salami, etc. Instead of preserved mince, purchase a piece of mincing meat and mince it at home, adding onions and herbs during the process. It tastes a lot better than preserved mince, and you avoid red colorings, nitrate, and taste enhancers. The recipes suggest small quantities of bacon for flavoring. You will be able to tolerate bacon in small amounts once you recover or markedly improve. Until that happy day, substitutes for bacon include homemade mincemeats with herbs and minced shellfish, e.g., mussels. Look up the herb and spice combinations used in commercial hamburger sauces, takeout chicken, sausages, and luncheon sausage. Children enjoy these herb and spice combinations when added to their home-cooked meat meals.

*Meats.* Whenever possible, buy a variety of free-range meats from a recommended supplier, thereby avoiding meat from confined animals raised on growth hormones. While you are ill and recovering, it is better to cook small pieces of meat rather than a large piece. If you fancy a larger portion of meat, cook it slowly in the oven or microwave so the heat will penetrate throughout. Wild rabbits are tasty and, wherever possible, are preferred to battery-raised chicken. Goat meat and venison is expensive, but you will not require large quantities. Meat two to three times a week and fish twice a week is a good rule during recovery. Do not forget to eat an average serving of free-range liver, kidneys, or sweet breads once or twice during the week. It is worth spending time cutting off all fat from lamb and sheep meat to reduce the strong flavor. Free-range goat meat, venison, rabbit, and other animal meats available locally should be rotated every ten to fourteen days.

*Warning:* Avoid beef from barn-fed cattle. Not only does it have undesirable antibiotics, antifungal chemicals, excess fat, reduced unsaturated fats, and low immunity levels, but the flesh contains growth hormones that are suspected of causing obesity and mold toxins that cause symptom flare-up in patients with CRC. Avoid pork and chicken livers. Pork meat should be avoided until you have recovered your remembered health.

Ask the local allergy support center for the address of fresh fish dealers, butchers, or meat companies supplying OWGG-free and preservative-free sausages and meat products.

*Cheeses and yogurt.* Until you recover remembered health, use plain cheeses such as colby, cheddar, gouda, edam, and local cheeses you know are mild and free of excess molds. Avoid colored cheeses. The plain cheeses retain some mold, but the level will not increase if the cheeses are stored in the freezer. Do not open a packet of cheese, take a portion, and leave it in the refrigerator, as it will always become infected with the molds that live in your refrigerator. Instead, purchase a plain local cheese without coloring and additives. Cut the cheese block into daily rations, wrap portions in wax paper, and freeze them. Those who have problems with CRC and other molds (e.g., asthmatics) should be careful, trying small quantities of plain cheeses, including cottage and sour cheeses, to see whether they react.

Milk is readily converted to yogurt when the friendly acidophilus bacteria change the lactose to lactic acid. *Candida* cannot ferment lactic acid. Use plain yogurt whenever you can. Fresh cottage and soft cheeses are safe if they are kept no longer than two to three days. The yogurt should be sweetened with stewed fruit or a sweetener. Avoid flavored commercial fruit and yogurt products. Women over forty-five years and men over sixty years need calcium supplements, in addition to the calcium they obtain from dairy foods.

*Sweeteners.* Cyclamates are very sweet chemicals. Our patients prefer liquid cyclamates to other sweeteners, such as saccharin and aspartame. Shop around, as a locally prepared cyclamate product may be considerably cheaper than the original brand. A problem with aspartame is the addition of lactose sugar. Purchase the cyclamate sweetener brand that does not include additional sugars. Cyclamates may break down during cooking and are best added to the dish or baked good by sprinkling a few drops before eating. Some allergic people will react to chemicals, e.g., MSG or one or more of the sweeteners. If you are affected, try to forget about your sweet tooth. Help is at hand, however, in the form of stevia extract, a natural sweetener that is popular in Japan. As a powder it is easy to use in baking. Sorbitol sugar is a sweetener in diabetic food products, but may cause diarrhea.

*Herbs and spices.* Dried herbs contain molds, but the small amounts you use may not affect you. If you have a garden and the energy, grow some fresh herbs. Spices should be rotated; avoid using the same herb or spice every day. Be aware that allergies to cinnamon, cloves, nutmeg, and allspice are common. Cinnamon is added to a wide range of preserved and processed foods. If you have IBS, chronic or intermittent diarrhea, indigestion due to CRC, *Giardia, Helicobacter,* or for no known reason, avoid chili, coffee, and the sweetener sorbitol. Yet, this is a world of opposites, and some people with diarrhea of unknown origin get relief from small doses of chili. Cautiously reintroduce coffee or chili to your meals as you begin to feel better. A coffee allergy can be a hidden cause of IBS, chronic mucous diarrhea, and strong-smelling flatulence. Diabetic jams contain pectin, usually derived from apples, and the sweetener sorbitol. The apple pectin affects those with OWGG allergies, and many people are sensitive to sorbitol.

*Beverages.* If you must drink beverages, use those with sweeteners. Avoid Diet Coke, as the chocolate and cola stimulate CRC activity in the bowel. If you can tolerate wine, drink bottle fermented whites. Maté substitutes for coffee and tea. Carob substitutes for chocolate, but there may be added sugar in the powder.

*Oils, vinegars, and butter.* Rotate a wide variety of vegetable oils, such as corn, soy, sunflower, safflower, olive, and flaxseed oil. Sesame oil may cause diarrhea. Do not use fermented vinegars of any type; substitute synthetic vinegar with 4 percent acetic acid. Use 1 ro 2 tsp of vinegar on the breakfast and evening meal vegetables. The acidic vinegar stimulates gastric secretion and digestion. Those with digestive problems should not drink during, or for 1 or 2 h after the meal to avoid diluting the gastric juices. Do not eat margarine, and be sparing of butter until you are on the way to recovery.

Monosodium glutamate (MSG) is FDA approved, but hundreds of clinic patients, especially CFIDS/ME patients, had problems with the additive. The FDA also approved aspartame (Equal) sweetener, which affected many clinic patients as well. If in doubt, do the elimination and provocation check on aspartame.

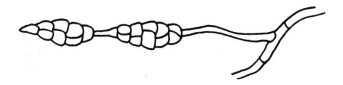

### Daily Meals Using the Recipe Index

*Breakfast*

Breakfast includes a choice of the following:

1. Fresh or stewed fruit with no added sugar
2. Porridges—either non-OWGGs based or nongrain carbohydrates
3. Cooked breakfast recipes
4. Breakfast breads and muffins

*Non-OWGG porridge.* All flours and grains are stored in the freezer to prevent mold growth. Freezing does not affect their texture.

Amaranth seed has been cultivated in Mexico for over 7,000 years. It makes a porridge with a grainy nutty flavor. It is high in mucin and other proteins, fiber, iron, calcium, and trace minerals. Amaranth flour becomes bitter unless it is stored in the freezer. Amaranth flour and seeds are said to decrease the number of parasites in the bowel. We suggest eating amaranth three times a week. Plant amaranth seed in your garden; the leaves are edible and nourishing, similar to spinach (**B4**).

Buckwheat is the seed of a plant of the rhubarb family. The soft, pyramid-shaped seeds are encased in a tough, dark brown sheath that is milled off to make groats. Buckwheat has good nutritional value, with 8 percent protein, Vitamin B complex, trace minerals, and, especially, calcium and dietary fiber. The roasted seed is called kasha, a traditional Russian and Middle Eastern food. The Japanese use buckwheat extensively, and their popular traditional food is *soba*. Buckwheat flour is used in baking. It has the quality of acting as a binder for bread, biscuits, cakes, pancakes, and fritters (**B5, B25**).

Quinoa (pronounced ′kēn-wä) is a tiny white to golden-colored seed, cultivated in South America for the last 5,000 years. It has a delicate taste and is easy to prepare. Before buying quinoa, ask if it has been debittered. It has high protein content, with an ideal balance of amino acids. It provides starch, sugars, and oil (high in linoleic acid); dietary fiber; minerals and B vitamins. Its uses are as a porridge (**B6**), and in baking, soups (**L30**), and desserts.

Quinoa grain has a naturally occurring bitter-tasting coating. Commercially, it is removed prior to sale, but there may be a small to moderate amount of bitter residue left on the grain. It is removed by rinsing the grain before cooking. If the bitter taste is not removed, the grain should be brought to a boil, the water drained, and the process repeated again until the draining water is clear; then fresh boiling water is added, and the quinoa is left to cook slowly for 30 min or more until it swells and becomes tender.

Maize, or corn, is another source of non-OWCG porridge. There are three varieties: dent corn, which supplies commercial cornmeal; sweet corn, the vegetable; and popping corn. Some of the many by-products are cooking oil and corn sweeteners. Finely ground cornmeal is maize/corn flour, medium-ground cornmeal is known as grits. Store both products in the freezer until use (**B7, L37**).

Tapioca is an important nongrain food crop of the wet tropics. The large roots are peeled and crushed, the toxic substance is allowed to dissipate in the air, and then the starch is washed out. The starch is dried to form pearls, flakes, and a fine flour. Tapioca flour is an easily prepared dessert base, and has a very beneficial effect on those under treatment for CRC. Tapioca is gelatinous and acts in a similar way to seaweed or agar-agar. Before World War II, it was widely used in institutions because of its gentle laxative action. The gelatinous material mixes with the mucus formed by the lining of the gut. The combination distances unfriendly gut organisms from the surface cells of the lining. Make it a rule to eat a tapioca dish two or three times a week (**B1**).

Sago starch, another nongrain product, is extracted from a tropical palm tree. It is a gelatinous food but is less effective than tapioca against bowel organisms. It is more pleasant to eat than tapioca, and one or two recipe dishes should be eaten every week (**B2, B3**).

Okra is a mucilaginous vegetable that is popular in warmer climates. Local mucilaginous foods may be available for you to use once or twice a week. Patients are convinced that the addition of mucilaginous foods to their diet is as effective as taking garlic, a very old remedy for CRC symptoms. We recommend fresh garlic or a garlic preparation be taken with one or more meals every day.

*Cooked breakfast recipes.* Take your choice from eight popular recipes (**B21-B28**). It is easy to modify some of the other cooked dishes for breakfast. Spend some time preparing four or five servings of three or four of your favorite cooked breakfasts and put them in the freezer. They can be quickly heated if you are in a rush to get to work. Do not keep leftover food from a frozen meal that contains meat or fish. The safest practice is to discard such leftovers.

Use frozen vegetables when fresh are expensive or in short supply. Select a mixture of frozen vegetables, beans, in particular, broad beans, and 1 tbsp of the chickpeas you cooked and froze. While preparing the evening meal, boil the frozen vegetables for 5 min, drain, and store in a container with a lid. For best results, do not throw frozen vegetables into the frying pan. Warm the oil and herbs in the pan, then add the cooked vegetables and leftover cold potato or pasta. Heat until hot, but not frizzled. Add diced leftover cold meat or fish and a choice of thin sauces. Fry for 2 to 3 min and serve. Do not boil more than three days' supply of frozen vegetables. For best results, prepare the night before.

*Breakfast breads and muffins.* Take your pick from a wide variety of plain, spiced, and tasty breads (**B10-B19, L39-L42**).

Toppings for toast and bread should include diabetic jams, but if you later develop diarrhea, suspect the unabsorbable sugar, sorbitol, or apple pectin. To make a fresh fruit jam, stew the fruit in its own juice. Prepare enough for four to five days, freezing any excess. Add a cooking gum, agar-agar, gelatin or stiff tapioca, or sago to gel the stewed fruit. All items are boiled to sterilize them. Do not use apple pectin. Apple, pear, and quince have wheatlike allergens (antigens) so exclude them during the three to four months of the exclusion diet. Commercial "just fruit" spreads without any other ingredients are available from health food outlets. For another topping, you can grind the selected nuts to a paste. Make enough nut butter to last a week.

## Lunch or Light Evening Meal

After a large breakfast, you may not need lunch. People who suffered allergy problems for years often wake up nauseated and cannot look at food until morning tea or lunchtime. After two to three weeks of OWGG exclusion, the breakfast recipes may not nauseate you. There are no OWGGs, sugar, or honey in the lunch recipes, so you will not get sleepy 1 or 2 h later. Lunch is the time to eat your daily salad, even though you may have little appetite after a good breakfast. If you cannot face a salad at lunch, have a salad before the evening meal. When possible, vary the salad greens. If you do not snack on nuts and seeds, be sure to add some freshly ground ones to your salads (**B21, B9-B20, L39-L41**).

*Soups.* Preparing homemade soups takes time, so make a large quantity and freeze the excess in meal-size portions (**L30-L32**). Take your hot homemade soup to work in a stainless steel thermos. Some of the commercial canned soups without modified starch may appeal to you. If you pressure-cook your vegetables, save the vegetable water and add to it a quarter of the volume of a canned soup concentrate.

*Salad dressings.* Those attending the clinic prefer simple dressings, so as not to smother the taste of greens, radishes, onions, etc. More elaborate dressings are useful when your greens are a few days old or you decide to change the dressings. You can make variations of the dressing (**L44**). Two more-complex salads are **L45** and **L46**.

*Breads.* Do not expect wheat-free bread to be soft, moist, and white without the use of wheat flour. Bread can be made many other ways. A wide variety of flours with better flavors and improved nutritional balance is available. Ensure that the flours are fresh and do not smell musty. Preparation of breads from ingredients takes 18 to 25 min. Wheat-free breads are best served fresh and hot, but they freeze well. Slice before freezing, wrap in wax paper in meal-size servings, and serve by toasting slices straight from the freezer. The texture of the mixtures is different, unless they contain banana "flour" (mashed banana), which can absorb quantities of water without becoming liquid. Wheat-free bread mixes need to be wet enough to make a sticky batter. These mixtures cannot hold all the carbon dioxide ($CO_2$) produced by yeast. Bicarbonate of soda and tartaric acid still need to be added to the mixture to make it rise. Use a non-OWGG homemade or commercial "wheat-free" baking powder. Non-OWGG bread mixtures require double the amount of baking powder.

The baking powder breads without egg are crumbly and drier. The liquids are added to the dry ingredients with as little extra mixing as possible. The structure of the dough forms as the wet and dry ingredients are mixed together. Do not overmix, as this will press much of the gas out of the mixture so that it will not rise on baking. Do not leave the wet mixture to stand at this point, or you will lose the light structure from the escape of $CO_2$. It must go straight into the heated oven. The ½ to 1 tsp of sugar in some recipes reacts with the starch during cooking and improves the texture, leaving the bread slightly sweet. Several commercial gluten-free bread and baking mixes are available. Check that they do not contain OWGGs. These mixes are expensive compared to the bread from recipes in the index. Buckwheat flour has a strong flavor, and similar to many non-OWGG flours, it should be combined with a plain-tasting flour in baking to improve the flavor of the final product. For savory dishes and baking, use pea and potato flour. For cakes and baking, use soy, potato, and corn flour (see recipes for bread machines, p. 289). Waffles are a change of bakery for lunch and a treat for children returning home after school.

*Snacks*

Commercial dried fruits are expensive and may contain preservatives, added sugar, and food colorings. Try different brands and countries of origin to find dried fruits and nuts that agree with you. Do not "pig out" on commercial popcorn or potato and corn chips with high fat contents. Make low-fat popcorn (**S72**) and potato skins (**S73**). These are popular with children. A microwave chip maker turns out fat-free potato and sweet potato chips. Prepare or buy corn and potato dips with low spice and pepper content. A dehydrator unit pays for itself by making tasty dried fruit, when in season. Check the unit's handbook to find a variety of fresh foods suitable for dehydrating. Store any excess in the freezer to prevent mold growth. More substantial snacks are pancakes (**B9**), flat breads (**L40-L42**), and waffles (**L33-L36**).

*Car trips.* Keep an airtight snack container in the car with puffed corn, soybeans, peanuts, nuts, seeds, and unsweetened banana chips. Should you attend a social function and there is nothing you can eat, you will be prepared. For longer car trips, take cans of fish or meat, peas or beans, and unsweetened pineapple or fruit. Do not drive on an empty stomach. **Note:** Keep a can opener, fork, and spoon in the glove box. More substantial snacks are (**S73-S77**).

*The Midday or Evening Dinner*

*Soups.* **D50-D51, L32.**
*Flat breads.* Flat breads are dipped in soup. Held in the mouth until soft, they enhance the flavors of wine (**L40-L42**).
*Pasta.* Popular non-OWGG pastas are 100 percent corn, bean, buckwheat, and quinoa flours (**D57**).
*Pizza crusts.* **D59, D60, D61.** *Beware:* Italian restaurants and takeout pizza places serve OWGG pastas and pizza crusts.
*Mexican meals.* Add Mexican ingredients of meat, cheeses, and beans to the corn tortilla recipe (**L38**). Refer to Mexican recipe books for a variety of foods. Your Mexican meal may not be authentic Mexican cuisine, but who cares, as long as the meal is tasty, a little different, and does not bring on your IBS or other symptoms. Beware of "wheaten 'corn' chips" masquerading as Mexican corn chips. Mexican restaurants are popular with OWGG-allergic people.
*The main course.* The recipes **D53-D56, L37,** and **L39** may be altered using other meats, herbs, and spices. We suggest you do not change the ingredients until you feel you are on the way to recovery and have increased energy. At first the cooked meals are simple, with little or no spices and herbs. Introduce more flavors and complexity as you begin to feel better.
*Vegetables.* Steamed vegetables are best, but do not overcook them. If hungry, eat a plate or more of mixed vegetables. I am not asking you to become a vegetarian. Large quantities of vegetables and their roughage encourage the return of friendly microbes to your bowel (refer to Ngaire's story, p. 239). You may have a hidden allergy to one or more vegetables. Suspect carrots, string beans, green peppers, and broccoli. The best way to detect a vegetable allergy is the five- to seven-day water fast (Collison and Hall, 1989; Hyde, 1992). The results have surprised some people (**D58, B24**).

**IK**  "Can you help me? My singing career is over! When I begin to sing I do not know if I will be a soprano or mezzo. I was trained as a soprano." Her nose, chest, IBS, and lethargy improved with OWGG exclusion, but her two voices persisted. Her favorite vegetable was carrot, and on testing with carrot provocation shots, the mezzo voice was neutralized to a soprano. Her partner's physician ridiculed carrot allergy. Her partner secretly added carrot juice to a stew. After the meal, she attended a charitable concert, began to sing, and out came the mezzo voice. She broke down and was taken home. The next day

I had an interesting telephone call from the husband. She went on to be a successful operatic soprano.

*Desserts and sweets.* For the first six to eight weeks, keep the desserts simple and avoid sugar and honey. Once your child has shown signs of recovery, try ice cream recipes **(D64-D66)**. If CRC and *Giardia* are diagnosed, eat tapioca, sago, and amaranth desserts and breakfasts three to four times a week. Tapioca and sago gel substitute for gelatin in dessert recipes **(D63, D64, D68)**.

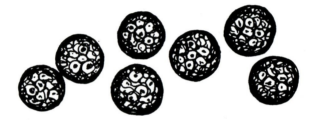

*Cooking Basics*

The following methods are included in the recipe index: thickening **(CB1)**, roux **(CB2)**, stocks **(CB3)**, baking powder without yeast **(CB4)**, and pie shell **(CB5, D59, D60)**.

## *THE RECIPE INDEX*

The recipe index for no Old World grass grains (OWGGs) is arranged to help those beginning their OWGGs food exclusion. The prefix **B** = breakfast; **L** = lunch; **D** = dinner, including desserts; **S** = snacks. Thickenings, roux, and stocks are lettered **CB.** As the exclusion proceeds and you gain more confidence, please choose any menu that takes your fancy for a particular meal. You may be hungry in the morning instead of at dinner time. Periods of hunger and nausea may come and go without any pattern. When you are well on the way to recovery, the normal daily eating pattern will return.

Sweeteners: choice of sweeteners and intensity of sweetness.

Measures for flour weights are as follows:

- 1 cup potato flour = 165 grams (g) (6 ounces [oz]); 2 cups potato flour = 330 g (12 oz)
- 1 cup buckwheat flour = 155 g (5½ oz); 1 cup pea flour = 105 g (3½ oz)
- 1 cup soy flour = 95 g (3¼ oz); 1 cup fine cornmeal = 105 g (3½ oz)

## Breakfast Recipes

### B1—Tapioca: Breakfast/Dessert (Preparation Time: 5 Min)

Allow 2 to 3 tbsp of "ball or pellet" tapioca per serving. It is better to prepare larger amounts of tapioca (e.g., 8 to 10 tbsp). The cooked tapioca will not ferment in the refrigerator unless fresh fruit is added.

• Soak in cold water overnight, or for 8 to 10 h • Drain the tapioca in a large strainer and run fresh water through it • Shake and replace in the saucepan • Add boiling water (1½ quarts [qt]) and place on the heating element • Bring to a boil and simmer until the mixture becomes clear and thickens (15 to 20 min) • While cooking, stir frequently with a metal spatula or cooking spoon to free tapioca from the saucepan and to prevent burning • Separate the quantity needed for the present serving; let the remainder cool before storing in the refrigerator • Add stewed fruit, canned crushed pineapple, diced fresh fruit (no apples or pears) to the serving • Other flavors to add include vanilla, aniseed, and hazelnut • Add sweetening, if needed, just before serving.

**Note:** Porridges are cooked in a microwave oven/Crock-Pot. The slow cooking improves the taste. Fill the pot to within 1½ inches (in) from the rim. This will allow the porridge to swell without overflowing, which is a sticky mess to clean up.

Quick tapioca is made from tapioca flour. Allow 2 to 3 tbsp per serving. Prepare enough for the meal.

• Mix with a little cold water, and then add hot to boiling water, stirring frequently • Add water for desired consistency • Add fruit or flavorings and sweeten before serving • Do not store in a refrigerator.

### B2—Sago (Preparation Time: 4 Minutes)

*Method.* Soak 2 tbsp per person or a larger amount, up to 10 tbsp, for additional meals • Place in a fine mesh strainer and wash; pick out discolored sago grains • Place in a saucepan and add 1 cup of warm to hot water for every 2 tbsp • Bring to a boil, then simmer • Stir frequently with metal spatula until the grains become a clear jelly (10 to 15 min) • Add fruit or flavorings and sweetener before serving • Use as a filler for other desserts.

### B3—*Fruit and Rhubarb Sago (Preparation Time: 5 Min)*

*Ingredients.* 2 tbsp sago per person • 1 cup hot tap water • 1 to 3 stalks of diced rhubarb or equivalent fruit • Sweetener, if required.

*Method.* Partially cook the fruit/rhubarb in the microwave or saucepan • Prepare sago as for recipe **B2** • When sago jelly forms, stir in the rhubarb • Place in the microwave (3 to 4 min) or saucepan • Serve with sweetener and acidophilus yogurt • Popular with kids, add stewed lemons/crushed oranges to sago.

### B4—*Amaranth Porridge (Preparation Time: 4 to 5 Min)*

*Method.* 3 tbsp amaranth seed per serving • Soak for 4 to 8 h • Wash thoroughly and drain • Place in saucepan and cover with water, i.e., 2 parts water to 1 part grain • Bring to boil for a few minutes • Drain water using a strainer or sieve • Add fresh boiling water and bring to a boil, then simmer for 20 to 30 min adding more water as it boils away • Stir with metal spatula • Turn off the heat when seeds have swollen and burst and the liquid should be thickened • The porridge should be soft and fluffy • Serve with stewed fruit and plain yogurt.

### B5—*Buckwheat Porridge (Preparation Time: 4 to 5 Min)*

*Method.* Allow 3 tbsp per person for a serving • Wash the grain and pick out any oat grains • Soak in warm water for 4 to 8 h and drain • Pour boiling water over the grains and bring to a boil for 1 to 2 min • Drain off the rhubarb-colored liquid • Replace with more boiling water and bring to a boil • Cook for 15 to 20 min, adding more water to retain the volume until the grains swell and fluff up, absorbing any free liquid • Stir with a metal spatula (see **B1)** • Serve with stewed fruit, in particular, black currants, apricots, and plain yogurt.

### B6—*Quinoa Porridge (Preparation Time: 4 to 5 Min)*

*Method.* 3 tbsp per person • Wash and soak 6 to 8 h, drain • Cover with boiling water, 1 part grain to 2 parts water • Bring to a boil, then simmer for 15 to 25 min • Stir with metal spatula • Cook until the grains become soft and puffy and the seed germ separates as a small white half-moon • Serve with stewed fruit and plain yogurt.

### B7—*Cornmeal Porridge and Italian Polenta (Preparation Time: 10 Min)*

*Ingredients.* 1 cup medium to coarse cornmeal • 4 cups water • Italian polenta • 1 cup grated mild cheese (optional).

*Method.* Mix the cornmeal in a large saucepan and bring to a boil, stirring constantly with metal spatula • Simmer on a low heat for about 20 min until cooked, continuing to stir at short intervals.

*Cornmeal porridge.* Allow to cool • To a warm serving, add stewed fruit, yogurt, crushed nuts, or other flavorings.

*Italian polenta.* To cooked cornmeal porridge, add half the cheese; mix in well • Turn into an oiled casserole dish • Sprinkle remaining cheese on top and bake at 350°F (180°C) for 15 min or until lightly browned on top • Serve with a spicy tomato sauce. *Variation:* Add 1 tsp of dried basil and some chopped onion.

### B8—Legumes (Dried Soybeans, Peas, Beans, and Lentils)

Beans contain a toxin that is destroyed by boiling, the high temperatures of pressure cooking, and baking. Use legumes in soups and stews. Legume flours are used in baking. Red and green lentils are rich in protein, iron, and zinc, with good levels of potassium and the vitamin B group. Red lentils are easier to cook. Mexican and Middle Eastern cookbooks will include bean and chickpea recipes. Red beans are introduced after two to three months. They may upset digestion and IBS. Cook large quantities of chickpeas and lima beans. After cooking, wash and shake off excess water, bag, and freeze. Add cooked beans to breakfast dishes.

| Legume<br>Quantity = 1 cup | Water for Soaking (cups) | Cooking Time (min) | Yield (cups) |
|---|---|---|---|
| Black beans | 4 | 90-120 | 2-2½ |
| Garbanzo beans (chickpeas) | 4 | 180 | 2 (approx.) |
| Great northern beans | 3½ | 120 | 2 |
| Kidney beans | 3 | 120-150 | 2 |
| Lentils (soak ½ h) | 3 | 30-40 | 2½ |
| Lima beans | 2 | 120 | 1½ |
| Soybeans | 4 | 180 | 2 |
| Split peas (soak ½ h) | 3 | 45 | 2 |

### B9—Pancake Batter (Preparation Time: 5 min)

*Ingredients.* 1 cup (4 oz/125g) flour • Pea and potato flour for savory pancakes • Soy and corn flour for sweet pancakes • ⅛ tsp salt • 1 egg • 1 cup milk or plain yogurt and water • Butter or oil for frying • Lemon juice • ½ to 1 tsp castor sugar.

*Method.* Sieve the flour and salt into a bowl, and make a well in the center • Beat the egg and stir into the flour • Gradually add about two-thirds of the milk, mixing well • Beat with a wooden spoon or plastic spoon for a few minutes to incorporate as much as air as possible • Heat a tiny piece of butter or a small amount of oil until it is hot • Pour a little of the batter (2 tbsp) and tilt the pan until the batter covers the bottom • Cook for 1 min • Toss, or turn with a spatula, and cook the other side • Sprinkle with lemon juice and sweetener • Roll up and serve hot. *Variations:*

1. Hot stewed fruit (1 to 3 tbsp) or jam spread on pancake before rolling up.
2. Roll up two or three spears of asparagus in each pancake and arrange them side by side in a shallow oven-safe dish. Make a cheese buck-wheat sauce and pour it over the pancakes. Sprinkle with spices or herbs and heat through at 350°F (180°C) for 15 min.
3. Fill with finely chopped cooked meats, sliced bananas, or 2 tbsp crushed pineapple. Reheat filled rolled pancakes in oven-safe dish.
4. Cooked diced chicken or salmon in sauce with cooked peas, as a filling and sauce.
5. Mashed, drained, or cooked canned or bottled apricots. Spread apricot mix over pancakes and place in layers in a oven-safe dish. Warm apricot syrup and pour over pancakes.
6. Sprinkle pancakes with flaked almonds and a few drops of almond essence. Reheat.

Gluten-free baking powder, see **CB4** (p. 288).

### B10—Cheese and Celery Bread (Preparation Time: 20 Min)

*Ingredients.* 2 cups flour, pea and potato • 3 tsp baking powder • ¼ tsp salt • 5 tbsp (2 oz/70 g) butter • 1¼ cup (6 oz/150 g) celery, finely chopped • 1 tbsp chives, finely chopped (optional) • ½ cup grated cheese • 1 egg, beaten • ½ cup milk, or plain yogurt and water • Pinch of cayenne pepper • 1 lightly greased loaf tin with nonstick paper on the bottom.

*Method.* Set the oven to 370°F (190°C) • Sift the flours, baking powder, and salt into a bowl; rub in the butter until the mix resembles bread crumbs • Stir in the celery, chives, and cheese • Beat egg, then add to dry ingredients, with a ¼ to ½ cup of yogurt to make a moist dough • Mix quickly, then put in a prepared loaf tin • Bake in a moderate oven 370°F (190°C) for 30 min, until golden colored and firm to the touch • Remove from loaf tin, cool, then slice and freeze • Sesame seeds and cheese can be sprinkled over the top before cooking.

### B11—Zucchini (Courgette) Quick Bread (Preparation Time: 15 to 20 Min)

*Ingredients.* 3 tbsp (40g) butter • 1 to 1½ cups grated zucchini • ½ of a small onion, grated (optional) • ½ cup grated cheese • 2 cups flour, potato and pea • 3 tsp baking powder • 1 tbsp chopped parsley or chives • Pinch cayenne pepper and/or marjoram • ½ tsp salt • 1 egg, beaten • ¼ cup plain yogurt and water.

*Method.* Grate the zucchini; chop or grate the onion • Grate the cheese • Sift the flours and baking powder with the seasonings • Rub the butter into the flours • Add the cheese, onion, and zucchini, and the chives and parsley • Add the beaten egg, yogurt, and water to dry ingredients • Mix quickly to make a moist dough • Put in a greased loaf tin • Sprinkle top with cheese and sesame seeds • Bake at 350°F (180°C) for 30 min • Turn out of the tin • Cool, slice, then freeze.

### B12—Cottage Cheese and Herb Bread (Preparation Time: 15 Min)

*Ingredients.* 1 cup potato flour • 1 cup pea flor • ¼ tsp salt • 3 tsp baking powder • 1 tbsp chives; pinch cayenne pepper, thyme, or marjoram • Half container (9 oz/250 g) cottage cheese • 2 eggs • ½ cup cool water.

*Method.* Beat 2 eggs until thick • Sift the dry ingredients • Mash or cream the cottage cheese • Mix all together with water until well moistened • Put in a well-greased loaf tin and bake for 30 min at 350°F (180°C) • Sesame seeds and grated cheese can be sprinkled on top before baking • Turn out, cool, slice, and freeze.

### B13—Miner's Corn Bread (Preparation Time: 15 Min)

*Ingredients.* 2 large eggs • 1 cup milk (approximate), otherwise plain yogurt and water • ¼ cup oil • ¼ tsp chili powder (more if desired) • 1 can whole kernel corn (10 oz/310 g), drained • 2 cups coarse cornmeal • 1 cup potato flour • 1 cup pea flour • 2 cups grated cheese • 3 to 4 tsp baking powder • ½ tsp baking soda.

*Method.* Combine the eggs, milk, oil, chili powder, and corn • In a separate bowl, combine the dry ingredients and cheese • Combine egg and corn mixture with the dry ingredients until just moistened; do not overmix • Turn into a 1 qt greased and lined loaf tin • Bake at 350°F (180°C) for

50 to 55 min, or until a toothpick comes out clean • Slice into ½ in slices • Corn bread is best eaten on the day it is baked. *Suggestion:* Grill one side of a slice, turn over, top the other side with a mild cheese and herb mix, and toast that side—suitable for children's snacks.

### B14—Farm Corn Bread (Preparation Time: 15 Min)

*Ingredients.* 1 cup fine cornmeal • 1 cup potato flour • ½ cup mashed cooked pumpkin • ¼ tsp salt • 1 tsp sugar • 2 to 3 tsp baking powder • Pinch cayenne pepper • ¼ tsp Vitamin C added to 1 beaten egg • ¼ cup grated mild cheese (optional) • 1 tbsp linseeds (optional) • ¾ cup plain yogurt and water • 1 tbsp butter, melted (optional) • ½ tsp guar gum.

*Method.* Sift dry ingredients into bowl • Rub in butter • Add pumpkin, egg, yogurt and water, vitamin C, and guar gum to make a moist dough • Put in a greased small loaf tin, lined • Sprinkle grated cheese and sesame seeds on top • Bake at 400°F (200°C) for 30 min, or until firm to touch and golden colored • Turn out, cool, slice, then freeze • For a lighter texture, fold in two stiffly beaten egg whites just before baking (use yolks in place of the egg in the recipe).

This loaf does not rise as much as other breads.

### B15—Buckwheat Banana Bread (Preparation Time: 15 Min)

*Ingredients.* 2 cups buckwheat flour • 3 tsp baking powder • ¼ tsp salt • ½ cup pumpkin seeds • ¼ cup walnut pieces • 2 bananas • ⅓ cup safflower/olive oil • ¼ tsp vitamin C • Vanilla essence • 2 tbsp linseed • ¾ cup cold water.

*Method.* Boil linseed for five minutes, then leave to cool • Sift the buckwheat flour into a bowl with the baking powder and salt • Grind the pumpkin seeds and shelled walnut pieces in a food processor • Transfer to bowl with dry ingredients • Process oil, vanilla, Vitamin C, and banana until smooth • Add dry ingredients and mix • Grease loaf tin, and put paper in base • Cook at 350°F (180°C) for 30 min or more, until light brown and firm to touch • Turn out, cool, slice, and freeze.

The loaf is not for toasting. For lunch, cover with cottage cheese and diabetic or homemade black currant jam for a sandwich.

### B16—Carrot and Orange Loaf (Preparation Time: 15 Min)

*Ingredients.* 2 medium carrots (200 g), peeled and roughly chopped • Rind of an orange (use a vegetable peeler) • 2 tsp sweetener/¼-⅛ cup sugar • ½ cup natural yogurt • 2 eggs • 1 cup soy flour • ¾ cup potato flour • 2 to 3 tsp baking powder • 1½ tsp cinnamon • 2 tsp spice • 1 cup raisins and/or sultanas (boiled, drained, and cooled).

*Method.* Place carrots and orange rind in food processor • Process until fine • Add sugar, yogurt, and eggs • Process until smooth • Lightly mix in the dry ingredients • Turn into greased loaf tin with baking paper lining the base • Bake for 1 h in moderate oven (350°F/180°C).

The success of this recipe varies, due to the season and freshness of the carrots.

### B17—Muffins (Preparation Time: 15 Min)

*Ingredients.* 1 cup potato flour • ¾ cup soy flour • 3 tsp baking powder • ¼ tsp salt • ¾ cup natural yogurt and water • 1 egg • 2 mashed kiwifruit • 1 tbsp lemon juice • or ¾ cup drained, unsweetened crushed pineapple (use pineapple juice instead of the water) • 1 tsp cinnamon, or equivalent nutmeg or allspice • 1 tbsp sugar • 2 tbsp melted butter. Makes 6 muffins.

*Method.* Preheat oven to 350°F (180°C) • Grease muffin tray • Melt butter • Sift flours and baking powder • Mix in remaining ingredients until moistened • Spoon into muffin tray • Bake for 25 min • Eat hot or cold, sliced, with butter or jam. *Variations:* ¾ cup blueberries, raspberries, or black currants adds excellent flavor to these muffins. Refer to other cookbooks for muffin recipe variations (substitute non-OWGG flours for the OWGG flours). Add a sprinkle of sweetener before serving (optional).

### B18—Lemon and Zucchini (Courgette) Muffins (Preparation Time: 15 Min)

*Ingredients.* 1 cup potato flour • ¾ cup soy flour • 3 tsp baking powder • 2 tsp lemon rind • ¼ tsp nutmeg or desired spice • Pinch salt • 2 tbsp sugar • ½ cup currants (preboiled, drained, and cooled) • 2 eggs • ½ cup natural yogurt and water (may need more) • 1 cup raw zucchini, grated.

*Method.* Combine flours, spice, baking powder, and salt • Add lemon rind, drained currants, beaten eggs, zucchini, sugar, and liquid to make a moist dough • Spoon into greased muffin tins • Bake at 370°F (190°C) for 25 min • Turn out and cool.

### B19— Savory Muffins (Preparation Time: 15 Min)

*Ingredients.* 1 egg • 1 cup natural yogurt and water • 7½ tbsp (3 oz/ 75 g) butter • 1 cup potato flour • ½ cup fine cornmeal, and ½ cup pea flour • 3 to 4 tsp baking powder • ½ to 1 tsp salt • ½ of a small onion, finely chopped, or 4 spring onions, or fresh herbs • ½ cup grated cheese. *Option:* 1 cup grated vegetables, e.g., carrots, sweet potato • ¼ to ½ cup bacon meat, without fat, for those on the way to recovery.

*Method.* Mix the egg, yogurt, and water • Melt butter • Cook the chopped bacon in a pan or in the microwave • Sift flours, baking powder, salt • Add the bacon and cheese • Make a "well" in the dry ingredients, then pour in the liquid ingredients; stir to dampen ingredients only • Half fill nonstick or lightly greased muffin tins • Bake in a preheated moderate oven 370°F (190°C) for 25 min, until golden brown • Serve warm with butter. Muffins freeze well.

### B20—Brown Buckwheat Cookies/Cakes (Preparation Time: 15 Min)

*Ingredients.* 1 large banana • 1 egg or egg substitute • ½ tsp vanilla • 3 tbsp sugar • ¼ to ½ cup yogurt and water • 4 oz (100 g) buckwheat flour • 4 oz (100 g) potato and soy flour • 1 tsp baking soda • ½ tsp cream of tartar • 2 oz (50 g) butter or oil • 2 oz (50 g) sultanas • ½ tsp spice or cinnamon.

*Method.* Bring sultanas to a boil, drain, and cool • Combine with egg or egg substitute • Add vanilla and sweetener • Sift dry ingredients together, then rub in butter • Mash banana • Add liquids, banana, sultanas, and yogurt with water to the dry ingredients • Mix to make soft dough • Spoon onto greased pans • Bake 15 to 20 minutes at 370°F (190°C) until lightly browned • When cool, wrap individual cookies in wax paper and place in freezer until needed.

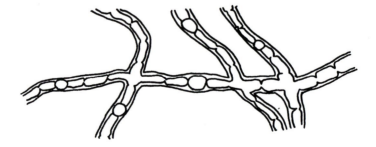

### B21—Salmon Cakes (Preparation Time: 10 Min)

*Ingredients.* 1½ cups mashed potatoes (no butter or milk) • 1 small can of sockeye salmon, or equivalent fresh cooked salmon • Salt and pepper to taste • 1 tbsp parsley.

*Method.* Mash or flake fish • Add parsley and fish to potato; mix well • Dust dried potato flour onto both hands and form tablespoonfuls of mixture into patties • Shallow fry both sides in oil. *Variation:* For sweet corn and potato cake, to the mashed potato, add 1 cup cooked corn (canned, fresh, or frozen) and ½ of a beaten egg.

### B22—Scrambled Egg (Preparation Time: 10 Min)

*Ingredients.* 1 egg • ⅛ tsp salt • 1 tsp butter • 1 tbsp milk or yogurt and water • 1 tsp chopped parsley.

*Method.* Beat the egg lightly with a whisk or fork • Add seasoning and milk • Heat the butter in a saucepan just until it begins to bubble • Add the egg mixture and cook gently on low heat • Draw wooden or plastic spoon over the base of the pan to form flakes • Remove from heat when almost set but still slightly moist; the heat of the pan will complete the cooking • Serve immediately on hot, toasted non-OWGG bread, garnished with parsley. *Variations:*

1. Cheese scramble: Add 2 tbsp grated cheese to egg mixture before cooking.
2. Bacon scramble (or other cooked meat): Add 1 tsp chopped or minced bacon (or other meat), with the fat removed, to the egg mixture and pour into a covered glass dish. Microwave, full power, for 1 min.
3. Sweet corn scramble: Add 1 tbsp cooked whole kernel or creamed corn to the egg mixture before cooking.

### B23—Omelette (Preparation Time: 10 Min)

*Ingredients.* 2 eggs • 1 tbsp cold water • ¼ tsp salt • Pinch pepper • 1 tbsp butter.

*Method.* Beat the eggs, water, and seasoning gently with a fork until well mixed, but not frothy • Heat the butter in a small omelette pan or a heavy frying pan, until just beginning to color • Pour in the egg mixture and stir lightly with a fork • Cook over moderate heat • Loosen the edges of the omelette with a spatula while cooking, and tilt the pan to allow the uncooked mixture to run underneath; use the spatula to stop the omelette from sticking to the pan's surface • When the underside is golden brown and the upper part still moist, fold the omelette away from the pan handle • Grasp the handle underneath and flip the omelette quickly onto a pre-heated plate • Serve with a tossed salad. *Variations:*

1. Herb omelette: Add 2 tbsp chopped parsley or fresh herbs to the egg mixture.
2. Bacon (or other cooked meat) omelette: Add 2 tbsp bacon (or other cooked meat), diced or minced, and fat removed, to the egg mixture, or later sprinkle the meat into the fold of the omelette.
3. Other omelette fillings are asparagus and corn, or 2 or 4 tsp of commercial savory beans, to make barbecue, Mexican, or Italian omelettes.

### B24—Bubble and Squeak (Preparation Time: 10 Min)

A traditional breakfast or lunch dish makes practical use of any left-overs, e.g., potatoes, sweet potatoes, mixed vegetables, meats, diced liver, and fish. The items can be used individually or bound together with egg. Use a good cooking oil and do not overheat. Vary the herbs, spices, and sauces.

*Ingredients.* Leftover cooked vegetables, meats, or fish • Salt and pepper to taste • Herbs • 1 egg per person (optional) • Soy sauce, clear fish/corn sauce.

*Method.* Dice the cold meat and vegetables • Beat the eggs and then stir them into the cold meat and vegetables • Melt 1 tbsp butter or heat the cooking oil, together with selected herbs and spices, in a frying pan. Add egg mixture • Fry over moderate heat for 10 to 15 min, turning after 5 min • Sprinkle with grated mild cheese • Alternative to cheese, 1 tsp soy sauce and/or clear fish/corn sauce • Turn the vegetables with a spatula • For a variation in flavor, add a few drops of Worcestershire sauce.

### B25—Fritters (Preparation Time: 10 Min)

*Ingredients.* 1½ tbsp pea flour • 1½ tbsp potato flour • ⅛ tsp salt • ½ tsp baking powder • 1 egg or egg substitute • herbs or spices • 1 tbsp of chopped bacon (fat removed) • 2 or 3 chopped cooked asparagus, or 1 finely grated raw carrot • ½ zucchini, grated, may be combined with carrot • 2 tbsp cooked whole kernel corn, or 2 to 3 tbsp creamed corn • 1 tbsp chopped parsley •1 tbsp chopped chives or spring onions.

*Method.* Sift dry ingredients into a bowl • Prepare fillings • Beat the egg with fork or beater • Heat 1 tbsp oil in small frying pan • Add chosen filling to dry ingredients, then mix in the egg • Drop spoonfuls into hot oil • Turn over carefully with a spatula when golden underneath and bubbles are breaking on the surface of the mixture • Cook the other side, then remove from pan, and drain on kitchen paper • Serve at once with non-OWGGs tomato sauce or fresh tomato.

### B26—Buckwheat Pilaf (Preparation Time: 10 Min)

*Ingredients.* 1 onion, chopped • ½ cup hazelnuts, chopped or ground • 1 cup buckwheat grains or groats • 2½ cups stock • 1 tsp herbs, fresh or dried • 2 tomatoes or 1 tbsp tomato purée • 1 to 2 cups cooked peas, or any mixture of vegetables.

*Method.* Fry onion and nuts gently in oil for 5 min • Rinse buckwheat in water, turn with onion and nuts, then add stock, tomato puree, and herbs • Simmer for 15 min (covered), then add vegetables • Heat through, fluff up, and check seasoning. *Option:* 2 cups of precooked buckwheat reduces simmering time.

### B27—Soybeans with Sardines (Preparation Time: 10 Min)

*Ingredients.* 1½ cups (12 oz) cooked soybeans • 10 sardines or 1 cup of salmon • ½ cup cottage cheese • 2 tbsp oil from the sardines (or butter) • 1 tomato • Pinch of salt and pepper • parsley.

*Method.* Flake fish with fork and fry in oil or butter for 3 min • Add soybeans and cottage cheese • Mix thoroughly and heat for 5 min over low heat • Season to taste, and garnish with sliced tomato and parsley.

### B28—Soybean and Carrot Pistou (Preparation Time: 10 Min)

*Ingredients.* ¾ cup (6 oz) cooked soybeans • 3 or 4 medium carrots • 2 to 3 garlic cloves • 4 tbsp tomato puree • ½ cup cooking oil • 1 cup grated cheese • 2 tsp basil.

*Method.* Scrub the carrots and slice • Cook until just tender • Crush the garlic and put in a blender with basil and tomato puree • Blend at low speed and add drops of oil until the mix begins to thicken • Add remainder of oil • Beat in the cheese and 3 or 4 tbsp of the soybean liquid • Mix the soybeans and carrots in a serving dish • Pour sauce over them and serve with a green salad.

## Lunch Recipes

### L30—Quinoa Corn Chowder (Preparation Time: 10 Min)

*Ingredients.* 2 cups vegetable or beef stock • ¼ cup quinoa, rinsed • ½ cup cubed potato • 2 tbsp diced carrot • ¼ cup chopped onion • 1½ cup whole kernel corn (cooked or canned) • 2 cups milk or plain yogurt and water • 1 tsp salt • ¼ cup chopped parsley. *Option:* Add 1 cup precooked quinoa to reduce simmering time.

*Method.* Simmer the quinoa, potato, carrot, and onion in the stock until tender (about 20 min) • Add the corn • Bring to a boil and cook for 5 min • Add milk and heat *just* to boiling • Season to taste • Garnish with parsley.

### L31—Spanish Soup (Preparation Time: 15 Min)

*Ingredients.* 6 oz (375 g) cooked beans (e.g., lima beans) • 1 onion, finely chopped • 2 tbsp chopped cooked meat or bacon • A small can of tomatoes, or equivalent, cooked • 2 tsp tomato paste • ½ tsp salt • 1 small potato, peeled and cubed • 1 to 2 bunches spinach • Precooked mince, spiced, or 2 tbsp salmon • Thickening, corn flour, or arrowroot.

*Method.* Thaw the cooked dried beans • Melt butter in saucepan and sauté onion and bacon • Add tomatoes, tomato paste, and chopped potato, then simmer for 10 to 15 min • Add beans and cook another 5 min • Add cooked spiced mince or salmon • Wash spinach, chop, then add to other ingredients in saucepan • Cook 5 more min • Thicken with maize corn flour dissolved in water.

### L32—Creamy Sweet Potato and Fish Chowder (Preparation Time: 15 Min)

*Ingredients.* White fish, fresh, or canned fish in spring water • 2 cups of flaked fish • ¼ tsp salt • 2 medium sweet potatoes, peeled and chopped • ½ of a small onion, peeled and chopped • 2 carrots, peeled and chopped • 3 cups water or beef stock • 2 tbsp chopped parsley • ½ cup plain yogurt.

*Method.* Poach the fish, or simmer gently in water for 15 min until it flakes easily; drain • Place the sweet potato, onion, carrots, water or stock in saucepan with salt • Simmer gently for 20 to 25 min or until the vegetables are cooked • Puree or mash until smooth • Add the flaked fish, parsley, and yogurt • Mix lightly, then reheat gently; the mixture could curdle and may need more water.

*L33—Basic Waffle Batter (Preparation Time: 15 Min)*

Follow the manufacturers' waffle-maker instruction booklet for helpful hints, safety, care, and use. If the booklet contains waffle recipes, modify to exclude your allergic foods.

*Ingredients.* 1 cup flour: for plain waffles, pea and potato flour; for savory waffles, cornmeal and a little buckwheat flour; for sweet waffles, soy and potato flours • 1 tsp baking powder • ⅛ tsp salt • 1 egg, separated (optional) • ¾ cup milk or plain yogurt and water • 5 tbsp (45 g) melted butter • Sweetener for sweet waffle mix.

*Method.* Preheat waffle maker • Sift flours into bowl • Add beaten egg, water and yogurt or milk, melted butter • Add sweetener for sweet waffles • Place about ½ cup of batter at a time onto base of waffle maker, spreading evenly over plate with a spatula • Close lid and cook, until waffles are golden brown and stop steaming, generally for 2 to 3 min • Makes 2 or 3 waffles.

*L34—Meat/Ham and Cheese Waffle (Preparation Time: 15 Min)*

*Ingredients.* See ingredients for **L33** • ½ cup cooked meat/ham, finely chopped, fat removed • ½ cup plain cheese, grated • 1 tbsp chopped chives or parsley, with other herbs, if desired.

*Method.* Cook as in **L33** • Add the chopped meat/ham, greated cheese, and herbs. *Variations:*

1. Ham, pineapple, and cheese waffle: Add ½ cup unsweetened crushed pineapple, drained.
2. Salmon waffle: Use ½ cup mashed salmon instead of the meat/ham, with 1 tbsp chopped parsley or chives.

*L35—Sour Cream Waffle (Preparation Time: 15 Min)*

*Ingredients.* ½ cup potato flour • ½ cup pea/soy flour • 1 or 2 eggs • 1 tsp baking powder • ½ to ¾ cup plain yogurt • ½ cup water • 5 tbsp (45 g) butter, melted • ¼ cup sour cream • 1 tbsp sugar/sweetener.

*Method.* Preheat waffle maker • Beat egg whites until stiff peaks form • Add sugar and beat again • In a bowl, stir together the egg yolks, yogurt, water, butter, and sour cream • Fold egg whites into batter mixture • Brush cooking plates with butter • Place ½ cup (approx.) batter at a time onto base of waffle maker, spreading evenly over plate with a spatula • Close lid and cook until waffles are golden brown, 2 to 3 minutes • Serve with sliced avocado or asparagus.

*L36—Fresh Fruit Waffles (Preparation Time: 15 Min)*

*Ingredients.* 1½ cups milk or yogurt and water • ⅓ cup melted butter or oil • 3 eggs • 1½ cups flour (equal parts soy, maize/corn flour, and potato) • 3 tsp baking powder • ¾ cup fruit (raspberry, blueberry, pineapple, strawberry, apricot).

*Method.* Preheat waffle maker • Put all the ingredients, except the fruit, into the food processor and process until smooth • Fold in the fruit (If no food processor, beat eggs, add sifted dry ingredients, oil or butter, then fruit; mix together) • Add 3 tbsp of batter, and cook the waffle till golden brown; fruit waffles need longer cooking • Serve with whipped cream and fruit or a fruit syrup.

*Berry topping.* Half cover fresh boysenberries/raspberries with cold water and bring to a boil and hold 1 min • Thicken with a little arrowroot or corn flour diluted with water • Add sweetener • Serve over sweet waffles • *Option: Orange syrup.* ⅔ cup orange juice • ⅔ cup water • ⅔ cup sugar • 3 tbsp butter. Boil sugar and water for 5 min; add other ingredients; boil for 1 min. Berry and orange or lemon toppings are favorites with children.

*L37—Grilled Polenta Wedges with Chili Vegetable Stew*
*(Preparation Time: 20 to 25 Min)*

*Polenta ingredients.* 1½ cups washed coarse cornmeal • 1 cup cold water • 1 cup boiling water or stock • ¼ tsp salt and a pinch nutmeg or desired spice • ¼ cup (30 g) cheese, grated.

*Stew ingredients.* 1 tbsp oil • 1 onion, finely sliced • ½ to 1 tsp crushed garlic • 2 tsp oregano • 2 cups (400 g) prepared green vegetables (e.g., sliced beans, sliced zucchini, broccoli florets, green pepper • 2 cups (400 g) tomatoes, in juice, pureed • Salt and freshly ground black pepper to taste.

*Method.* Polenta • Mix the cornmeal with the cold water in a bowl, stirring well • Stir this into the pot of boiling water • Cook over low heat, stirring constantly, until thick and sticky (approx. 5 min) • Remove from heat and stir in the seasonings and cheese • Place on a greased oven tray, and with wet hands, pat out a rectangle ½ in thick • Cut into large wedges • Grill on either side for 5 min • *Sauce:* Heat the oil in a fry pan, and sauté the onion till soft • Add the garlic, oregano, and vegetables; cook for 2 min • Add the tomatoes and simmer for 7 to 10 min • Season well • Place the polenta on a plate • Top with the vegetable stew • Serve with a bowl of grated cheese.

## L38—Tortillas

*Ingredients.* 1½ cups flour (pea, potato, and maize/corn flour) • 1 cup cornmeal, medium grind • 1 cup warm water.

*Method.* Sift flours into a large bowl • Make a well in the center; gradually add warm water • Using a knife, mix to a firm dough • Turn dough onto lightly floured (potato flour) surface • Knead dough until smooth, about 3 min • Divide dough into required portions • Roll out between lightly floured waxed paper, until paper-thin • Keep in paper till ready to cook • Heat a heavy frying pan or griddle • Place one tortilla in a dry pan • When the edges begin to curl slightly, turn and cook the other side; a few seconds on each side is sufficient • Clean pan with absorbent paper towel before reusing • Tortillas soften on standing • Tortillas keep fresh for a week in an airtight container • Warm briefly in oven or microwave before serving. Stale tortillas can be fried in butter or oil. *Options:* Break tortillas into pieces and serve with dips • Make burritos with a filling of meat and cheese or beans.

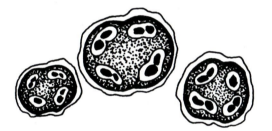

## L39—Zucchini (Courgette) Slice (Preparation Time: 15 Min)

*Ingredients.* 2½ (13 oz/375 g) medium zucchinis • 1 onion • 2 to 3 tbsp cooked minced meat • Grated carrot • 1 tsp baking powder • ½ cup oil • 4 eggs (or use egg substitute) • 1 cup grated cheese • Salt and pepper • ½ tsp curry powder • 1 cup flour (pea, potato, lentil, cornmeal) — ¼ to ⅛ tsp curry • ¼ cup canned crushed pineapple.

*Method.* Cut the ends of the zucchini • Grind in food processor with onion and carrot • Sift dry ingredients into bowl • Grate the cheese and add to flour mixture • Combine oil and egg and beat with a fork • Thaw the meat and add to ingredients in bowl • Make a well in the center of the dry ingredients and add puree of vegetables and egg/oil mixture • Stir well, then pour into greased quiche dish • Bake at 350°F (180°C) for

40 min until the mix has risen and is golden • Cuts easier when cooled and set. Variations of grated vegetables can be used.

### L40—Chapatis, Indian Pancakes (Preparation Time: 20 Min)

*Ingredients.* 1¾ cups pea and potato flour • ¼ tsp salt • 4 tbsp butter, melted • ½ to ¾ cup warm water.

*Method.* Sift flours and salt into bowl • Mix in melted butter • Gradually mix in sufficient warm water to form a soft dough • Knead well for 5 min • Leave to stand for 10 to 15 min • Divide mixture into six equal portions • Roll out each portion between waxed and floured paper into a thin round pancake • Grease and heat a griddle or frying pan • Add a chapati to griddle and cook until small blisters appear on the surface • Turn and cook the other side, till light brown.

There is no rising agent in chapatis. Make a batch, separate with wax paper, and freeze. Defrost for a packed lunch or snack. Use sweet or savory fillings. The best chapatis are round, of equal size and thickness, and evenly cooked.

### L41—Buckwheat Spice Bread (Preparation Time: 15 Min)

*Ingredients.* 2 cups buckwheat flour • 1½ cups soy flour • 2 tsp cream of tartar • 1½ tsp baking soda • ½ tsp salt • 4 tsp mixed spice • 2 tsp oil • 1 cup sultanas • 2½ cups water.

*Method.* Sift and mix buckwheat, soy, baking soda, cream of tartar, salt, and spice • Add water and oil, then sultanas, and mix well with dry ingredients • Line loaf tin with cooking paper and oil to grease • Pour mixture into tin • Cook in preheated oven at 400°F (200°C) for 30 to 50 min • When cooked, a skewer should come out dry. *Option:* Place mixture in muffin tins and cook.

### L42—Quick and Easy Flat Bread (Preparation Time: 15 Min)

*Ingredients:* 1 large banana • ²⁄₃ cup grated carrot, or 1 cup (100 g) tofu • 1 egg • ¼ cup milk or plain yogurt and water • 1 ¾ cup (150 g) soy flour • 1¾ cup (150 g) potato flour • 1 tbsp corn flour • 1 tsp cream of tartar • 1 tsp bicarbonate of soda • ½ tsp tartaric acid, or 2½ tsp baking powder • ⅛ tsp salt • 3 tbsp (25 g) olive oil • 1 tsp sugar or choice of sweetener.

*Method:* Beat the banana/carrot/tofu to a smooth puree with the milk and egg (best done in a blender) • Sift the dry ingredients into a bowl

• Mix the oil into the puree mixture • Line a 9 in (25 cm) baking dish with nonstick baking paper • Fold the flour ingredients into the puree; do not overmix nor leave to stand, as you will lose the light structure to the bread dough • Spread the mixture in baking pan to a 1 in (2.5 cm) depth • Bake in a preheated oven at 420°F (220°C) for 30 to 40 min • Bread is done when skewer inserted in center comes out clean. *Variations:* Add 1 to 4 tsp tomato puree to the blended mixture • Replace olive oil with ²/₃ cup grated cheese in carrot-based loaf • Replace corn flour with cornmeal.

The method of cooking makes a lot of difference to the bread. Cook in a shallow tray rather than a loaf tin. Makes a tasy, soft bread with a crisp, golden crust. Flat bread is best eaten when warm or on the day it is baked. Slice and freeze any excess.

### L43—Bean Salad (Preparation Time: 10 Min)

*Ingredients.* 2 cups (250 g, approx.) mixed cooked dried beans, frozen beans, or a small can of four-bean mix • 2 cups (250 g, approx.) green beans (cooked, drained, and cooled) • 2 stalks celery, chopped • 1 small onion, finely chopped and cooked • 1 cup cooked whole kernel corn (frozen or canned).

*Method.* Mix all ingredients together in a bowl • Combine 2 tbsp olive oil, salt and pepper, and lemon juice as a dressing, or use **L44**.

### L44—Yogurt Salad Dressing (Preparation Time: 5 Min)

*Ingredients.* 2 cups (250 ml) natural yogurt • 1 tsp lemon juice • Chopped chives • Pinch of salt • Pinch of French or German mustard.

*Method.* Mix all ingredients together well • Chill before serving.

### L45—Potato Salad (Preparation Time: 10 Min)

*Ingredients.* 2 medium potatoes, diced (2 cups/250 g) • ¼ tsp salt • 1 small onion (finely chopped) or spring onion • 2 tbsp chopped cooked meat or fish • 1 stalk celery • 1 tbsp chopped fresh herbs (parsley, chives, mint, or chervil) • ½ clove garlic, crushed (optional) • 2 tbsp cooked whole kernel corn (optional) • 4 tbsp yogurt dressing.

*Method.* Peel the potatoes; boil in salted water till just tender • Cool and dice • Mix together the salad ingredients • Garnish with salad greens • Serve with cold meats, egg or cheese dishes.

### L46—Coleslaw (Preparation Time: 10 Min)

*Ingredients.* 2 cups finely shredded cabbage • 1 medium carrot, grated • 1 to 2 stalks celery, finely sliced • 1 small onion, finely chopped (optional) • 1 tbsp chopped parsley • ¼ to ½ cup oil dressing.

*Method.* Mix all the ingredients together • Add the dressing (olive oil, lemon juice, salt and pepper) • Toss lightly and chill • Turn into a salad bowl, rubbed with a cut clove of garlic • Garnish with parsley, and serve with either hot or cold meats, savory meats, or savory dishes. *Variations:* Add 1 to 2 tbsp nuts, flour or chopped; 1 to 2 tbsp sultanas or raisins; 1 green pepper, sliced, diced, or in rings; 1 orange, segmented, cut in pieces; or ¼ cup unsweetened pineapple pieces.

### L47—Cheese and Herb Sauce (Preparation Time: 10 Min)

*Ingredients.* 1 tbsp polyunsaturated oil, safflower or soybean • 2 tbsp buckwheat or corn flour • 1 cup nonfat milk • 3 tbsp grated cheddar cheese • 3 tbsp finely chopped fresh herbs (e.g., parsley, chives, thyme, basil).

*Method.* Heat oil in a saucepan • Add the flour and mix to a paste • Gradually add the milk, while heating and stirring continuously for 3 to 4 min or until the sauce thickens • Add the cheese and herbs • Serve with vegetables, pasta, fish. *Option:* Prepare in microwave. In a microwave bowl blend the oil, flour, and cheese • Gradually add the milk, stirring until smooth • Cook on full power for 3 to 4 min, stirring once during cooking • Add the herbs and mix well.

### L48—Tree Tomato Chutney (Preparation Time: 10 Min)

*Ingredients.* 4 tree tomatoes • 1 small onion • 1 tbsp brown sugar or sweetener.

*Method.* Peel and finely chop the tree tomatoes and onion • Mix together the tree tomatoes, onion, and brown sugar/sweetener. Serve with cold meats, fish, or chicken • Makes more than one cup.

### Dinner and Dessert Recipes

### D50—Sweet Potato Soup (Preparation Time: 10 Min)

*Ingredients.* 1 tbsp butter • 1 small onion, finely chopped • ½ clove garlic, crushed • 2 medium sweet potatoes, peeled and cubed (2 cups/250 g)

— 2 cups beef or chicken stock (1 cup frozen stock and 1 cup water) • ¼ tsp ground nutmeg • ½ tsp salt • 1 stalk celery, chopped • 1½ oz plain yogurt.

*Method.* Melt the butter, then sauté the onions and garlic in a saucepan • Add the sweet potato, stock, celery, and salt • Simmer gently for 20 min (approx.) until tender • Mash with potato, or liquidize in a food processor, then return to the saucepan • Stir in the yogurt, nutmeg, and parsley • Reheat, but do not boil • Serve with pinch of nutmeg and grated cheese. *Variations:*

1. Use pumpkin in place of sweet potato to make pumpkin soup.
2. For a flavor change, add 2 tsp concentrated orange juice, or equivalent.

### D51—Sweet Corn Chowder (Preparation Time: 15 Min)

*Ingredients.* 2 medium potatoes, cut into small cubes (2 cups/250 g) • ½ to 1 cup cubed pieces of fish fillet • ½ onion • 1 stalk celery (washed, trimmed, and chopped) • 1 can sweet corn or frozen corn • ½ cup plain yogurt • 1 cup stock • ¼ tsp salt • 1 tbsp corn flour • 2 tbsp cold water • 1 tbsp fresh parsley, chopped.

*Method.* Put stock in saucepan • Add chopped onion, cubed potato, celery, corn, and cubed fish fillet • Bring to a boil, then let cook gently for 15 to 20 min, until potato is tender (may need frequent stirring) • Blend corn flour in water till smooth, then stir ingredients into saucepan • Add yogurt and parsley just before serving.

### D52—Plum Pork (Preparation Time: 20 Min)

*Ingredients.* 4 lean pork butterfly steaks (16 oz/500 g) • 2 cups stewed or canned plums • 1 medium orange • 1 medium onion, roughly chopped • ½ tsp ground cinnamon • 1 tbsp maize/corn flour • Pinch of freshly ground black pepper • 2 tbsp water.

*Method.* Remove all visible fat from the meat, and cut each steak in half • Brown the meat in a nonstick frying pan • Place the browned meat in a casserole dish • Add the plums, grated rind and juice from the orange, onion, cinnamon, and pepper • Cover and bake at 320°F (160°C) for 1½ h • Drain the juice from the casserole into a small saucepan • Mix the corn flour and water into a paste • Add to the juice and heat gently until thickened • Arrange pork and plums on a serving dish and top with the sauce • *Option:* Prepare in the microwave. Brown the meat and prepare casserole as instructed • Cover and cook on 70 percent power for 25 min • Let stand for 5 min • Thicken the drained juices on full power for 2 to 3 min.

### D53—Fish with Tomato-Cheese Crust (Preparation Time: 15 Min)

*Ingredients.* 2 medium fish fillets, or equivalent flaked fish from home baking or steaming (see p. 251) • 1 medium tomato, peeled, seeded, finely chopped • 2 tsp tomato paste • ¼ tsp ground cumin (optional) • ¼ tsp ground coriander (optional) • ⅛ tsp ground pepper (optional) • 1 tsp lemon juice • 2 tsp butter, melted • ½ cup grated cheddar cheese • ¼ cup fresh corn bread crumbs.

*Method.* Preheat oven to 350°F (180°C) • Brush a 12.5 × 9 in (32 × 28 cm) oven tray with melted butter or oil • Place chopped tomato in a small bowl • Add onion, tomato paste, cumin, coriander; mix well and set aside • Combine lemon juice, butter, and pepper in a separate small bowl • Place fish fillets on a prepared tray; brush each with lemon mixture and top with tomato mixture • Sprinkle with combined cheese and non-OWGG bread crumbs • Bake 15 min or until fish flakes are tender when tested with a fork • Serve hot with accompanying salad and warmed tortilla.

### D54—Chili Bean Mince (Preparation Time: 10 Min)

*Warning:* Chili is not suitable for those with indigestion or irritable bowel symptoms.

*Ingredients.* 10 to 12 oz (300 g) lean minced beef • 1 large onion • 1 tsp herbs or spices, or ¼ tsp chili powder • ¾ cup water • 16 oz (450 g) can mild flavored beans (may be substituted for equivalent can of kidney beans or frozen lima beans) • ¼ cup tomato paste.

*Method.* Heat the oil in saucepan • Sauté the onion for 3 to 4 min or until softened • Add the mince and herbs or spices • Continue sautéing until the mince is browned • Add the water and beans; simmer gently for 15 to 20 min • *Option:* Prepare in microwave. Cover and cook the oil and onion on full power, 2 to 3 min • Add the mince and herb or spice powder • Cook on 70 percent power for 4 to 5 min or until the mince is browned • Reduce the water to ¼ cup • Add the water and mild flavored beans Cover and cook on 70 percent power for 4 to 5 min. The filling is suitable for pancakes, taco shells, pizza, over cooked potato or sweet potato slices, or with pasta. Top with sour cream or yogurt and grated mild cheese.

*D55—Cottage Pie (Preparation Time: 15 Min)*

*Mashed potato topping ingredients.* 3 medium potatoes • ½ tsp salt • 1 tbsp butter • 3 to 4 tbsp milk • Shake pepper.

*Filling ingredients.* 2 medium onions, chopped • 1 to 2 medium carrots, grated or diced • 2 tomatoes, skinned and diced • ½ to 1 tbsp tomato paste (optional) • 8 oz (250 g) minced beef • ½ tsp salt.

*Method.* Put minced meat in dry frying pan and cook on moderate to high heat, stirring frequently until lightly browned • Sprinkle with 1 tbsp potato or pea flour • Add onion while cooking the meat • Add salt and pepper, and water to just cover the meat • Add carrots and tomatoes, and tomato paste • Simmer for 20 to 30 min stirring occasionally, and add more water if necessary • Transfer to casserole dish • Boil the potatoes • When cooked, drain and mash with milk and butter • Pile over the meat mixture, and smooth out • Sprinkle with mild grated cheese • Bake at 350°F (180°C) until golden brown.

*D56—Baked Fish (Preparation Time: 5 Min)*

*Ingredients.* 1 medium white fish fillet • ½ stalk celery • ¼ onion, chopped (optional) • Parsley • ½ of a lemon.

*Method.* Preheat oven to 350°F (180°C) • Line a medium-sized casserole dish with foil, with enough to overlap fish and seal • Place the cleaned fish on the foil in the dish, squeeze the lemon over the fish, and add chopped celery and onion • Fold foil over and pinch edges together • Bake in oven for 20 to 25 min until the fish flakes easily when tested with a knife • Lift fish and other ingredients on to plate. • Decorate with parsley and serve with yogurt and salad. • For a larger meal, combine with **L37**.

*D57—Meat and Leek Pasta (Preparation Time: 10 Minutes)*

*Ingredients.* ½ cup (4 oz) corn, buckwheat, or bean dry pasta, or corn dry spaghetti • 1 tbsp oil • 2 dsp of diced, cooked meat or bacon, if tolerated • ¼ clove of garlic, chopped • 1 medium leek, finely sliced • ¼ cup grated cheese • 1 tbsp chopped parsley • ½ cup plain yogurt • 1 avocado, diced (optional).

*Method.* Cook the pasta according to the manufacturer's instructions • Heat the oil in a frying pan; add the cooked meat or bacon • Stir in the garlic and cook for 30 sec • Leeks are cooked until softened, or boiled separately • Mix in the cheese, yogurt, and avocado. • Season with salt and pepper • Thoroughly toss the drained pasta and serve immediately. For a larger meal, combine with **L38** or **D58**.

### D58—*Sweet Potato and Pumpkin Stir-Fry Vegetables* (*Preparation Time: 15 Min*)

*Ingredients.* ½ of a medium sweet potato or white potato • 5 oz (150 g) pumpkin, peeled, or rutabaga, celery, and zucchini for variety • 1 tbsp olive, soy, or other vegetable cooking oil • 2 to 3 tsp of diced meat, flaked fish, or bacon, if tolerated • A little garlic, chopped, or 1 tbsp chopped onion • Grated cheese, chives, or parsley sprinkled on top before serving.

*Method.* Cut the vegetables into bite-sized chunks • Boil the potato, pumpkin, or other vegetables until tender • Heat the oil in a small frying pan • Add the diced meat or fish and garlic; sauté for 2 to 3 min • Add the pumpkin and potato and stir-fry for 4 to 5 min, or until the vegetables are cooked and lightly browned • Sprinkle the cheese, parsley, or chives on top • Serve immediately.

### D59—*Pizza (Preparation Time: 20 Min)*

*Dough ingredients.* 1 cup flour, pea and potato (lentil and cornmeal will give a change in flavor) • 1 tsp baking powder • ¼ tsp salt • 3 tbsp olive oil or soybean oil • 4 tbsp milk or plain yogurt and water.

*Filling/topping ingredients.* 2 tbsp tomato paste • ½ cup cheese, grated • 2 tbsp onion, chopped • 2 tbsp cooked meat, chopped • ½ cup grated zucchini • 3 cups grated cooked asparagus or other vegetable, e.g., celery (baked beans are a simple pizza filling) • 2 medium tomatoes, sliced • 2 eggs or 2 tbsp cottage cheese • Salt and pepper to taste.

*Method.* Sift flour, baking powder, and salt into medium bowl • Measure oil and liquid into a cup • Preheat oven to 400°F (200°C). • Make a firm dough by adding liquid to the dry ingredients • Spread dough over the pie plate • Spread tomato paste on base before adding filling • Spread the fillings over the dough, then add the tomato slices and grated cheese • Beat eggs together with fork, or use cottage cheese; add salt and pepper • Pour the beaten eggs over the pizza before placing it in the oven • Bake for 10 min, then reduce heat to 350°F (180°C), and cook for another 15 to 20 min (place a pan under the pizza plate, as the eggs can leak off the pizza). This pizza freezes well. It can be used for packed lunches and served cold or reheated in the microwave or oven.

### D60—*Nut Seed Crust (Preparation Time: 15 Min)*

*Ingredients.* ¾ cup cashew nuts • ¼ cup sesame seeds • ¼ cup tapioca or arrowroot starch • ½ tsp cinnamon (optional) • Pinch salt • 3 tbsp boiling water.

*Method.* Grind the nuts in a blender with 1 tbsp water or oil • Add the sesame seeds, starch, and seasonings and stir well • Add boiling water and stir until the mix forms a ball, or use a blender • Grease a 9 in (23 cm) plate • Flatten dough out to cover base, using wet fingers • Bake at 350°F (180°C) for 20 min • Filling for vegetable pie (mixture of cooked, seasoned, and mashed vegetables) is placed on the dough during the last 15 min of cooking • Sprinkle cheese and diced cooked meats on top.

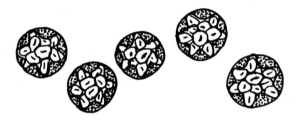

### D61—Potato Pastry (Preparation Time: 15 Min)

*Ingredients.* 1 egg • 2 tbsp water • 1½ cups mashed potato (see under Method) • 1¼ cups maize/corn flour (pea flour is an option) • ½ cup powdered milk • Salt and pepper to taste.

*Method.* Combine egg and water with potatoes and mix well • Combine flour, powdered milk, seasonings • Stir into potato mixture; knead lightly • Roll pastry either between two pieces of waxed paper to required size, or just spread base out in dish and roll the top cover between the waxed paper • Pour in desired precooked filling, e.g., mince with vegetables, thickened with arrowroot • Cover with remaining pastry, vent, and glaze with milk • Bake in preheated oven at 400°F (200°C) for 20 to 30 min (if using a very moist filling, precook pie shell for 15 min). For best results, potatoes should be steamed, then mashed, without adding any liquid or butter.

### D62—Apricot Shortcake (Preparation Time: 15 Min)

*Ingredients.* 4 tbsp butter • 4 tbsp sugar (or choice of sweetener) • 1 egg or egg substitute • 1 cup flour (soy, potato, corn) • 1 tsp baking powder • 1 tbsp milk, or 1 tbsp plain yogurt and 2 tbsp water • 1 can apricot halves with own juice.

*Method.* Cream butter and sugar or sweetener; gradually beat in egg or egg substitute • Sift flour and baking powder • Add to cream mixture with yogurt to make soft dough • Spread half of mixture in greased pie dish • Cover the base with the apricot halves • Spread remaining mixture on waxed paper, then invert over apricots • Bake for 30 min at 350°F (180°C).

### D63—Gelatin Desserts (Preparation Time: 5 to 10 Min)

*Ingredients.* 1 envelope or 3 tsp gelatin • ½ cup (150 ml) hot water • 1 cup (300 ml) cold unsweetened canned fruit (e.g., pineapple or apricot), or equivalent of fresh fruit, cooked or raw, or frozen berry fruit • 2 tbsp lemon juice • Choice of sweetener.

*Method.* Add gelatin to hot water, and stir until dissolved • Stir in the fruit and syrup • Add the sweetening • Place dessert in the refrigerator or freezer till set. *Variations:*

1. Fruit whip: Leave the jelly till thickening • Beat with an egg beater until very thick and foamy • Place in a serving bowl, and leave to set.
2. Fruit sponge: Leave the jelly until thickening • Beat with an egg beater until thick and foamy, gradually adding a beaten egg white.

### D64—Basic Ice Cream, No Eggs or Grain (Preparation Time: 15 Min)

*Ingredients.* 3 oz full cream milk powder • 3 oz cold water • 3 oz sugar • 2 tsp gelatin • ¼ cup water • 2 cups milk • Vanilla to flavor.

*Method.* Soak gelatin in ¼ cup water and stand over hot water until dissolved • Beat dried milk into cold water • Add milk, sugar, and vanilla • Combine with gelatin and freeze overnight or until firm • Beat again, until double its bulk, and return to freezer to set.

### D65—Ice Cream or Cake Topping, No Sugar (Preparation Time: 10 Min)

*Ingredients.* 1 cup of cream • 1 cup fresh or frozen fruit of choice • Juice of half a lemon • Choice of sweetener.

*Method.* Mash the chosen fruit • Squeeze juice from lemon • Beat the cream till thick • Stir in the fruit and sweetener • Place in the freezer • When partly frozen, whip with a fork, then refreeze.

### D66—Kiwifruit Ice Cream (Preparation Time: 15 Min)

*Ingredients.* 1 cup mashed kiwifruit (6 large kiwifruit) or selected fruit • 5 oz castor sugar • 3 eggs, separated • 1¼ cups whipped cream.

*Method.* Peel and mash fruit; leave some lumpy pieces • Stir in half the sugar and let stand for 15 min • Separate eggs; beat yolks and remaining sugar over hot water until thick and creamy • Cool • Beat whites until stiff • Fold both into the fruit with the whipped cream • Freeze quickly, until mushy, then stir, and freeze until solid.

### D67—*Yogurt Popsicles ® (Preparation Time: 10 Min)*

*Ingredients.* 1 cup (225 g) frozen orange juice concentrate, or 3½ cups (910 g) fresh or frozen strawberries • 2 cups (460 ml) plain yogurt or soft silken tofu.

*Method.* Puree the fruit in a blender • Add the yogurt or tofu and blend again • Transfer to Popsicle® molds and freeze overnight or until firm • Insert Popsicle® sticks for handles when mixture is semifirm.

### D68—*Synthetic Sweetened Jam (Preparation Time: 10 Min)*

*Ingredients.* 1½ tsp gelatin • 1½ tbsp cold water • 3 cups of fruit or berries • Choice of sweetener, to taste.

*Method.* Soften the gelatin in cold water • Add to the fruit and heat slowly in a saucepan, stirring constantly until the mixture boils • Remove from stove and mix in the sweetener to taste • Pour into heated containers and seal.

### Snack Recipes

### S70—*Mexican Corn Dip (Preparation Time: 15 Min)*

*Ingredients.* 1 onion, chopped • 1 tbsp oil • 1 red or green sweet pepper (optional) • ½ to 1 tsp ground cumin • ½ to 1 tsp oregano • 14 oz (440 g) canned baked beans, thickened with corn flour, or home-cooked lima red beans • 1 tbsp tomato paste.

*Method.* Cook the onion in oil until lightly browned and transparent • Add the chopped pepper, cumin, and oregano • Cook 12 min longer • Separate beans and mash • Add mashed beans and sauce, re-heat. *Options:* Use with corn chips or raw vegetables, as a filling for corn bread or crispbreads, or thin down and serve hot over corn or buckwheat pasta.

### S71—*Potato Chips, Potato Wedges, and Corn Chips*

Purchase plain, organic flavored chips. Serve with non-OWGG taco sauce or a spicy pasta sauce.

### S72—Popcorn (Preparation Time: 3 Min)

*Ingredients.* ¼ cup popping corn • Microwavable oven bag • 1 tbsp butter and salt to taste.

*Method.* Place the butter and corn in the oven bag • Loosely twist the open end of the bag and place in the oven • Cook on full power for 2½ to 3 min or until most kernels are popped. *Variations:*

1. Curried popcorn: Add 1 tsp curry powder to the popcorn bag and mix well.
2. Sweet and spicy popcorn: Add 1 tbsp brown sugar and 1 tsp cinnamon to the popcorn bag and mix well.
3. Raisin popcorn: Add 1 tsp cinnamon and ½ cup raisins/sultanas to the bag.

### S73—Potato Skins (Preparation Time: 10 Min)

*Ingredients.* 2 large potatoes and 1 large sweet potato • 2 tbsp polyunsaturated oil • 3 tsp paprika.

*Method.* Make a thick peeling of the potato and sweet potato, $1/3$ in thick • Brush the peels with the oil and sprinkle with paprika • Bake at 425°F (220°C) for 50 to 60 min or until crunchy and golden brown • Place the potato and sweet potato centers in water for later use.

### S74—Cheese Sticks (Preparation Time: 15 Min)

*Ingredients.* 1 cup flour, pea and potato • ½ tsp salt • Pinch cayenne pepper • Pinch cumin • $1/8$ tsp baking powder • ½ cup grated cheese • 2½ tbsp water • 3 tsp sesame seeds (optional) • 6 tbsp (50 g) butter.

*Method.* Lightly grease an oven tray • Cut or rub the butter into the dry ingredients • Add the grated cheese • Mix well • Sprinkle water on the mixture and mix with a knife to bind ingredients together lightly • Chill for 10 min • Roll into an oblong $3/16$ in thick 6 in wide • Sprinkle with sesame seeds and lightly press them on • Crosscut the oblong in strips $3/16$ in wide • Transfer to oven tray using spatula and keep the strips separate • Bake at 400°F (200°C) for 10 to 15 min or until golden brown • Cool on a wire rack.

### S75—Coconut Crispettes (Preparation Time: 15 Min)

*Ingredients.* 12 tbsp (100 g) butter • ½ cup (125 g) sugar • 1 tbsp carob powder or cocoa • 2 tbsps boiling water • ¾ cup flour, soy and potato • 1 tsp baking powder • ¾ cup coconut.

*Method.* Cream butter and sugar • Add carob, mixed with boiling water • Spoon in the sifted flours and baking powder, then the coconut • Put in spoonfuls on oven tray; flatten with a fork • Bake 15 to 20 min at 350 °F (180°C).

### S76—Bird Seed Bars (Preparation Time: 15 Min)

*Ingredients.* 1 cup sesame seeds • 1 cup sunflower seeds • 1 cup coconut • 1 cup chopped cashews • 1 cup sultanas, boiled and drained • 12 tbsp (2 oz/100 g) butter • 1 tsp vanilla essence • ½ cup brown sugar or preferred sweetener.

*Method.* Heat the sesame and sunflower seeds, coconut, and cashews in a dry pan on low heat, stirring constantly until lightly browned • Mix with sultanas • Heat butter in saucepan, add vanilla essence and sweetener or sugar, then pour over the mixture • Mix well • Press into dish, so it is ¾ in thick • When nearly cold, cut into bars • Can be frozen, but may crumble.

### S77—Currant Biscuits (Preparation Time: 20 Min)

*Ingredients.* 2 cups flour, a mix of soy, potato, and maize/corn flours • 4 ozs (100 g) butter • 4 ozs (100 g) sugar, or preferred sweetener • 2 oz (50 g) currants • ½ tsp cinnamon or spice • 1½ tsp baking powder • Grated rind of half a lemon • 1 egg or egg substitute • Plain yogurt for mixing.

*Method.* Cream butter and sweetener or sugar, then add egg and beat • Bring currants to a boil, drain, then cool • Sift dry ingredients together • Grate the lemon rind • Add currants, and dry ingredients to mixture • Roll out on maize/corn floured board to ¼ in thickness; cut into rounds with fluted cutter • Bake 15 min at 300 to 325°F (160 to 180°C).

### Cooking Basics

### CB1—Arrowroot Thickening (Preparation Time: 5 Min)

Arrowroot is a fine-grained starch that is easily digested and excellent for thickening gravy. Add it to a hot meat liquid just before serving, and do not overcook. Use 1 tbsp arrowroot with 2 tbsp water to make a paste. Add this to gravies. More is required for arrowroot desserts, which need fruit flavoring and sweetener.

*Note:* Explore the texture and taste of other flours made from taro, lotus root, water chestnut, sesame, and artichoke.

## CB2—Basic Sauce (Roux Method) (Preparation Time: 2-3 Min)

*Ingredients.* 1 tbsp butter with 1 tbsp buckwheat flour, in 1 cup liquid, for thin sauce • 2 tbsp butter with 2 tbsp buckwheat flour, in 1 cup liquid, for medium sauce • ½ tsp salt • Pinch pepper.

*Method.* Melt the butter over a low heat, then remove from heat • Stir in the flour, ½ tsp salt, and a pinch of pepper with a wooden spoon • Mix until evenly blended to form a roux • Reheat gently for 1 to 2 min, making sure that the roux does not brown • Remove from the heat • Add about ¼ cup milk, and beat until smooth • Gradually stir in the rest of the milk • Return to heat and bring slowly to a boil, stirring constantly • Reduce heat and simmer for 2 to 3 min.

## CB3—Beef Stock (Preparation Time: 5 Min)

*Ingredients.* 2 pieces of shinbone or 16 oz (1 kilogram [kg]) of meaty beef marrowbones • 1 bay leaf or pinch each of marjoram and thyme • 1 tbsp parsley • Juice from half a lemon • 1 medium onion, sliced   • 1 small carrot, peeled and sliced lengthwise • Celery leaves • Water to cover bones.

*Method.* Place the bones and water in a pressure cooker and simmer gently for 15 min • Remove any scum that forms on the surface • Add the remaining ingredients and cook under 15 pounds (lbs) pressure for 45 min • Cool • Strain the stock and leave to go cold, then remove the solid fat from the surface • Freeze the stock in small quantities for later use in soups, stews, and sauces. *Option:* Cook in Crock-Pot/saucepan; simmer gently for 2 to 3 h, adding water as it boils away. *Variations:*

1. Chicken stock: Follow the same recipe using a chicken carcass instead of the beef bones.
2. Fish stock: Follow the same recipe using fish bones and trimmings instead of beef bones.

## CB4—Yeast-Free Baking Powder (Preparation Time: 2 Min)

*Ingredients.* 2 tsp cream of tartar • 1 tsp baking soda • ¼ tsp arrowroot (a larger quantity is kept in a screw-top jar).

**Note:** Knead the dough as little as possible. Yeast-free baking powder acts quickly, so put the mixture into the baking tin and into a hot oven as soon as possible to stop the $CO_2$ bubbles from escaping.

## CB5—*Cornmeal Pie Shells (Preparation Time: 10 Min)*

*Ingredients.* 1 cup maize/corn flour • ½ cup fine cornmeal • ¼ cup unrefined sunflower oil (or butter) • ½ cup water (approx.).

*Method.* Preheat oven to 425°F (220°C) • Mix the corn flour and cornmeal together in a bowl • Cut or rub butter into dry ingredients, to a breadcrumb-like consistency, or mix the oil into the flour • Sprinkle the water on gradually, stirring it in thoroughly with a fork (only enough water so mixture sticks together to form a soft dough) • Press the dough straight into the oiled pie dish, to even depth • Shell can be fully baked, partly baked, or filled unbaked • To bake "blind," prick base with fork, then put layer of dried beans on top to keep shell flat, and bake for 10 min • For fully baked shell, remove beans after 10 min and bake for another 10 min until crisp and lightly colored • Makes 9 in (22 cm) pie crust. Use the same recipe for pie crust top.

## CB6—*Soy Milk (Preparation Time: 5 Min)*

*Ingredients.* 4 cups (2 l) water • 1 cup soybean flour.

*Method.* Add water to flour • Mix the flour, first, with a little of the water to make a smooth paste, then add the balance of the water, and boil for 5 min, watching that it does not catch on the saucepan • Strain through a cloth. Make small batches rather than a large quantity. Use in place of ordinary milk in baking.

### *Bread Machine Recipes*

If you have a bread machine, try the following recipes, or modify them for baking, to make tasty non-OWGG breads. Ensure the non-OWGG flours are fresh, with no hint of mold smell. Locate a supply of fresh yeast or "active" yeast granules. Keep the products in the refrigerator before use. Non-OWGG breads need extra protein from, for example, eggs, milk, cottage cheese, dried milk powder, buttermilk powder, and food gums. These ingredients aid the rising of the bread and support it after baking. The carbon dioxide from the action of yeast and ingredients such as bicarbonate is trapped when the protein coagulates during baking. Be careful with the kneading phase of the cycle because too much kneading allows the $CO_2$ to escape, resulting in a disappointing "flat" loaf.

> "Bread makers can increase your popularity with the local bird po-
> pulation. I reckon the birds got the first eight flat loaves before my

persistence and innovation paid off with acceptable loaves. Trouble was, the birds kept coming back, so I took pity on them and have had regular feeding appointments for the last three years. Early on my daughter asked me, 'Are the birds like you? Do they get sick when they eat real bread?' To find out, she fed them real bread and they ate it. Her class heard all about the birds and mummy at the morning talk session."

The latest bread machines turn out better non-OWGG loaves than the earlier models. You still need to be persistent with trials and innovation until you learn the secret of successful OWGG loaves.

Select a bread machine with a powerful motor and strong blade, as the non-OWGG doughs are stiffer and stickier than wheaten dough. Look for a machine without a "second punch down and second rising program." Recent models feature a rapid cycle of 15 min kneading, a rest period of an hour, and then the baking begins. All non-OWGG loaves tend to be flat on top.

These bread recipes require cooking gums, which aid the rising of bread and support it from collapsing after baking. Gums hold moisture and improve the texture of OWGG breads. Xanthan gum powder is a good substitute for wheat gluten. Most bread and risen baking items contained in the recipe index require eggs (or egg substitute), producing a richer cakelike texture and an attractive crust. The less expensive guar gum, derived from a plant seed, works just as well, but it has a high fiber content and, for some people, a laxative effect. Use ¼ to ½ tsp for each cup of flour. (*Warning:* Food Poisoning). The time delay cycle is never used with dough mixes containing eggs. Bacteria that may be in the eggs will multiply and produce their toxins if the dough or ingredient mix is not baked after the hour allowed for the yeast to ferment.

Ingredients that improve flavor and texture include vitamin C powder, white imitation vinegar (4 percent acetic acid), and tapioca flour. If the taste is not to your liking, try adding butter or a vegetable oil. The fats increase crumbling, yield a softer crust, and prolong the staying qualities. If you have an additional allergy to dairy and beef protein or lactose intolerance, substitute soy flour for dried milk and buttermilk powders. Use "active" yeast granules or, better still, obtain fresh baking yeast blocks. Salt is added to slow down the rate of yeast fermentation. Take care with the quantities of yeast, salt, and sugar. The yeast ferments the sugar to form $CO_2$ gas. The three ingredients make a delicate balance to encourage fermentation and produce the $CO_2$ and the rising of the dough during baking. If you are not satisfied with the bread's texture and appearance, dissolve a teaspoon of unflavored gelatin (derived from cow and vegetable) in some warm water and add it to the mix.

*Method.* Put dry ingredients—flours, cooking gums, sugar, salt, half vitamin C, seasonings, flavoring, and milk powder—in bowl and add butter and oil • Mix well • Measure egg substitute in cup, add water, and beat with fork • Beat eggs in measuring cup • Add vinegar, softened butter/or oil, egg substitute, and 1 cup warm water • Place liquids in the baking pan of the bread machine, add mixed dry ingredients, and sprinkle the yeast granules on top • Put baking pan in the bread machine and secure it • Set program for rapid, or set the baking control "light" and the control to start • After the first few minutes of kneading, check that the dough has a consistency similar to batter • If it appears too dry, add water, 1 tsp at a time, up to 2 tbsp • Use a rubber spatula to aid the mixing of all ingredients • When the dough is of the right consistency and sticky to the touch, it will swirl around the machine with a definite raised area on top • If the dough is smooth on top, it is too moist; add a little of the flour mix until it reaches the right consistency • Check to see that the mix will not overflow; spoon off any excess before the baking cycle starts • When baking is completed, remove, cool on the stand, slice, and bag or wrap excess bread and place in the freezer.

### *BM1—Plain or Herb Bread (Preparation Time: 15 Min)*

*Ingredients.* 1½ cups potato flour • 1 cup buckwheat, pea, or fine lentil flour • ¼ cup soy flour • ½ cup tapioca flour • ¼ cup milk powder • 2 tsp gum • 1½ tsp salt • 1 to 2 tsp yeast granules • 2 to 3 tbsp sugar • 1 tsp egg substitute with 2 tbsp warm water • 2 eggs • ½ tsp imitation vinegar • 3 tbsp softened butter • ¾ to 1 cup warm water • ¹/₁₆ tsp turmeric (optional) • 1 tbsp grated onion • 2 tbsp fresh herbs.

### *BM2—Corn Bread (Preparation Time: 15 Min)*

*Ingredients.* 1 cup potato flour • 1¼ cups finely ground cornmeal • ¼ cup soy flour. • ½ cup tapioca flour • ¼ cup milk powder • 1½ tsp salt • 2 tsp guar gum • 2 to 3 tsp yeast granules • 2 to 3 tbsp sugar • 2 eggs (3 eggs if egg substitute is not used) • 1 tsp egg substitute in 2 tbsp warm water • 3 tbsp softened butter • Pinch cayenne pepper • ½ tbsp vinegar • 1 cup lukewarm water • ½ cup precooked kernel corn • ½ cup grated cheese (optional) • 1 tbsp fresh garden herbs.

### BM3—Buckwheat and Sultana Bread (Preparation Time: 15 Min)

*Ingredients.* ½ cup tapioca flour • 1¼ cup buckwheat flour • ¼ cup soy flour • 1¼ cup potato flour • ¼ cup milk powder • 1 tsp salt • 1½ tsp guar gum • 2 to 3 tsp yeast granules • 2 to 3 tbsp sugar • 3 tbsp softened butter • 2 eggs • 1 tsp egg substitute in 2 tbsp warm water • 1 cup sultanas • 2 tsp mixed spice • ½ to 1 cup warm water.

### BM4—Egg Substitute and Lactose-Free Bread (Preparation Time: 15 Min)

*Ingredients.* ½ cup soy flour • 1½ cups pea or fine lentil flour • ½ cup tapioca flour • 1½ cups potato flour • ¼ cup buttermilk powder • 1½ tsp salt • 1 tsp baking soda (optional) • 2 tsp xanthan gum • 2 tsp sugar • 2 to 3 tsp yeast granules • 3 tbsp softened butter • ½ tsp vinegar or vitamin C crystals • 5 tsp egg substitute in 10 tbsp warm water • 1¾ cup warm water. *Variations:* Add 1 tbsp onion flakes or finely chopped onion, ¾ cup finely sliced celery, or ½ cup grated cheese.

### BM5—Apricot Almond Bread (Preparation Time: 15 Min)

*Ingredients.* 1½ cups potato flour • 1 cup soy flour • ½ cup maize/corn flour • ½ cup tapioca flour • 1½ tsp salt • 2 tsp guar gum • 3 tbsp softened butter • 2 eggs • 1 egg substitute in 2 tbsp warm water • ½ tsp vinegar • 2 to 3 tbsp sugar • 2 to 3 tsp yeast granules • ½ tsp almond essence • ¾ cup chopped dried apricots • ¾ cup apricot nectar with hot water added to make 1 cup.

### Pasta and Sausage Machine Recipes

Indulge your appetite and taste buds with non-OWGG sausages, pastas, and savory sauces. Explore the variety of commercial non-OWGG pastas, avoiding the rice and millet mixes, until you are much better or have recovered. Non-OWGG sausages may be unobtainable. A sympathetic butcher may process sausage mince as a bulk buy, but if colorings or preservatives are added, it is best to make your own sausages. If you prefer organic foods and enjoy a variety of flavors in your pastas and sausages, consider purchasing a pasta and sausage machine. As with bread machines, be careful in your choice. Some patients prefer the old hand-operated models of mincers and extruders.

Commercial minced meat may contain traces of a previous batch of sausage meat containing OWGGs. If commercial meat minces are unsuitable, do your own mincing, to exclude the colorings and preservatives. A cooperative butcher may agree to make up a bulk order of mixed minced meat according to your instructions. Ask the butcher to process your order before the meat is used for commercial sausage mince. On receiving the bulk order, divide into smaller portions and place in the freezer. Retain a quantity to make into sausages, without delay. An alternative is to process the entire bulk order into sausages and place them in the freezer.

*Pasta method.* Follow the appliance instructions • Begin with a mix of half the ingredients as a trial batch of the recipe • Substitute the non-OWGG flours; add egg or egg substitute • Mix for one minute • Add more flour or water to obtain the "crunchy" consistency • Extrude the desired pasta shape into a colander • Place in prewarmed oven, 212°F (100°C), for 15 min or in microwave oven, on defrost setting, for 2 to 3 min • Pasta shapes are heated to reduce water content • Place pasta in single layers to be dried to prevent shapes sticking together • Store in freezer bags. Frozen pasta keeps for six months.

*Meal preparation.* Cook pasta in salted water with 1 tbsp olive oil added • Boil for 1 to 2 min • Strain off water and rinse with hot water • Serve with savory sauces or in a salad.

*Useful hints.* (1) Egg substitute does not produce as good a pasta as eggs. (2) Guar or xanthan gum and other available gums are necessary for adhesion of the ingredients. (3) Use larger nozzle shapes until you devise a satisfactory pasta mix. (4) Use vegetable or fruit colorings as a plain potato/tapioca pasta, on cooking, has a clear color and tacky consistency. (5) If you like the taste of amaranth and quinoa flours, use 1 to 2 tbsp to replace the other flours in the recipes.

*Sausage method.* Read and follow the appliance instructions • Place minced meats, seasonings, flours, water, and other ingredients in a bowl and mix thoroughly, or place mixture in the bowl of the sausage machine and blend thoroughly • Extrude the mixture into sausage casings • Twist every 6 in (15 cm) to form individual sausages • Finish by tying knots at the ends of the skins • Cook on the day of preparation or freeze excess sausages • Precook sausages for a meal in the microwave on high, 1½ to 2 min; cut one or more sausages to determine if thoroughly cooked. Sausages may be baked, grilled, pan-fried, crumbed, or barbecued. Pay attention to hygiene during the preparation of sausages and clean the machine thoroughly, checking that no meat particles remain. *Option:* Leftover sausage mix can be converted into rissoles; dip in seasoned egg, roll in non-OWGG bread crumbs, soy flakes, or pea flour, and cook.

### PM1—Corn Pasta (Preparation Time: Mixing and Extruding, 20 Min)

*Ingredients.* ¾ cup finely ground cornmeal • 1 tbsp tapioca flour • 1 tbsp finely ground lentil flour (optional) • 1 egg • 1 tbsp olive oil • Carrot juice to half load mark • ½ tsp salt • ¼ tsp xanthan gum.

### PM2—Buckwheat Pasta (Preparation Time: 20 Min)

*Ingredients.* 1 cup buckwheat flour • 1 tbsp tapioca flour • ¼ tsp xanthan gum • ½ tsp salt • 1 egg • 1 tbsp olive oil • Tomato juice to the half load mark.

### PM3—Plain Pasta (Preparation Time: 20 Min)

*Ingredients.* In pasta machine cup measure: 1 tbsp tapioca flour • 1 tbsp lentil flour • ¾ cup pea flour or ¾ cup potato flour • ¼ tsp guar gum • ½ tsp salt • 1 egg • 1 tbsp olive oil • Spinach juice and puree to half load mark.

### SM1—Bratwurst Sausages

*Ingredients.* 12 oz (750 g) minced pork • 6 oz (350 g) minced beef • ¼ tsp allspice • 2 tsp caraway seeds (optional) • 2 tsp diced fresh mixed herbs (sage, thyme, rosemary, parsley) or ½ tsp dried mixed herbs • ½ tsp salt • Pepper to taste • 2 tbsp cold water • 2 tbsp pea or soy flour (optional) • 1 grated clove, and alternative flavor.

### SM2—Beef and Tomato Sausages

*Ingredients.* 5 oz (325 g) minced beef • 4 oz (100g) belly pork • 1 tbsp tomato puree or paste • 2 tsp diced fresh herbs (thyme, parsley, chives) or ½ tsp dried mixed herbs • Pinch coriander • Salt and pepper to taste • 1 to 2 tbsp soy flour may be added.

### SM3—Chipolata Sausages

*Ingredients.* 5 oz (325 g) minced pork • 3 to 4 oz (100 g) belly pork • 3 tbsp potato or pea flour • 2 oz (50 ml) water • 1 small pinch each of dried coriander, pimento, grated nutmeg • 1 tbsp diced fresh thyme and parsley • Salt and pepper to taste.

# Saga's End

Before this book fades away into appendixes and index, have you satisfied your interest in latent viruses? Multiple latent virutherapy is no mere "add on" therapy to conventional and alternative medicine. The additional treatment bonus for some is small; for others, significant, even large; and some lucky patients experience spectacular improvement in health, regaining what had been lost for many years.

> "Before I attended the Virutherapy Clinic, I was resigned to taking drugs—forever—so I could cope with my job and living. Latency treatment gave me a new start in life."
>
> A patient who suffered
> from asthma and bronchitis
> and responded to latency therapy

# Appendixes

## APPENDIX I: HIGHLIGHTS
## FROM "LATENCY IMMUNITY AND THERAPY—
## A CLINICAL STUDY"

The following are highlights from an anecdotal study of 297 patients with unexplained chronic fatigue of over two years' duration:

1. Patients received little or no relief from conventional and alternative therapies. The majority of patients suffered fluctuating fibromyalgia, which cleared or was relieved by latency therapy. The latent causes of unexplained chronic fatigue, lack of motivation, and fibromyalgia were similar or identical.
2. All patients provoked to EBV testing. The majority recollected or discovered they had a past history of glandular fever infection, either confirmed by laboratory testing or clinical diagnosis. EBV was the principal cause of chronic fatigue in 200 people. It frequently provoked, and later relieved, fibromyalgia symptoms.
3. The principal viruses of the other 97 people were as follows: hepatitis, 21; influenza, 17; cytomegalovirus, 11; poliomyelitis, 11; rubella, 6; for a total of 66. Secondary viruses, excluding EBV associated with the previous five viruses, numbered 135 of 193. EBV and the five principal viruses are responsible for the majority of latency symptoms described in *CFIDS, Fibromyalgia, and the Virus-Allergy Link.*
4. Response to latency therapy: 47 percent reported 80 to 100 percent recovery. Many of those in the recovery group of 50 to 80 percent were in the top 75 to 80 percent. Prompt control of relapses is a feature of latency therapy.
5. Laboratory tests for recent EBV antibodies were taken from 281 patients in the year before attending the clinic. Fourteen were posi-

---

For more information, see Duncan, R. B. (1999). Latency immunity and therapy: A clinical study of latent Epstein-Barr virus incidence in 297 idiopathic chronic fatigue patients with plausible hypotheses. *Journal of Chronic Fatigue Syndrome* 5(2): 77-95.

tive for recent or ongoing EBV infections. Nearly all were young people, ages 12 to 18.

6. Treatment consisted of a principal virus and, on average, five secondary viruses and EBV. All patients on testing provoked to CRC dilutions and received effective treatment vials. Successful treatment vials were given for *Giardia,* 164, and *Helicobacter,* 98.

7. The predominant food allergy was OWGGs, 221. The other commonly used allergic foods were dairy/beef, 71, and poultry, 55.

8. Prior infections that may have contributed to the chronic fatigue, lack of motivation, and, possibly, fibromyalgia were severe postviral infection, 175, and severe vaccination reactions occurring within eight weeks of receiving the dose, 16. (Table 7, p. 86 of the article, has Rubella numbers as a principal and secondary virus transposed. The correction is principal virus, 6; secondary virus, 10.)

### Two Tables from the Article

TABLE A. Results of Combined Allergy and Latency Therapy

| Improved by preliminary work-up | 252 |
|---|---|
| Improved by ML Virutherapy | 238 |
| Recovery less than < 50% | 49 |
| Recovery less than < 80% | 76 |
| Recovery between 80% and 100% | 139 |
| Failures | 33 |
| Poor compliance | 20 |
| EBV testing positive, declined therapy | 12 |

TABLE B. Viruses Used for ML Virutherapy (297), *Giardia, Helicobacter* Effective Therapy (262)

| Virutherapy less than < 4 viruses | 76 |
|---|---|
| Virutherapy less than < 7 viruses | 121 |
| Virutherapy less than < 12 viruses | 96 |
| Virutherapy less than < 16 viruses | 4 |
| *Giardia* effective | 164 |
| *Helicobacter* effective | 98 |

## Summary

Eighty to 100 percent recovery was achieved by 46.7 percent of patients. A few of those in the 50 to 80 percent group were in the top 75 to 80 percent. Table 1, p. 83, of the article, gets to the basics of CFIDS/ME immunology. There were only 14 positive laboratory antibody tests out of 267 patients who took a test in the year before attending the clinic. Research into CFIDS/ME continues to depend on responses of the blood and cellular immunity systems. Because results in the form of effective therapies are disappointing, the surmise (hypothesis) of latent immunity is advanced in the hope that it may redirect some of these efforts toward clinical anecdotal investigations. The article reports encouraging results achieved by a low-cost therapy.

It could be that "scientific medicine" requirements may be inappropriate and do not accommodate latency illnesses. Scientific medicine and its accompanying statistics do not produce convincing results or conclusions for some fields of clinical medicine such as food allergies, CRC, and the functional, subjective symptoms and illnesses, including those receiving psychological therapies. Alternative medical therapies, homeopathy, electro-medical, acupuncture, and herbal medicines may not conform to "scientific" medicine.

The latency immunity concept suggests new causes for psychological, functional, neurotic symptoms of allopathic medicine and certain symptoms and remedies of alternative medicine. The concept depends on future latency immunity clinical studies.

## APPENDIX II—CLINIC QUESTIONNAIRE©

### *ALLERGY • MULTIPLE LATENT VIRUS • PETROCHEMICAL*

### Questionnaire and History

Circle "YES" to significant or meaningful questions. Underline the option you experience.

V = Virus. CRC = *Candida*-Related Complex.

**ONSET OF CONDITION:**
Began gradually . . . . . . . . . . . . . . . . . . . . YES
Suddenly . . . . . . . . . . . . . . . . . . . . . . . . YES
V After overseas trip . . . . . . . . . . . . . . . . YES
V Childhood infection . . . . . . . . . . . . . . . . YES
V Vaccination . . . . . . . . . . . . . . . . . . . . . YES
V Food poisoning . . . . . . . . . . . . . . . . . . . YES
V Glandular Fever . . . . . . . . . . . . . . . . . . . YES
Any other suggestions . . . . . . . . . . . . . . . . YES

**DISCUSSION OF ONSET—RELAPSES:**
Began gradually . . . . . . . . . . . . . . . . . . . . YES
Suddenly . . . . . . . . . . . . . . . . . . . . . . . . YES
Once a day . . . . . . . . . . . . . . . . . . . . . . . YES
Once a week . . . . . . . . . . . . . . . . . . . . . . YES
Once a month . . . . . . . . . . . . . . . . . . . . . YES
Once a year . . . . . . . . . . . . . . . . . . . . . . YES
Duration—minutes . . . . . . . . . . . . . . . . . . YES
Duration—hours . . . . . . . . . . . . . . . . . . . . YES
Duration—days . . . . . . . . . . . . . . . . . . . . . YES
Duration—whole season . . . . . . . . . . . . . . YES
Occur during day . . . . . . . . . . . . . . . . . . . YES
Occur during night . . . . . . . . . . . . . . . . . . YES
Afternoon . . . . . . . . . . . . . . . . . . . . . . . . YES
Morning . . . . . . . . . . . . . . . . . . . . . . . . . YES
During meals . . . . . . . . . . . . . . . . . . . . . . YES
During sports . . . . . . . . . . . . . . . . . . . . . . YES
During vacations . . . . . . . . . . . . . . . . . . . YES

Cause of relapses . . . . . . . . . . . . . . . . . . . .
What stops relapses . . . . . . . . . . . . . . . . . . .

**HEAD SYMPTOMS:**
1. Frequent headaches . . . . . . . . . . . . . YES
   Migraines . . . . . . . . . . . . . . . . . . . . YES
2. V Constant head pain every day . . years. YES
3. Headache behind eye . . . . . . . . . . . . YES
   Stiff neck . . . . . . . . . . . . . . . . . . . . . YES
4. Other types . . . . . . . . . . . . . . . . . . . YES

5. Do you get sleepy for no reason . . . . . YES
6. Difficult to concentrate . . . . . . . . . . . YES
   to think correctly . . . . . . . . . . . . . . . . YES
7. More tired than others . . . . . . . . . . . YES
   Unexplained fatigue . . . . . . . . . . . . . . YES
8. Duration of fatigue . . . . . . . . . . . . . . YES
9. Do you get convulsions or fits . . . . . . . YES
10. V-CRC Do you get cold in bed and
    cannot warm-up . . . . . . . . . . . . . . . . YES
11. Cold hands and feet . . . . . . . . . . . . . YES
12. V-CRC Do you feel cold during hot
    weather . . . . . . . . . . . . . . . . . . . . . . YES
13. Do your hands and feet swell badly . . . YES

**VIRUS SYMPTOMS:**
14. V Do you perspire excessively at
    work / in bed / after meals . . . . . . . . . YES
15. V-CRC Perspiration smells musty (M) /
    chemical (CH) / animal-like (AML) . . . . YES
16. V Do you have bad breath (halitosis)
    constant / variable / M / CH / AML . . . . YES
17. V-CRC After waking in the morning does
    the bedroom smell M / CH / AML . . . . . YES
18. V Do you itch when you sweat . . . . . . . YES
19. V-CRC Saunas make your perspiration
    smell M / CH / AML . . . . . . . . . . . . . . YES
20. V Do saunas bring on symptoms you
    know . . . . . . . . . . . . . . . . . . . . . . . . YES
21. V-CRC Sauna symptoms last for
    hours . . . . . . . . . . . . . . . . . . . . . . . . YES
22. V Do you have — restless sleep . . . . . YES
    — insomnia . . . . . . . . . YES
23. V Do you sleep long hours and wake
    tired . . . . . . . . . . . . . . . . . . . . . . . . . YES
24. V-CRC Are your dreams frequent /
    infrequent / vivid / fearful / pleasant /
    unpleasant / repetition of same dream . YES
25. V-CRC Do you have muscle cramps /
    bruising pain / restless limbs . . . . . . . . YES

26. V Do cramps occur asleep in bed / after exercise / for no apparent reason . . . . . YES
27. V Childhood virus infections that were worse than other children
    a. . . . . . . . . . . . . . . . . . . . . . . . . . . . .
    b. . . . . . . . . . . . . . . . . . . . . . . . . . . . .
    c. . . . . . . . . . . . . . . . . . . . . . . . . . . . .
    d. . . . . . . . . . . . . . . . . . . . . . . . . . . . .
28. V Have you had or been suspected of:
    a. Glandular fever      b. Hepatitis
    c. Dengue               d. Herpes
    e. Chicken Pox          f. Shingles
                            or v. zoster   YES
29. V A severe undiagnosed viral infection in the past . . . . . . . . . . . . . . . . . . . . YES
30. V Venereal herpes—do not answer, but tell the physician in confidence . . . . . . YES

**NEUROTIC FUNCTIONAL SYMPTOMS:**

31. V Do you experience distorted vision / dull vision / change of or loss of color vision / what you look at gets smaller / larger / twisted . . . . . . . . . . . . . . . . . . . . . . . YES
32. V Do you experience terrifying visual images while awake / asleep . . . . . . . . YES
33. CRC Do you get tired / sleepy while driving the car . . . . . . . . . . . . . . . . . YES
34. CRC Do you bloat for no apparent reason / after meals . . . . . . . . . . . . . . YES
35. V-CRC Do you cry for no apparent reason. .YES
36. V-CRC Do you feel your moods and symptoms are being manipulated by toxins or viruses . . . . . . . . . . . . . . . . . . . . YES
37. CRC Do you feel you are like a puppet . YES
38. Do your limbs feel bruised and painful . YES
39. Do your limbs often feel as heavy as lead . . . . . . . . . . . . . . . . . . . . . . YES
40. CRC Do you crave sugar / honey / chocolate / coffee / tea / alcohol / drugs. YES
41. CRC Do you get itching / or grumbling pains / or sudden knife-like pains in the rectum/anus . . . . . . . . . . . . . . . . . . YES
42. CRC Do you get grumbling pains in right / left side of groin . . . . . . . . . . . . . . . . YES
43. Do you expel gas frequently, mild smell / strong / like rotten eggs . . . . . . . . . . . YES
44. V-CRC Have you depression / deep depression / cannot continue with living . YES
45. V Is your smell and taste poor / enhanced / distorted / normal . . . . . . YES
46. V-CRC Is your skin exceedingly sensitive to touch or to needle prick . . . . . . . . . . YES
47. V-CRC You cannot stand people touching your skin . . . . . . . . . . . . . . . . . . . . . YES

48. V Do you avoid crowds because of close contacts . . . . . . . . . . . . . . . . . . . . . . YES
49. V-CRC Your skin sensitivity is coldness / burning / itching / tingling / crawling sensation / electric / pins and needles / numbness / dull pain or aching . . . . . . YES
50. CRC Have you been diagnosed as having candidiasis / *Candida*-related complex / *Giardia* / *Helicobacter* / bowel molds / bowel microbes . . . . . . . . . . . . . . . . YES
51. Has CRC / *"Candida"* treatments aggravated symptoms ("die-off") and then improved symptoms . . . . . . . . . . . . . YES
52. Have you used nystatin / amphotericin B / Nizoral / Diflucan / other drugs . . . . . . . YES
53. Has an influenza infection aggravated or brought on some/many of the above symptoms . . . . . . . . . . . . . . . . . . . . YES

**CEREBRAL SOMATIC SYMPTOMS:**

54. V-CRC Inability to "get-up and get going" . . . . . . . . . . . . . . . . . . . . . . . YES
55. V-CRC Sleeping pattern change to 4-5 a.m. to 12-1 p.m. . . . . . . . . . . . . . YES
56. V-CRC Have you muscle aching / weakness / localized spasm / muscle knots or pressure points / trigger spots / muscle twitching or fibrillation . . . . . . . . . . . . YES
57. Neck muscle pain . . . . . . . . . . . . . . . YES
58. Low back pain— enlarged or tender lymph glands in neck / armpits / groin . . . . . . YES
59. V Do you experience memory defects / poor recall / duration . . . . . . . . . . . . . YES
60. V-CRC Do you experience "spaced out" / elated periods . . . . . . . . . . . . . . . . . YES
61. V-CRC Do you have for no apparent reason depression / moodiness . . . . . . YES
62. Do you sigh for breath (air hunger) have hyperventilation attacks (overbreathing) . . . . . . . . . . . . . . . YES
63. V-CRC Do you get skin tingling / numbness / burning / skin color change— blue / white / red . . . . . . . . . . . . . . . YES
64. V Do you have recurrence of itchy vesicles / shingles . . . . . . . . . . . . . . . . . . . . . YES
65. Have you recently consulted a psychiatrist . . . . . . . . . . . . . . . . . . YES
    Have you recently consulted a psychologist . . . . . . . . . . . . . . . . . . YES
66. CRC Have you taken long courses weeks / months of the following drugs— corticosteroids / NSAIDs / antibiotics / synthetic vitamin A drugs . . . . . . . . . YES

67. CRC Did past nystatin therapy courses aggravate (die-off) headaches / poor memory / irritability / moods / depression / muscle aches / vaginal discharges / skin rashes ...................... YES
68. Were you diagnosed as having *Giardia* / *Helicobacter* / bowel fungi / bowel microbes ...................... YES
What treatments were given ............

## NASAL SYMPTOMS:
69. Does the inside of your nose itch / pain  .. YES
70. Does your nose block often ......... YES
71. Do you get headaches when your nose blocks ...................... YES
72. Do you have postnasal drip ......... YES
73. Have you had polyps removed from your nose ....................... YES
74. Do you get hay fever from pollinosis / from cut grass ..................... YES
75. Do you often blow out mucus—clear / yellow / green / crusts / clear watery discharge .................... YES
76. Have you been treated for sinus trouble— drugs / operation ................ YES
77. Do you seem to get frequent colds / flu.  YES
78. When you catch a cold/flu, does it seem to hang on for weeks / months ....... YES

## THROAT:
79. Do you have frequent itching of the palate or back of the throat .............. YES
80. Do you often have a sore throat on waking that goes away during the day ....... YES
81. Do people tell you that you snore or sleep with open mouth ................. YES
82. Do you have to clear mucus from your throat in the morning upon waking .... YES
83. Do you clear your throat frequently .... YES
84. Do you get hoarseness or huskiness of the voice at times even though you have no cold .................. YES
85. Do you get ulcers on the mouth / tongue / lips ......................... YES
86. Does your tongue feel swollen / sore / coated / excessively red / shapes like maps ...................... YES
87. Is your mouth usually dry due to drugs / diabetes .................... YES
88. V Do you get persistent sore throats on the back wall / sides of the throat ........ YES

## CHEST:
89. Do you cough frequently—a bark / a whoop / rough or deep down / dry cough  . YES
90. Is chest mucus with coughing clear / yellow / green / contains tiny black spots .. YES
91. Asthma—do you use or have you used corticosteroids (cortisone) inhaler / gas propelled / powder capsules ........ YES
92. Do you have frequent attacks of bronchitis / other chest condition ..... YES
93. What other drugs are you taking for your chest ........................

## EARS:
94. Are you bothered with itching of the ear canals ..................... YES
95. Do you have frequent ear pain ...... YES
96. Do you get a sensation of pressure or fullness or water in one or both ears at times ...................... YES
97. Do you have variable/distorted deafness in one or both ears .............. YES
98. Do you get attacks of vertigo / dizziness / floating / veering / rotation. Intermittent / continuous .................... YES
99. Do you get noises or ringing in your ears at times ...................... YES
100. Do you have hearing that at times is normal, at other times distorted .... YES
101. V Did influenza or a virus infection damage your balance / hearing ...... YES

## EYES:
102. Do your eyes itch—which parts ...... YES
103. Do your eyes water often .......... YES
104. Do your eyes become irritated at times . YES
105. Do you often suffer from bloodshot eyes ........................ YES
106. Does the skin of your eyelids become reddened and swollen ........... YES
107. Is the lower lid swollen / colored blue/black (shiners) .............. YES
108. Do you usually wear dark glasses .... YES
109. Do your eyes often have a thick ropy secretion that causes the lids to stick together in the morning ........... YES

## SKIN:
110. Did or do you have acne, face / chest / back ......................... YES
111. Do you suffer from eczema or any other chronic skin eruption ............. YES

112. CRC Do you sometimes suffer from
hives . . . . . . . . . . . . . . . . . . . . . . . YES
113. Are you bothered with itching of the skin . YES
114. Do you sometimes get swelling of certain
parts of the skin for no apparent reason . . YES
115. Does contact of your skin with certain substances cause a rash or "breaking out" . . YES
116. Do you suffer from nail infections / softness
/ breaking / chipping . . . . . . . . . . . . . YES
117. Your hair has split ends / thin in patches /
breaks easily / is very oily / is very dry / is
falling out . . . . . . . . . . . . . . . . . . . YES
118. Does your skin blister easily . . . . . . . . YES
119. Does your skin sweat/perspire a lot—
which areas . . . . . . . . . . . . . . . . . . . YES
120. Have you ever had a rash from any drug
you took by mouth / applied to your skin /
was given by injection or shot . . . . . . . YES
121. As far as you know, are you sensitive to
any of the following drugs—aspirin / sulfa
drugs / penicillin / Aureomycin / tetracycline /
iodine / phenol / nose drops / laxatives /
sedatives / codeine / morphine / or any
other drugs . . . . . . . . . . . . . . . . . . . YES

## STOMACH AND INTESTINES:
122. Do you often belch or have bloating after
meals . . . . . . . . . . . . . . . . . . . . . . YES
123. Do you suffer from indigestion following
meals . . . . . . . . . . . . . . . . . . . . . . YES
124. List any foods that you feel disagree
with you every time you eat them . . . . . . . .
. . . . . . . . . . . . . . . . . . . . . . . . . . . .
. . . . . . . . . . . . . . . . . . . . . . . . . . . .
125. Do you have periods when your appetite
is poor . . . . . . . . . . . . . . . . . . . . . YES
126. Do you suffer a lot from periods of diarrhea
/ Do you have diarrhea every day . . . . YES
127. Do you ever pass mucus or blood
in your motions . . . . . . . . . . . . . . . . YES
128. Do you suffer from constant constipation
or bouts of constipation . . . . . . . . . . . YES
129. Do you have a regular pattern of two
to three days constipation and one day
of diarrhea . . . . . . . . . . . . . . . . . . . YES
130. Do you get cramping pains in your lower
abdomen . . . . . . . . . . . . . . . . . . . . YES
131. Have you ever been diagnosed as mucus
colitis / colic / Crohn's disease / regional ileitis YES
132. Do you have gall bladder disease /
ulcerative colitis . . . . . . . . . . . . . . . . YES
133. Have you had an acute pain in the abdomen,
together with hives and itching skin . . . YES

## FOOD HISTORY:
134. Do you suspect any food that causes
or aggravates your condition . . . . . . . . YES
135. Are there any foods you dislike . . . . . . YES
136. Are there any foods that you overindulge
in or eat frequently because you like them
or they help your well-being . . . . . . . . . YES
137. Are there foods that you find difficult
to digest . . . . . . . . . . . . . . . . . . . . . YES
138. Are there foods that cause nausea,
vomiting, diarrhea, heartburn, belching,
gas in the stomach, cramps, hives, skin
rashes, headache . . . . . . . . . . . . . . . YES
139. Do you usually eat or nibble between
meals . . . . . . . . . . . . . . . . . . . . . . YES
140. Do some foods quiet you down or help
you go to sleep . . . . . . . . . . . . . . . . YES
141. Do you take more than two alcoholic
drinks a day . . . . . . . . . . . . . . . . . . . YES
142. Do you drink more than six cups of tea
or coffee a day . . . . . . . . . . . . . . . . . YES
143. Are you on any type of diet at present . . . YES
144. Is your appetite poor . . . . . . . . . . . . . YES
145. Have you lost weight lately . . . . . . . . YES
146. Do you gain weight easily . . . . . . . . . YES

## INHALANTS HISTORY:
Does your trouble begin or is it aggravated when:
147. The house is being cleaned or swept . . YES
148. The bed is being made or the mattress
is being turned . . . . . . . . . . . . . . . . . YES
149. The first cold snap of autumn arrives . . YES
150. When you are at dusty places, e.g.,
theaters, churches, halls, supermarkets,
grocery stores, department stores,
libraries, your bedroom . . . . . . . . . . . YES
151. Home alterations are under way . . . . . YES
152. While walking or outside near trees, bushes,
or forests, in the sunset gloaming period . . YES
153. You go into a damp house, a damp
basement, shed, or cellar . . . . . . . . . . YES
154. You enter a closet where there are old
stored shoes, unused luggage, gloves,
or other leather goods . . . . . . . . . . . . YES
155. You eat cheese, mushrooms, melons,
or drink beer . . . . . . . . . . . . . . . . . . YES
156. You sit on old overstuffed furniture . . . . YES
157. When you use paper nasal tissue . . . . YES
158. You open a freshly printed folded
newspaper . . . . . . . . . . . . . . . . . . . YES
159. In nightclubs or other smoky places . . . YES
160. You are in company with people who use
a lot of powder or perfume . . . . . . . . . YES
161. You are near to a pet or animals . . . . . YES

## CHILDHOOD HISTORY:

Did you have:

162. Nasal (hay fever) or sinus problems ... YES
163. Recurrent ear infections / frequent "colds" / or sore throats ............ YES
164. Asthma or bronchitis or a lot of coughing . YES
165. Stomach problems—colic / diarrhea / vomiting / appendicitis ............ YES
166. Skin problems—eczema / hives / rashes .. YES

## FAMILY HISTORY:

167. Do you have blood relatives with allergies. . YES
168. Are these relatives one or both of your parents ...................... YES

## PREVIOUS TREATMENTS:

169. As far as you know, do you have an infection in any part of your body not listed on the questionnaire ......... YES
170. Have you ever had operations for your condition ..................... YES
171. Have you ever had treatment for your allergic condition before. If so please list it ........................ YES
172. Have any of the treatments or drugs prescribed given prolonged relief. If so, which drugs ................... YES
173. At the present time are you taking medicine for your condition ......... YES
174. Sexual desire—normal / poor / absent— If confidential inform physician later ... YES

## FOR WOMEN ONLY:

175. Are your menstrual periods usually painful....................... YES
176. Have you PMT / endometriosis / midcycle pain ........................ YES
177. Are your periods irregular / scanty / excessive ................... YES
178. Have you had any female operations .. YES
179. Have you been told you have a laceration or erosion of your womb or that you need to be cauterized ................ YES
180. Are you experiencing menopause .... YES
181. Have you finished menopause ...... YES
182. Are you taking hormone shots at the present time .................. YES
183. Are you using the pill / cannot tolerate the pill....................... YES
184. Are you pregnant .............. YES
185. Past pregnancies—felt well during pregnancy / felt awful / felt toxic / allergies aggravated / allergies cleared ... YES

186. Do you have frequency of urination at night ..................... YES
187. Do you pass pinkish urine after physical activity ...................... YES
188. V Have you recurring kidney/bladder infection / burning on passing urine ... YES
189. V Do you get a low pelvic pain, like bearing down ................. YES
190. Do you suffer loin or kidney pains .... YES
191. V Do you suffer pain, left side at lower edge of chest ................. YES

## FOR MEN ONLY:

192. Do you have trouble starting your stream when urinating ................. YES
193. Have you ever been told you have infection in your prostate gland ............ YES
194. Do you have periods of hours or a day when your urine smells very strongly .. YES

## ECOLOGY (ENVIRONMENT):

195. Is your home old ............... YES
196. Is your house damp ............. YES
197. Do things mildew easily around the house ...................... YES
198. Near your house is there a factory space / an animal pen or henhouse / a swampy area / lots of trees ....... YES
199. Anything you suspect as being a possible cause of your symptoms in your house and surrounding areas ........... YES
200. Is your house heated by open gas heaters / electric units / open fireplaces / central heating system with ducts .......... YES
201. Do you have plants in the house or in window boxes ................. YES
202. Do you use insect sprays or powders / moth repellents in the home ........ YES
203. Do you keep house cleaning chemicals in the kitchen / or perfumes and powders in the bedroom ................. YES
204. Do you keep any books or magazines that gather dust in the house ........ YES
205. Do you have any stuffed birds or trophies in the house .................. YES
206. Are there any fumes or smells continuously or frequently present about or around the house ................... YES
207. Is there any place in the house where you have symptoms regularly ....... YES
208. Is there any type of business enterprise carried out in your home ........... YES
209. Are you engaged in any hobby in your home ..................... YES

210. Do you have symptoms at work or school . . . . . . . . . . . . . . . . . . . . . YES

211. Is the place where you work—dusty / smoky / damp / open windows / air-conditioned / centrally heated . . . . . . . YES

212. Are there any fumes / gases / smokes / chemicals / or odors where you work . . YES

213. Do you come in contact with grain dusts / animal feeds / paints / varnishes / floor dust / or powders / any other product . . YES

214. Insecticides/pesticides/herbicides used at work . . . . . . . . . . . . . . . . . . . . . YES

**YOUR PRINCIPAL COMPLAINTS IN ORDER OF SEVERITY AND DURATION:**

Years/Months

215a. . . . . . . . . . . . . . . . . . . . . . . . . . . . . . .

215b. . . . . . . . . . . . . . . . . . . . . . . . . . . . . . .

215c. . . . . . . . . . . . . . . . . . . . . . . . . . . . . . .

215d. . . . . . . . . . . . . . . . . . . . . . . . . . . . . . .

215e. . . . . . . . . . . . . . . . . . . . . . . . . . . . . . .

**FURTHER QUESTIONS TO ASK PHYSICIAN OR NURSE:**

## LATENT VIRUS PROVOCATION AND NEUTRALIZATION

RT. GRIP ............. KILO          PEAK FLOW .................          LT. GRIP ............. KILO

| LT. | PEAK FLOW | RT. | LT. | PEAK FLOW | RT. | LT. | PEAK FLOW | RT. |
|-----|-----------|-----|-----|-----------|-----|-----|-----------|-----|
| 7 3 0 -5 | 1 | | | 9 | | | 17 | |
| 7 3 0 -5 | 2 | | | 10 | | | 18 | |
| 7 3 0 -5 | 3 | | | 11 | | | 19 | |
| 7 3 0 -5 | 4 | | | 12 | | | 20 | |
| 7 3 0 -5 | 5 | | | 13 | | | 21 | |
| 7 3 0 -5 | 6 | | | 14 | | | 22 | |
| 7 3 0 -5 | 7 | | | 15 | | | 23 | |
| 7 3 0 -5 | 8 | | | 16 | | | 24 | |

*Note:* The shaded numbers represent the order of inoculations. On average, the duration of each inoculation is 15 min, with twelve to sixteen inoculations given during a 4 h session.

# Bibliography

Health book shops stock a bewildering array of allergy, nutrition, CRC, petrochemical toxicity, and related recipe cookbooks. Over 150 titles were assessed as part of developing this book, and the following titles were selected for added practical and informative support of *CFIDS, Fibromyalgia, and the Virus-Allergy Link.* They are popular with clinic patients. If some of the titles are not available, contact your physician's office or local support group for similar books, better suited to the treatment you are receiving and the region where you live.

At first, many patients will be unable to read or remember what they read or heard. As you gradually recover, spend time learning about your illness and why some treatments help you. Where do you start? You have only so much energy and time when ill. Instead of reading cover to cover, identify the relevant sections of the books using their indexes. Photocopy useful pages to help your memory, and in case you later suffer a relapse.

If you cannot find answers to your questions, put them to the professionals at the clinic. Before purchasing a book, determine its relevancy to your illness because the person recommending the book may suffer or have suffered from different symptoms and causes. Remember, recovery is 85 percent your understanding and complying with treatment and 15 percent your physician's experience and therapies.

## References for Patients

Brostoff, J. and L. Jamlin (1989). *Food Allergy and Intolerance.* London: Bloomsbury Publishing.

Callem, J. (1993). *Getting the Most Out of Your Vitamins and Minerals.* New Canaan, CT: Keats Publishing.

Collison, D.R. and T. Hall (1989). *Why Do I Feel So Awful?* London: Angus Robertson.

Crook, W.G. (1995). *The Yeast Connection and the Woman.* Jackson, TN: Professional Books.

Crook, W.G. (1996). *The Yeast Connection Handbook.* Jackson, TN: Professional Books.

Crook, W.G. and M.H. Jones (1989). *The Yeast Connection Cookbook.* Jackson, TN: Professional Books.

Davies, S. and A. Stewart (1989). *Nutritional Medicine.* London: Pan Books.

Duncan, R.B. and J.R. Smith (1993). *The Hidden Viruses Within You.* Wellington, New Zealand: Viroprint.

Eades, M.R. and M.D. Eades (1998). *Protein Power.* New York: Bantam Books.

Feltner, A.G. (1990). *Viruses, Agents of Change.* New York: McGraw-Hill Publishing.

Galland, L. (1988). *Superimmunity for Kids.* New York: Bantam Books.

Garrett, L. (1995). *The Coming Plague.* New York: Penguin.

Gittleman, A.L. (1993). *Guess What Came to Dinner?* New York: Avery Publishing.

Goldstein, J.A. (1993). *Chronic Fatigue Syndromes.* Binghamton, NY: The Haworth Press, Inc.

Golos, N. and F. Golos (1983). *If This Is Tuesday, It Must Be Chicken.* New Canaan, CT: Keats Publishing.

Gottschall, E. (1994). *Breaking the Vicious Cycle.* Baltimore, Ontario, Canada: Kirkton.

Hamilton, G. (1999). Inside trading. *New Scientist* 2192: 42-46.

Heller, R. (1992). *The Carbohydrate Addict's Diet.* London: Cedar.

Huggins, H.A. (1993). *It's All in Your Head, Mercury Amalgams and Illness.* New York: Avery Publishing.

Hyde, B.M. (Ed.) (1992). *The Clinical and Scientific Basis of ME/CFS.* Ottawa, Ontario, Canada: Nightingale Research Foundation.

Lewis, S.K. and L. Blakeley (1996). *Allergy and* Candida *Cooking Made Easy.* Coralville, IA: Canary Connect Publications.

Mandell, M. (1979). *The Five Day Allergy Relief System.* New York: Pocket Books.

Mansfield, J. (1997). *The Asthma Epidemic.* London: Thorsons.

McTaggart, L. (1996). *What Doctors Don't Tell You.* London: Thorsons.

Miller, J.B. (1989). *Relief at Last.* Springfield, IL: Charles C Thomas.

Rapp, D. (1992). *Is This Your Child? Discovering and Treating Unrecognized Allergies.* New York: William Morrow and Company.

Rapp, D. (1996). *Is This Your Child's World? How You Can Fix the Schools and Homes That Are Making Your Children Sick.* New York: Bantam Books.

Rousseau, D., W.J. Rea, and G. Enwright (1988). *Your Home, Your Health, and Well-Being.* Point Roberts, WA: Hartley and Marks.

Schmid, R.S. (1994). *Native Nutrition.* Rochester, VT: Healing Arch Press.

Shepherd, C. (1989). *Living with ME.* London: Heinemann.

*Townsend Letter for Doctors and Patients* (Published ten times annually). Port Townsend, WA: J. Collins (Ed.), Publisher.

Webster, R. (1996). *Why Freud Was Wrong.* London: Fortuna Press.

Winderlin, C. and K. Sehnert (1996). *Candida-Related Complex.* Dallas, TX: Taylor Publishing Company.

Wright, J.V. (1990). *Healing with Nutrition.* New Canaan, CT: Keats Publishing.

## *References for Medical Professionals*

Anderson, M., J. Handley, L. Hopwood, S. Murant, M. Stower, and N.J. Maitland (1997). Analysis of prostate tissue DNA for the presence of the *H. Papillomavirus* by polymerase chain reaction, cloning, automated sequencing. *Journal of Medical Virology* 52: 8-13.

Buchwald, D., R.L. Ashley, T. Pearlman, P. Kith, and A.L. Komaroff (1996). Viral serologies in patients with chronic fatigue and chronic fatigue syndrome. *Journal of Medical Virology* 50: 25-30.

Engelhard, V.H. (1994). How small cells process antigens. *Scientific American* 271(2)(August): 44-51.

Hansen, H. (1996). *Papillomavirus* eye infections—A major cause of human cancers. *Biochemica et Biophysica Acta* 1288: f55-f78.

Mehlhop, P.D., M. Van de Rijn, A.B. Goldberg, J.P. Brewer, V.P. Kurup, T.R. Martin, and H.C. Oettgen (1997). Allergen induced bronchial hyper-reactivity and eosinophyllic inflammation occur in the absence of Ig E in a mouse model of asthma. *Proceedings of National Academy of Sciences, USA*: 1344-1349.

Skaloot, F. (1993). Double blind when healing is a gamble. *The Sun* (Chapel Hill, NC), 215(November): 6 pp.

## Petrochemicals and Xenochemicals

Collison and Hall, 1989; Feltner, 1990; Goldstein, 1993; Hamilton, 1999; Mandell, 1979; Mansfield, 1997; Miller, 1989.

## Recipes and Cookbooks

Collison and Hall, 1989; Crook and Jones, 1989; Feltner, 1990; Gittleman, 1993; Huggins, 1993; Hyde, 1992; Webster, 1996; Wright, 1990.

## Textbooks and Journals

Gottschall, 1994; Golos and Golos, 1983; Heller, 1992; Lewis and Blakeley, 1996; Mansfield, 1997; Shepherd, 1989.

# Indications for Multiple
# Latent Virutherapy

Order of frequency of symptoms seen at the clinic:

1. Unexplained mental and muscle tenseness, lack of motivation
2. Unexplained fatigue and sleeping disorders
3. Chronic sinusitis—sinus headache and ear symptoms, such as fullness
4. Recurring "flu infections" or "flulike symptoms" not controlled by repeated antibiotic courses or immunization
5. Skin conditions of one year or longer duration requiring frequent hydrocortisone or corticosteroid topical drug therapy
6. Indigestion, bloating, pain, and "colitis" symptoms (e.g., irritable bowel syndrome)
7. Headaches, migraines, and constant head pain (one that never goes away); considerable side effects from headache medications
8. Recurring eye irritation, mild infection, and visual disturbances
9. Kidney and bladder problems (e.g., urinary tract infections, urgency, pain on passage, and water retention)
10. Depression, moods, sleep disorders, and feelings of being manipulated like a puppet by unknown causes
11. Memory and recall defects, fearful dreams, and "spacing out" mind states
12. Variable pain and weakness of muscle groups, localized muscle spasms, e.g., pressure points or "knots"; chronic low back, shoulder, and neck pain that does not respond to conventional therapies
13. Asthma controlled by symptom suppression inhaled corticosteroids and cromolyn drugs, with sticky, often colored chest mucus
14. In children, variable deafness and sticky mucus in the middle ear, with or without ventilation tubes; failure to learn and reduced physical activities
15. Difficult to manage "overactivity" in children and teenagers, with or without long-term drug therapy
16. CFIDS/ME affecting adults, teenagers, and children, with constant or fluctuating symptoms of nine months or longer duration

# Recipe List

## Bread Machine Recipes

BM1     Plain or Herb Bread
BM2     Corn Bread
BM3     Buckwheat and Sultana Bread
BM4     Egg Substitute and Lactose-Free Bread
BM5     Apricot Almond Bread

## Breakfast Recipes

B1     Tapioca Breakfast Dessert
B2     Sago Breakfast Dessert
B3     Fruit and Rhubarb Sago
B4     Amaranth Porridge
B5     Buckwheat Porridge
B6     Quinoa Porridge
B7     Cornmeal Porridge and Italian Polenta
B8     Legumes
B9     Pancake Batter
B10     Cheese and Celery Bread
B11     Zucchini Quick Bread
B12     Cottage Cheese and Herb Bread
B13     Miner's Corn Bread
B14     Farm Corn Bread
B15     Buckwheat Banana Bread
B16     Carrot and Orange Loaf
B17     Muffins
B18     Lemon and Zucchini Muffins
B19     Savory Muffins
B20     Brown Buckwheat Cookies
B21     Salmon Cakes
B22     Scrambled Egg
B23     Omelette
B24     Bubble and Squeak

B25    Fritters
B26    Buckwheat Pilaf
B27    Soybeans with Sardines
B28    Soybean and Carrot Pistou

## Cooking Basics

CB1    Arrowroot Thickening
CB2    Basic Sauce (Roux Method)
CB3    Beef Stock
CB4    Yeast-Free Baking Powder
CB5    Cornmeal Pie Shells
CB6    Soy Milk

## Dinner and Dessert Recipes

D50    Sweet Potato Soup
D51    Sweet Corn Chowder
D52    Plum Pork
D53    Fish with Tomato-Cheese Crust
D54    Chili Bean Mince
D55    Cottage Pie
D56    Baked Fish
D57    Meat and Leek Pasta
D58    Sweet Potato and Pumpkin Stir-Fry Vegetables
D59    Pizza
D60    Nut Seed Crust
D61    Potato Pastry
D62    Apricot Shortcake
D63    Gelatin Desserts
D64    Basic Ice Cream
D65    Ice Cream or Cake Topping, No Sugar
D66    Kiwifruit Ice Cream
D67    Yogurt Popsicles®
D68    Synthetic Sweetened Jam

## Lunch Recipes

L30    Quinoa Corn Chowder
L31    Spanish Soup
L32    Creamy Sweet Potato and Fish Chowder
L33    Basic Waffle Batter

L34  Meat/Ham and Cheese Waffle
L35  Sour Cream Waffle
L36  Fresh Fruit Waffles
L37  Grilled Polenta Wedges with Chili Vegetable Stew
L38  Tortillas
L39  Zucchini Slice
L40  Chapatis, Indian Pancakes
L41  Buckwheat Spice Bread
L42  Quick and Easy Flat Bread
L43  Bean Salad
L44  Yogurt Salad Dressing
L45  Potato Salad
L46  Coleslaw
L47  Cheese and Herb Sauce
L48  Tree Tomato Chutney

## Pasta and Sausage Machine Recipes

PM1  Corn Pasta
PM2  Buckwheat Pasta
PM3  Plain Pasta
SM1  Bratwurst Sausages
SM2  Beef and Tomato Sausages
SM3  Chipolata Sausages

## Snack Recipes

S70  Mexican Corn Dip
S71  Potato Chips, Potato Wedges, and Corn Chips
S72  Popcorn
S73  Potato Skins
S74  Cheese Sticks
S75  Coconut Crispettes
S76  Bird Seed Bars
S77  Currant Biscuits

# Index for Medical Professionals

# General Index

Viruses, 117, 118, 125, 140, 141
  latent
    antibodies not provoked by, 137
    asthma and, 42
    the gut and, 181
    provocation neutralization and
      diagnosis of, 142
    symptoms of, 171
Virutherapy
  detoxing using, 187
  muscles and, 81, 82
  fear and reassurances about, 141,
    142
Vitamin A, 75
Vitamin B complex, 165, 186, 223,
  225
Vitamin B12, 165
Vitamin C, 75
Vitamin E, 225
Vitamin K, 224

Waffles, 219, 222
Warning notes on drug packages,
  196, 197
Warts, skin, 110

Water/fluid retention (oedema), 95,
  98
Weight control from OWGGs
  exclusion diet, 184
Weight loss, 169
Wheat. *See* Old world grass grains
  (OWGGs)
Wheaten cornflour, 167
Wholemeal and bran, 165
Whooping cough, 107, 109, 113
Wine tasting, 198
Withdrawal symptoms (foods), 163,
  184, 214
Wright, Jonathan V., 196

Xenodetoxing, 139
Xenopetrochemicals
  autodetoxing of, 180
  CFIDS/ME women and, 192
  home ecology and, 157
  inability to detox, 186
  treatment failures from, 153

Zinc, 75, 79, 234, 235